Communication in Autism

Trends in Language Acquisition Research

TiLAR publishes monographs, edited volumes and text books on theoretical and methodological issues in the field of child language research. The focus of the series is on original research on all aspects of the scientific study of language behavior in children, linking different areas of research including linguistics, psychology & cognitive science.

For an overview of all books published in this series, please see
http://benjamins.com/catalog/tilar

Volume 11

Communication in Autism
Edited by Joanne Arciuli and Jon Brock

Communication in Autism

Edited by

Joanne Arciuli
University of Sydney

Jon Brock
Macquarie University

John Benjamins Publishing Company

Amsterdam / Philadelphia

The paper used in this publication meets the minimum requirements of the American National Standard for Information Sciences – Permanence of Paper for Printed Library Materials, ANSI Z39.48-1984.

Library of Congress Cataloging-in-Publication Data

Communication in autism / edited by Joanne Arciuli, Jon Brock.

p. cm. (Trends in Language Acquisition Research, ISSN 1569-0644 ; v. 11)

Includes bibliographical references and index.

1. Autistic children--Language. 2. Communicative disorders in children--Treatment. 3. Language disorders in children--Treatment. 4. Autistic children--Means of communication. 5. Autism in children--Complications. I. Arciuli, Joanne, editor of compilation. II. Brock, Jon (Jonathan Peter) editor of compilation.

RJ506.A9C66 2014

618.92'85882--dc23 2014004004

ISBN 978 90 272 4400 0 (Hb ; alk. paper)

ISBN 978 90 272 7032 0 (Eb)

John Benjamins Publishing Co. · P.O. Box 36224 · 1020 ME Amsterdam · The Netherlands

John Benjamins North America · P.O. Box 27519 · Philadelphia PA 19118-0519 · USA

Table of contents

An introduction to communication in autism

Current findings and future directions

Joanne Arciuli & Jon Brock
University of Sydney / Macquarie University

Ever since Leo Kanner's original description of autism in 1943, impaired communication has been considered one of its central features. Autism has been defined and diagnosed in terms of communication impairment, co-occurring with qualitative abnormalities of social interaction and restricted and repetitive behaviours and interests. With an estimated prevalence of 1 in 88 (Baio 2012), it represents one of the more common disorders associated with communication impairment.

The emphasis on different aspects of communication in autism has shifted considerably over the years. In the late 1960s and early 1970s, severe disorder of speech and language was considered necessary for a diagnosis of autism (e.g. Creak 1964) with some researchers implicating language impairment as its primary cause (e.g. Churchill 1972; Rutter & Bartak 1971). Although impaired communication remains one of the core criteria for a diagnosis of autism, current diagnostic guidelines, such as the fifth edition of the Diagnostic and Statistical Manual of Mental Disorders (DSM-5), emphasise nonverbal communication and pragmatic conversational deficits, whilst allowing for the full range of individual variation in linguistic competence. Even high-functioning individuals with age-appropriate language skills struggle in conversational settings and may have difficulty with turn-taking and knowing how much information to provide.

In terms of the more structural aspects of language, variation is as extreme as it could possibly be. Some individuals have age-appropriate language, with a small number having exceptional language skills; others have little or no spoken language and are considered, according to current terminology, to be 'minimally verbal'. In between these two extremes are individuals who, although possessing some spoken language skills, experience significant linguistic impairments, particularly relating to phonology (the sound-system of language) and/or grammar (the rules for combining words). Structural language impairment in individuals with autism has sometimes been conceived as a separate comorbid dysfunction. However, it should be remembered that many studies deliberately screen out participants with autism who do not have a verbal IQ within the normal range. Those that take a more representative sample typically report language scores that are, on average, well below age-appropriate levels (e.g. Kjelgaard & Tager-Flusberg 2001; Lincoln, Courchesne, Harms & Allen 1993). Even though structural language deficits are neither universal across the spectrum nor specific to autism, the strong association with autism needs to be considered by any complete account of the disorder.

Research on the communication skills and difficulties of autistic individuals serves two broad and complementary purposes. From a practical viewpoint, understanding the causes of communication impairment is an essential part of developing and improving the therapies and interventions administered to autistic individuals aimed at improving their communication skills. Clearly, the heterogeneity of communication skills mentioned above indicates that the most appropriate interventions and communication strategies will vary on an individual basis. This heterogeneity represents a major challenge to autism research in general and is a recurring theme in many of the chapters here. Research on communication in autistic individuals also assists in identifying strategies by which non-autistic individuals may improve their own communication skills when interacting with people on the autism spectrum. Communication is, after all, a two-way street.

A second and perhaps less obvious benefit of research on autistic communication is to further our understanding of the mechanisms of human communication. When studying typical development, it can be difficult to tease apart different causal influences, because there is less variation or the variation is highly intercorrelated (children who are good at one thing tend to be good at other things). The natural variation within developmental disorders such as autism provides a critical test of theories of language and communication. In many ways individuals with autism are the 'exceptions' that test the 'rule'.

The chapters in this book reflect these two complementary objectives. They are a mix of review articles and empirical studies and, together, provide comprehensive coverage of both the practical and the theoretical aspects of autistic communication. One point of note is that, in keeping with the field more generally, our authors utilise somewhat different terminology when referring to individuals with autism. The recent introduction of DSM-5 (APA 2013) has brought official recognition to the term 'Autism Spectrum Disorder'. However, most of the research reported or reviewed here was conducted under the fourth edition of the DSM, which distinguished between Autistic Disorder, Asperger's Disorder, and Pervasive Developmental Disorder Not Otherwise Specified, To further complicate matters, practitioners (and some parents) tend to advocate the use of person-first language, referring to 'people with autism'. In contrast, the individuals themselves tend to prefer the adjectival description, 'autistic', in recognition of the fact that autism is a part of who they are. Notwithstanding the heterogeneity *within* autism, the reader should in general assume that these terms all refer to members of the same population. We chose to use the term 'autism' in our title and in this introductory chapter. We use this term in its broadest sense acknowledging that autism is a spectrum of disorders.

The 5 sections and 10 chapters of this volume are briefly outlined below. Section 1 focuses on symbolic communication, in particular, prelinguistic and assisted communication. Chapter 1 is a review of prelinguistic communication in autism by Keen. This chapter explores different forms of prelinguistic communication that can be seen in infants with autism, and the methods that can be used to assess this communication (e.g. interview protocols, naturalistic observations, and structured observations). Keen discusses how prelinguistic communication can be shaped/replaced/augmented in a way that assists the individual to move towards more effective communication, emphasising the important role of the adult communicative partner during this process. The issue of joint attention and interventions designed to enhance joint attention are an important focus in Keen's review.

Chapter 2, by May and Dymond, focuses on communication interventions for autistic individuals with 'emerging' language skills, outlining the behaviourist principles that underpin the Applied Behavioural Analysis (ABA) approach. More specifically, they propose strategies for improving the generalisability of learning word associations and provide preliminary evidence for the efficacy of these strategies from single case and small group studies. Aside from the potential practical utility of this research, May and Dymond argue that evidence from autistic individuals has led to a reshaping of behaviourist theories in general, thereby illustrating the important interplay between theory and practice in autism research.

Section 2 contains 3 chapters on oral language. In Chapter 3, Roberts reports an investigation of echolalia – the rote repetition of phrases out of context that is a commonly noted feature of language in autism, particularly for individuals in the early stages of language development. For many years, echolalia was seen as a problem behaviour that had to be 'extinguished' before proper language acquisition could begin. Roberts supports an altogether different view – that echolalia is in fact an important staging post on the route to language. Her longitudinal data from children with autism indicates a strong association between children's developing language abilities and the quality of their echolalia. Interestingly, children with specific language impairment (SLI) show a similar pattern, although the extent of echolalia is much lower.

The relationship between autism and SLI is further explored in Chapter 4. As Taylor and colleagues point out, some have argued that the language phenotypes of autism and SLI represent "a theoretically significant aetiological overlap". However, others have argued that the kind of overlap observed in autism and SLI does not result from shared causes. Taylor, Maybery and Whitehouse review behavioural, neurological, and molecular genetic studies contrasting the two disorders. They discuss the inconsistent findings across these studies and suggest avenues for future research.

Chapter 5 is a review article examining prosody. In this chapter Arciuli notes that atypical prosody has been observed in some individuals with autism since the early descriptions provided by Kanner (1943). There is evidence indicating that atypical prosody gives an impression of oddness that can impede social inclusion; yet, because we know little about the causal mechanisms underpinning this atypical prosody in individuals with autism, it is difficult to design effective remediation strategies. Research on the potential causal mechanisms underpinning atypical prosody in individuals with autism has encouraged investigation of similarities and differences with other non-autistic populations, such as individuals with childhood apraxia of speech (CAS), thereby deepening our understanding of this aspect of human communication more generally.

Section 3 includes research on literacy. In Chapter 6, Brock and Caruana revisit a seminal article by Frith and Snowling (1983) that investigated reading ability in individuals with autism. They note that subsequent studies have broadly supported Frith and Snowling's conclusion that many individuals with autism have particular difficulty understanding the meaning of sentences and larger sections of text. However, consistent with the heterogeneity discussed above, more recent literature highlights that reading ability is highly variable in children with autism, particularly in relation to understanding the meaning of sentences. Essentially, this research on autism converges on the same conclusions as research on other non-autistic populations; namely, that reading comprehension is a joint function of decoding skills and oral language comprehension abilities. This is an example of the mutual benefit of language research in typically and atypically developing populations.

Chapter 7, by Jacobs and Richdale, picks up nicely on this point in reporting a large empirical study of reading ability in 168 school-aged children aged 6–8 years. Amongst the results reported in this chapter are regression analyses examining predictors of reading accuracy (decoding) and of reading comprehension in children with autism versus peers without autism. On the whole, the data reveals that the predictors of reading ability are similar across the two groups.

Section 4 contains chapters on 'higher level' language. In Chapter 8, Stirling and colleagues provide a detailed review of the literature on narrative skills in children with autism. Narratives provide an extraordinarily rich source of information about the way individuals with autism use language to represent the world and their experiences. Narrative skill also touches on some of the pragmatic aspects of language with which even the most able autistic individuals have difficulty. Stirling et al. note that this field of research is still coming to grips with many challenges of methodology and interpretation. Stirling et al. conclude that there is much potential for furthering our understanding of autistic language and its relation to other aspects of cognition by examining narrative skills.

Chapter 9 sees Rendle-Short exploring similar conceptual and methodological issues in relation to the conversational skills of two 8-year-old children with autism. Rendle-Short points out that the success of an interaction cannot easily be defined as correct or incorrect. Her analysis reveals that while these two children show competencies in some aspects of their interactions there is evidence of pragmatic difficulties (e.g. associated with initiating topics). She argues that the conversational partner can play an important role in providing structure and predictability to enhance effective interactions.

Finally, Section 5 consists of a single chapter examining what might be considered a 'distal' cause of language impairment in autism. Hollier and colleagues review research that has examined the role of prenatal testosterone in the development of later language skills – a relationship that may perhaps be mediated by testosterone's influence on language lateralisation. The evidence is fairly indirect at present, but the chapter is a further reminder that cognitive and linguistic development can be influenced by events and environments from the earliest moments in development.

Hollier et al.'s final chapter highlights a recurring theme in this volume, namely, the importance of taking a multidisciplinary approach to understanding the communication difficulties associated with autism. Our authors are experts in a range of fields, including psychology, linguistics, and speech-language pathology. Their work is informed by neuroscience, genetics, and education. Their chapters showcase a wide array of methods currently being used in research in this area and should encourage readers to think about the many facets of communication and reflect on how these facets might be related. For instance, how does the presence of echolalia (Chapter 3) or atypical prosody (Chapter 5) impact upon the success of conversational interactions (Chapter 9)?

The volume makes a contribution in more specific ways too; for instance, the individual differences approach recommended in Chapters 6 and 7 is timely given the failure to identify autism-specific deficits in reading ability. Indeed, a recent meta-analysis of 36 studies of reading comprehension in autism has concluded that "Having ASD alone does not predict reading comprehension deficits" (Brown, Oram-Cardy & Johnson 2013: p. 932). Having noted this, we agree with commentators such as Hulme and Snowling (2009) that there is scope for researchers to explore more fully particular aspects of reading comprehension in individuals with autism; for example, with regard to the many different forms of inferencing. In a recent study Norbury and Nation (2011) found that a diagnosis of autism predicted 10% unique variance in comprehension when inferencing ability is the outcome measure. Furthermore, it is important to remember that reading comprehension in individuals with autism has often been explored using materials that have minimal social content and do not place high demands on decoding. Norbury and Nation (2011) pointed out that the stories they used in their recent study were pitched at children aged 7–8 years even though their participants with autism were teenagers. They suggest it is "highly likely that even the most linguistically able participants with ASD will need support to develop reading comprehension" (Norbury & Nation 2011: p. 207).

While the chapters in this volume cover a wide array of communicative abilities, there are some omissions. In particular, while some chapters refer to aspects of auditory processing (e.g. pitch tracking in Chapter 5), our volume does not include comprehensive coverage of auditory processing in individuals with autism. There is reason to believe that individuals with autism may experience atypical auditory processing. We direct readers to a recent review by O'Connor (2012) that concluded that there are a diverse range of auditory abnormalities seen in individuals with autism and that processing difficulties appear to be increased when it comes to complex stimuli and speech. We think it is important for those working in the area of communication in autism to carefully consider the role of auditory processing, especially in the diagnosis and remediation of communication difficulties in this population.

Also, we acknowledge that the research presented in our volume is based on speakers of English. We agree with recent commentators that there is a pressing need for cross-linguistic investigation of communication in autism, and in neurodevelopmental disorders more generally (Norbury & Sparks 2013). The world's languages differ in fundamental ways. Norbury and Sparks provide the example of an English-speaking child who fails to acquire tense marking (such as '-ed' signifies past tense) by the time they start school, and, consequently, may be diagnosed with a language impairment. Importantly, Norbury and Sparks point out that verb morphology might not be an effective marker of impairment in all languages and/or may exhibit a different developmental trajectory across languages. The case of atypical prosody in autism is a more specific illustration of this point. To date, everything we know about atypical prosody in autism comes from studies of English. While some languages use prosody in ways that are similar to English, other languages have different prosodic systems. It would be valuable to know whether speakers of languages other than English who have autism also exhibit atypical prosody, and, if so, whether their atypical prosody is an impediment to social acceptance as it is for English speakers. Importantly, evidence of atypical prosody in individuals with autism who speak languages other than English can assist in determining the extent to which causal mechanisms might be psychosocial and/or physiological as opposed to language-specific.

Finally, our volume is somewhat limited in that most of the content relates to children with autism. By comparison with the strong research focus on children with autism, there is a striking lack of research on adults with autism. For example, the lack of research on interventions and outcomes during adulthood has been highlighted recently (e.g. Bishop-Fitzpatrick, Minshew & Eack 2013; Howlin & Moss 2012). Although autism is widely acknowledged to be a condition that affects individuals throughout their lives there have been reports that some individuals can improve or perhaps even 'recover' over time (e.g. Helt, Kinsbourne, Pandey, Boorstein, Herbert & Fein 2008). In fact, there has been relatively little research that has tracked individuals from childhood to adulthood. This gap in the research is evident when it comes to the lifespan trajectory of communicative abilities in this population. We hope that there will be increased research effort in this area allowing us to determine the profiles of communicative abilities of individuals with autism as they transition from childhood to adulthood.

In closing, we would like to thank the many individuals who have contributed to this book, including our authors, anonymous reviewers, and series editors. The idea for the book arose from a workshop held in Sydney, supported by the Human Communication Science Network (HCSNet) which was funded by the Australian Research Council. The workshop brought together researchers and research students, educators and clinicians, and interested members of the public. We hope that this volume provides a continuation of the dialogue established at that meeting and provides a helpful resource on basic and applied research in the area of communication in autism.

References

American Psychiatric Association. (2013). *Diagnostic and Statistical Manual of Mental Disorders, Fifth Edition (DSM-5).* Arlington, VA: American Psychiatric Publishing.

Baio, J. (2012). Prevalence of Autism Spectrum Disorders – Autism and Developmental Disabilities Monitoring Network, 14 Sites, United States, 2008. *Morbidity and Mortality Weekly Report, 61*(SS03), 1–19

Bishop-Fitzpatrick, L., Minshew, N., & Eack, S. (2013). A systematic review of psychosocial interventions for adults with autism spectrum disorders. *Journal of Autism and Developmental Disorders, 43,* 687–694.

Brown, H., Oram-Cardy, J., & Johnson, A. (2013). A meta-analysis of the reading comprehension skills of individuals on the autism spectrum. *Journal of Autism and Developmental Disorders, 43*(4), 932–955.

Churchill, D. (1972). The relation of infantile autism and early childhood schizophrenia to developmental language disorders of childhood. *Journal of Autism and Childhood Schizophrenia, 2,* 182–197.

Creak, M. (1964). Schizophrenia syndrome in childhood: Progress report of a working party. *Cerebral Palsy Bulletin, 3,* 501–504.

Frith, U., & Snowling, M. (1983). Reading for meaning and reading for sound in autistic and dyslexic children. *British Journal of Developmental Psychology, 1*, 329–342.

Helt, M., Kinsbourne, M., Pandey, J., Boorstein, H., Herbert, M., & Fein, D. (2008). Can children with autism recover? If so, how? *Neuropsychology Review, 18*, 339–366.

Howlin, P., & Moss, P. (2012). Adults with autism spectrum disorders. *Canadian Journal of Psychiatry, 57*, 275–283.

Hulme, C., & Snowling, M. (2009). *Developmental Disorders of Language Learning and Cognition*. Malden, MA: Wiley-Blackwell.

Kanner, L. (1943). Autistic disturbances of affective contact. *Nervous Child, 2*, 217–250.

Kjelgaard, M.M., & Tager-Flusberg, H. (2001). An investigation of language impairment in autism: Implications for genetic subgroups. *Language and Cognitive Processes, 16*, 287–308.

Lincoln, A.J., Courchesne, E., Harms, L., & Allen, M. (1993). Contextual probability evaluation in autistic, receptive developmental language disorder, and control children: Event-related brain potential evidence. *Journal of Autism and Developmental Disorders, 23*, 37–58.

Norbury, C., & Nation, K. (2011). Understanding variability in reading comprehension in adolescents with autism spectrum disorders: Interactions with language status and decoding skill. *Scientific Studies of Reading, 15*(3), 191–210.

Norbury, C., & Sparks, A. (2013). Cultural issues in understanding neurodevelopmental disorders. *Developmental Psychology, 49*(1), 45–58.

O'Connor, K. (2012). Auditory processing in autism spectrum disorder: A review. *Neuroscience and Biobehavioral Reviews, 36*, 836–854.

Rutter, M., & Bartak, L. (1971). Causes of infantile autism: Some considerations from recent research. *Journal of Autism and Childhood Schizophrenia, 1*, 20–32.

SECTION 1

Symbolic communication

CHAPTER 1

Prelinguistic communication

Deb Keen
Griffith University

For children with autism, the development of intentional and symbolic communication can be a challenging process and some children remain at the prelinguistic stage of communicative development for extended periods. During this time, they rely on communicative behaviours that can be difficult for others to understand and interpret. Communicative forms can be subtle and idiosyncratic and may represent more than one communicative function. This can lead to frustration for the child and the communicative partner who may struggle to understand the meaning of the child's behaviour. Many communication breakdowns can result and with the child's limited skills to repair these breakdowns, behaviours can escalate to problematic forms. Research has shown that children with autism have higher rates of problem behaviour which limits opportunities for engagement and learning and for participation in the community. Improving our knowledge and understanding of prelinguistic behaviours may help to reduce problem behaviours and can inform interventions to support these children to communicate their needs and wants more effectively. This chapter explores our current understanding of the prelinguistic communicative forms and functions of children with autism and identifies gaps in our knowledge base and areas in need of further research. The author draws on her work in functional communication and prelinguistic behaviours and communicative repairs.

Children with autism experience differences in their communicative development compared to their typically developing peers. Communication impairments can be extensive and may include, to varying degrees, language, gesture, and pragmatics. Language outcomes for children with autism are extremely varied, with some children demonstrating precocious language skills while others never acquire the use of functional speech (Wetherby & Prizant 1992). Communicative impairments generally appear at an early age and are often the trigger for parents to consult with paediatricians and other health professionals about their child's development. Initially, parents may seek an assessment of their child's hearing, suspecting that this may explain the child's lack of response to auditory stimuli such as not responding to their name when called. These investigations may take place well before other developmental difficulties are identified and a diagnosis of autism received.

Critical to language development for all children is the emergence of intentional and symbolic communication which occurs for typically developing children around the age of 9–12 months (Wetherby, Warren & Reichle 1998). Prior to the onset of these important milestones in communicative development, an infant's behaviour may be interpreted by a caregiver as meaningful even when the behaviour is reflexive or is in response to an environmental stimulus but has no apparent communicative function. At around 5 to 6 months, infants begin to communicate with their caregivers about objects and events (Adamson & Chance 1998). By the end of their first year of life, infants become much more intentional in their communication and can engage in joint attention where they can reference themselves, caregivers and objects in a triadic relationship (Tomasello 1995). This period of development has been referred to as the illocutionary stage (Bates, Camaioni & Volterra 1975) and is marked by the development of more coordinated communicative behaviours. At this time, shifts in eye gaze between an object and a communicative partner may be combined with other forms of communication such as vocalisations and pointing, increasing the clarity of the child's message to the communication partner. These behaviours signal the onset of joint attention which refers to the use of behaviours such as pointing, showing and coordinating looks between objects and people in order to share attention with others. Joint attention can begin as early as 3 to 9 months of age (Mundy, Gwaltney & Henderson 2010).

Joint attention

Impairments and delays in the onset of joint attention are one of the earliest indicators of autism (Wetherby, Watt, Morgan & Shumway 2007). Research has shown that children with autism initiate joint attention (e.g. direct parent's attention to a favourite toy) and respond to other's bids for joint attention (e.g. follow a parent's pointing gesture) less than their typically developing peers (Charman 1998; Mundy & Crowson 1997). In summarizing the past 30 years of research in the area of joint attention and autism, Mundy et al. (2010) made the following observations:

> Children with autism display fewer joint attention behaviours compared to children with and without developmental disabilities; as early as 15–18 months, infants at risk for autism often display fewer acts of both responding to and initiating joint attention; over the course of development deficits in the tendency to initiate joint attention remain more robust than deficits in responding to the joint attention bids of others; and early interventions that increase joint attention have cascading effects on subsequent social learning (pp. 409–410).

Deficits in these areas, particularly in responding to joint attention bids, have been linked to poorer language outcomes (Luyster, Kadlec, Carter & Tager-Flusberg 2008). Furthermore, the responsiveness of caregivers to a child's focus of attention has also been associated with later language outcomes for children with and without disabilities (Siller & Sigman 2002; Yoder, Warren, McCathren & Leew 1998). Adults may respond to a child's joint attentional focus in a number of different ways. Yoder et al. (1998) examined three classes of adult responsiveness: non-linguistic contingent responses, linguistic contingent responses to the child's or infant's focus of attention, and linguistic contingent responses to the child's or infant's communicative act.

Non-linguistic contingent responses acknowledge the child's behaviour through the imitation of facial expression, imitation of children's play, and exact or reduced imitation of children's vocalizations. This type of responsiveness is thought to facilitate exploratory behaviour and contingency learning. While these responses appear to add little linguistic information to the child's behaviour, they appear to facilitate aspects of later levels of communication or language (Yoder et al. 1998).

Linguistic contingent responses to the child's focus of attention involve comments and directives about the child's focus of attention. There is empirical research to show that, for children with Down syndrome and typically developing children, linguistic contingent responses facilitate noun usage (Harris, Kasari & Sigman 1996). The third class of responsivity is linguistic contingent responses to the child or infant's communicative act. This form of responsivity adds linguistic information to the child's behaviour and may include linguistic mapping where the adult interprets what the child might mean by their communicative behaviour (Warren, Yoder, Gazdag, Kim & Jones 1993). Interestingly, mothers are more likely to linguistically map their child's communicative behaviours when they are intentional (Yoder, Warren, Kim & Gazdag 1994).

The importance of how an adult communicative partner responds to the communicative behaviour of children with autism has led to the development of interventions that focus not only on the communication of the child but also the sensitivity and responsiveness of the communication partner (usually the caregiver). Previous studies have reported success in teaching joint attention skills such as pointing and eye gaze to children with autism but the skills have often failed to generalise beyond the researcher to parents or teachers (Whalen & Schreibman 2003). In a recent study, Kasari et al. (2010) conducted a randomized controlled study to teach joint engagement behaviours to toddlers with autism. An intervention group comprising 19 caregiver/toddler dyads was compared with a wait-list control group which did not differ significantly from the intervention group on chronological age, mental age, developmental IQ, ethnicity, birth order, or caregiver's age and education. The intervention was mediated by the caregivers and individualized to the developmental readiness of the child. Parents were involved during play routines where they could follow the child's interests, as well as maintain and expand on their play activities. In total, there were 24 caregiver-mediated sessions over an eight week period with a follow-up one year after intervention was completed. The researchers found that the intervention group made significant improvements compared to the wait-list control group in targeted areas of joint engagement. The children demonstrated improvements in their responsiveness to joint attention and their diversity of functional play acts. Skills were maintained at follow-up. Studies such as these provide some evidence that although joint attention deficits are evident early in the development of children with autism, early intervention may ameliorate some of these deficits. It remains to be seen whether these interventions can also impact on the cascading effects on subsequent social learning to which Mundy et al. (2010) have referred.

While advances are being made in communication interventions, the developmental delays and difficulties in communication experienced by children with autism mean that some of these children may remain at the prelinguistic or pre-intentional stage of development for prolonged periods. This is a significant challenge for children with autism who, in the absence of more symbolic forms of communication, must rely on informal and often idiosyncratic ways of expressing their needs and wants. It is equally a challenge for the child's family and educators to try and interpret the function of these informal modes of communication. These attempts by children to communicate may not always be successful and this leads to breakdowns in communication.

Communication breakdowns

There are a number of ways in which breakdowns in communication can occur. The most common indicators of breakdown are requests for clarification, ignoring the communicative attempt, or a wrong response (Brady, McLean, McLean & Johnston 1995). A request for clarification, such as asking "What?" or "Do you want…?" is perhaps the most obvious indication that a breakdown has occurred. The breakdown is followed by a clear message from the adult that the child's message is unclear and the question posed by the adult creates an opportunity for the child to respond. This contrasts with ignoring the attempt, when there is no verbal or nonverbal acknowledgement of the child's behaviour and it may be unclear to the child whether the adult has ignored the behaviour on purpose (e.g. not wanting to give the child a sweet when the child whines) or merely that the behaviour has been overlooked (Brady et al. 1995). A wrong response signals a misunderstanding of the communicative message behind the child's behaviour. This may occur when, for example, a child points to a toy to request and the adult responds as if it were a comment by saying "Yes, that's a nice toy". Many children with autism are at increased risk of communicative breakdowns due to impairments in joint attention and reliance on prelinguistic forms of communication that may be ambiguous and difficult to understand (Keen 2003).

When a breakdown in communication occurs, children may attempt to repair the breakdown, protest or abandon the attempt to communicate (Golinkoff 1986). A communicative repair is defined as the attempt to persist in the communication attempt and to modify or revise the communication signal when this occurs (Wetherby & Prizant 1993). In order to do this, a child needs to recognize that the breakdown has occurred and to understand the needs of the communicative partner. This ability usually emerges around 12 months of age. The child must then enact the repair by repeating, modifying or changing their initial signal (Alexander, Wetherby & Prizant 1997). Communication repairs can be viewed from a developmental and an environmental perspective (Meadan, Halle, Watkins & Chadsey 2006).

From a developmental perspective, the type of repair used appears to change as the child's communication skills develop, with repetitions more common in children transitioning from the prelinguistic stage and repairs involving modification or changes becoming more prevalent as language competence develops (Alexander et al. 1997). There has been only a limited amount of research investigating the development and use of repair strategies for children with autism at the prelinguistic stage of development. As part of a larger study involving 120 typically developing children, Alexander et al. (1997) investigated the repair behaviours of six children with Pervasive Developmental Disorders (PDD), four of whom were at the prelinguistic stage and two in the early one-word stage of development. They found that these children with PDD tended to use more modifications than repetitions to repair, which differed from the pattern of the typically developing children. Similar to the typically developing children, however, the group with PDD used gesture to repair more often than other forms of nonverbal communication. These results suggest that children with autism may follow a different developmental trajectory in some areas of repair behaviour than their typically developing peers.

Recent research has considered environmental variables that may, in addition to developmental considerations, influence the repair behaviour of children with autism. Meadan et al. (2006) examined environmental influences on the repair strategies of two young children with autism with limited expressive language. They found that both participants attempted to repair the majority of communication breakdowns that occurred and that repair strategies varied across children, activities, and type of breakdown. One child, for example, pointed to the location of a missing puzzle piece during a puzzle activity and this was interpreted as a request. Pointing was used more frequently in this activity to repair breakdowns compared with other activities. This suggested that pointing in this activity was a more effective way for this child to convey his meaning than other behaviours he used to repair such as vocalising and reaching.

Interest in the use of repair strategies by children with autism has extended to examining whether there may be a relationship between communicative breakdown, repair and challenging behaviour. It has been known for some time that many challenging behaviours serve a communicative function (Durand & Carr 1991). Some researchers have suggested that challenging behaviour occurs as a form of protest or frustration in response to a failed attempt to communicate (Brady et al. 1995; Wetherby, Alexander & Prizant 1998). This proposes that the challenging behaviour occurs at the time of the communicative breakdown but is not an attempt to repair the breakdown. Another view is that some forms of challenging behaviour are a type of repair strategy (Halle, Brady & Drasgow 2004; Keen 2003, 2005). Alexander et al. (1997) observed that when children in their study with Pervasive Developmental Disorder or hearing impairment repaired a breakdown, they sometimes used gestures and vocalizations that were more emphatic and exaggerated. Keen (2005) found a similar pattern in some of the children with autism who participated in her study of repair strategies, hypothesising that some challenging behaviour may represent a repetition of an initial communicative behaviour with increased prosody. Further work is needed to explore this possible connection between repairs and problem behaviour as the outcomes of such research may have significant implications for interventions that target both communication and challenging behaviour.

Potential Communicative Acts

For children with autism which is accompanied by significant language impairments, it can be unclear whether their behaviour is both communicative and intentional (Iacono, Carter & Hook 1998). According to Wetherby and Prizant (1989), the following behaviours may be used as indicators of intentionality: (a) alternating eye gaze between goal and listener; (b) persistent signalling until the goal is accomplished or failure indicated; (c) changing the signal quality until the goal has been met; (d) ritualizing or conventionalizing the form of signal within specific communicative contexts; (e) awaiting a response from the listener; (f) terminating the signal when the goal is met; and (g) displaying satisfaction when the goal is attained or dissatisfaction when it is not. While these indicators may have some utility in practice, intentionality is something that must be inferred as it cannot be directly measured and applying these criteria of intentionality to children with autism can be problematic. For example, alternating eye gaze may be absent in some of these children, but this may not necessarily mean that these children are preintentional communicators (Granlund & Olsson 1999; Iacono et al. 1998).

The term Potential Communicative Acts (PCAs) has been used to describe informal or unconventional forms of communication frequently used by children with autism who have severe communication impairments or may be in the early stages of developing more intentional and symbolic forms of communication (Sigafoos et al. 2000). PCAs are behaviours that a communicative partner may interpret as communicative but where it is unclear whether the child is using them intentionally to communicate with that partner.

A priority for children who have severe communication impairments and communicate in these unconventional ways is to develop more symbolic and intentional forms of communication. Interventions to assist these children to achieve this goal may be informed through a better understanding of the nature of PCAs and to this end, a number of techniques have been used to identify PCAs used by these children. These techniques fall into three categories: interview protocols, naturalistic observations and structured observations.

Interview protocols

Detailed information about a child's communicative abilities can often be acquired from those who know the child best such as caregivers and teachers. Interviews of caregivers and teachers can be a useful way of gathering this type of information and a number of interview protocols have consequently been developed. These protocols are generally based on taxonomies of pragmatic communicative function (Cirrin & Rowland 1985; Coggins & Carpenter 1981; McLean & Snyder-McLean 1987). In the 1970s, prelinguistic communicative acts began to be categorized as proto-imperatives or proto-declaratives (Bates et al. 1975). Proto-imperatives refer to the child's intentional use of the listener as an agent or tool in achieving some end (requests). Proto-declaratives relate to the child's preverbal attempts to direct an adult's attention to some event or object (comments). During the 1980s, more detailed categorical systems were developed. A representative sample of these taxonomies of pragmatic functions is presented in Table 1.

These taxonomies have much in common with each other although there are some differences in terminology and in the specificity of the categories. For example, McLean and Snyder-McLean (1987) refer to seven different types of requesting while most other taxonomies refer to three. The work done by these researchers in determining taxonomies of pragmatic functions has underpinned the development of interview protocols for prelinguistic communicators which enable us to gain information about a child's communicative forms and their corresponding communicative functions. One such interview protocol for assessing the informal

Table 1. Taxonomies of pragmatic functions (reproduced with permission from Keen, 2001)

(Halliday 1975)	(Dore 1975)	(Coggins & Carpenter 1981)	(Cirrin & Rowland 1985)	(McLean & Snyder-McLean 1987)	(Butterfield 1991)
Instrumental	Labelling	Comment on action	Request action	Request object	Request object
Regulatory	Respecting	Comment on object	Request object	Request instrumental action	Request action
Interactional	Answering	Request for action	Request information	Request non-instrumental action	Reject
Personal	Requesting action	Request for object	Direct attention to self	Request attention to other	Protest
Heuristic	Requesting	Request for information	Direct for communication	Comments	Direct attention to self
Imaginative	Calling	Answering	Direct to object	Request attention to self	Direct attention to others
	Greeting	Acknowledging	Direct to action	Request cessation/reject/avoid	Response to name
	Protesting	Protesting	Answer	Request information/feedback	Response to greetings
	Practising		Protest	Initiation	Request for information
				Answer	
				Reply/acknowledge	
				Social convention/greeting	
				Expressive	

communication skills of children with severe communication impairment was developed by Schuler et al. (Schuler, Peck, Willard & Theimer 1989). The protocol provides a list of 23 behaviours that could be forms of communication such as facial expressions, aggression and crying, together with five possible communicative functions that could be associated with those forms: request affection/interaction; request adult action; request an item; protest; and comment. To help ascertain whether the informant who knows the child well believes any of the identified behaviours are communicative, they are asked questions in relation to each communicative function. For example, they may be asked how the child lets them know they want something to eat (request) or what the child would do if their favourite toy was taken away (protest).

Along similar lines, the Inventory of Potential Communicative Acts (IPCA) was developed as an interview-based assessment inventory. The IPCA can be used to systematically gather information from informants familiar with the child about behaviours they believe are used by the child to convey a particular message (Sigafoos et al. 2000). The IPCA prompts informants to indicate how the child communicates across 10 communicative functions through a series of 53 questions. Informants are assisted to think about a wide range of possible communicative forms through a detailed list of behaviours which they are given prior to the commencement of the interview. The IPCA also includes a useful matrix that shows the communicative forms mapped against the behaviours that informants have interpreted as communicative.

Naturalistic observations

Naturalistic observation has been an important tool in the assessment of a child's communicative behaviour as it takes into account the variability of this behaviour across settings and contexts (Iacono, Waring & Chan 1996). Environmental variables that may influence the frequency and type of communicative behaviour observed include the presence of different communicative partners, the activities in which the child is engaged and so forth. Naturalistic observation data is therefore often collected in a variety of contexts to provide a more comprehensive profile of communicative frequency, form and function (Halle 1993). While often yielding rich information about a child's communication, coding observational data can be very time consuming and there is a risk that some forms and functions may not be observed due to a lack of opportunity in the naturalistic setting.

Structured observations

Although less naturalistic, structured observations provide a way of systematically sampling a child's prelinguistic communication (Wetherby & Prutting 1984;

Wetherby, Yonclas & Bryan 1989). Situations can be structured to elicit certain behaviour from the child in relation to different communicative functions. Such situations, labelled communicative temptations by Wetherby and Prutting (Wetherby & Prutting 1984), can provide a quick and efficient means of gathering information in an objective way about the child's communication. Examples of communicative temptations to elicit requesting behaviour include eating a desired food in front of the child and not offering any, or putting a desired object/food in a hard to open container and giving the child the container. Communicative temptations can be very effective in sampling communication and have been incorporated into the Communication and Symbolic Behavior Scales (CSBS) which is a standardised assessment that evaluates the communication and symbolic abilities of children with a functional communication age between 6 months and 2 years (Wetherby & Prizant 2002).

Each of the three assessment techniques described above has limitations when used on its own and it is desirable to combine at least two of the techniques to ensure a more comprehensive communication profile of the prelinguistic communicator. In one study, Keen and colleagues (Keen 2001; Keen, Sigafoos & Woodyatt 2005) used a combination of the three different assessment approaches to identify the PCAs of eight children with autism aged 3–7 years. Initially, the child's teacher and parent were interviewed using the IPCA. This was followed by the use of both naturalistic and structured observations of the children to determine whether the observational data could verify the interview data. The interviews showed that for each child, both informants were interpreting a range of behaviours used by the child as communicative. The informants also associated the behaviours with a range of communicative functions from requesting to more developmentally advanced functions involving joint attention such as commenting. Functions requiring joint attention such as commenting and requesting information are not commonly found in children with autism (McArthur & Adamson 1996). Keen (2001) suggested, however, that her results may have been an artefact of the interview protocol (IPCA). In the IPCA, teachers and parents were asked how the child let them know that they were in pain (commenting) and a typical response was that the child cried. The crying was interpreted by the informant as a comment on the child's state. However, rather than being a true comment made intentionally by the child, the crying may have been a response to pain and elicited without communicative intent. Commenting and requesting information were not functions that were evident in any of the children in the study during structured and naturalist observation sessions. Differences were also found between the reports of the child's parent and teacher on the IPCA. On average, teachers and parents agreed on the presence of communicative functions 76% of the time and on communicative form only 9% of the time. One example of disagreement on communicative form occurred when one of the participants (Beth) wanted someone to be near. Beth's mother reported that Beth would cuddle her whereas the teacher reported that Beth would run toward her and bump into her.

It has been argued that children are sensitive to contextual variables and one of these variables of particular importance to communication is the communicative partner (Meadan et al. 2006). The partner may have an impact on both frequency and type of communication and interaction patterns may be built up over time as the child develops a shared history with each communication partner (Tomasello, Conti-Ramsden & Ewert 1990). In Beth's case, the mother likely reinforced the cuddling as a means of seeking comfort but this behaviour was probably received differently in the school setting. Beth's alternate way of seeking comfort at school through bumping into people was recognised by her teacher as a way to be near others, but was also perceived as problematic. Identifying the pragmatic communicative function of behaviours such as this can contribute to the development of appropriate intervention for children like Beth to teach an alternate way of seeking comfort in the school setting.

For children who rely on unconventional and less symbolic means to communicate, it is likely that their communicative forms will perhaps be even more context specific as they rely on people and objects in their environment to convey their message. Consider a child at home who wishes to communicate to his mother that he is hungry. He takes his mother by the hand and leads her to the refrigerator, placing her hand on the refrigerator handle. In a classroom setting devoid of refrigerators or food items, and without other means to communicate, the hungry child may struggle to find a way to make his needs understood.

Following the use of the IPCA, Keen and colleagues attempted to verify some of the behaviours that teachers had interpreted as forms of communication on the IPCA by using naturalistic and structured observations (Keen 2001; Keen et al. 2005). The naturalistic observations took place while the child was engaged in three different activities that were part of the normal classroom routine and were repeated across different times and days of the week. Sessions were videotaped and coded for communicative form and function. Structured observations also took place in the child's classroom. Samples of behaviours interpreted by teachers on the IPCA as communicative and representing a number of different pragmatic communicative functions were chosen for each child. The child was then presented with communicative opportunities that were designed to elicit a communicative act related to the chosen functions. For example, a communicative opportunity to request food involved the teacher sitting opposite the child during snack time with the child's food in sight but out of reach. For both the naturalistic and structured observations, communicative forms and functions were compared to those identified by the teacher informant on the IPCA to determine the degree of similarity.

Results indicated that 14% of the communicative forms identified by teachers were identical to those found using naturalistic observations and 70% for structured observations. However, partial agreement was also found using naturalistic observations for 63% of the communicative acts identified by teachers. During structured observations, partial agreement of up to 100% occurred whereby the teacher stated that the child used two behaviours simultaneously to request (e.g. reach and vocalise) but during observations, the child used only one (e.g. reach).

The results from these studies demonstrate the benefits of using different approaches to document the PCAs of children with autism. These assessments can show that parents and teachers do interpret PCAs as communicative and that further evidence of these PCAs can be gathered through naturalistic and structured observation. Identification of these PCAs can provide important information about the child's preferred modes of communication and can help guide the development of appropriate interventions.

Communication interventions and PCAs

It is unlikely that there will be a single intervention that will be appropriate for all children who are using PCAs to communicate although the goals of intervention will be the same across children using PCAs. That is, it is desirable to support these children to become more intentional and symbolic in their communication, thereby decreasing the frequency of communicative breakdowns and increasing the clarity and flexibility of their communication. Increasing the use of more symbolic forms of communication that represent the full range of communicative functions could lead to more effective and efficient communication that enhances the quality of life for individual children and their families. A detailed discussion of communication interventions is beyond the scope of this chapter. There is an extensive literature that investigates the use of augmentative and alternative communication for children with autism and/or severe communication impairments (e.g. Beukelman & Mirenda 2005; Mirenda, Iacono & Light 2009; Reichle, Beukelman & Light 2002; Sigafoos, Arthur-Kelly & Butterfield 2006). However, it is important to consider how the material presented in this chapter to date can inform intervention practices more generally. To this end, some intervention guidelines are outlined below that consider communicative forms used by children who rely on behaviours that may be idiosyncratic, unconventional or problematic.

These guidelines or 'decision rules' emanated from a study, conducted by Keen (2001), investigating the replacement of PCAs with new, more symbolic forms. These rules are based around an initial determination about whether the PCA form used by the child is problematic or socially inappropriate and are presented in Figure 1. Problematic forms may include behaviours such as screaming, hitting or spitting. Socially inappropriate forms may include grabbing or autistic leading where a child leads an adult by the hand to a desired object. A child using these forms would be well placed to benefit from an intervention that replaced the behaviours with more conventional or socially appropriate behaviours that could convey the same message. Keen et al. (2001) used a replacement intervention approach similar to functional communication training whereby challenging behaviour was replaced with more appropriate forms of communication (Durand 1993; Durand & Carr 1991). Through the replacement intervention, as the child acquired the new, more conventional behaviour, the use of the existing problematic form decreased. While this was an effective intervention for problematic

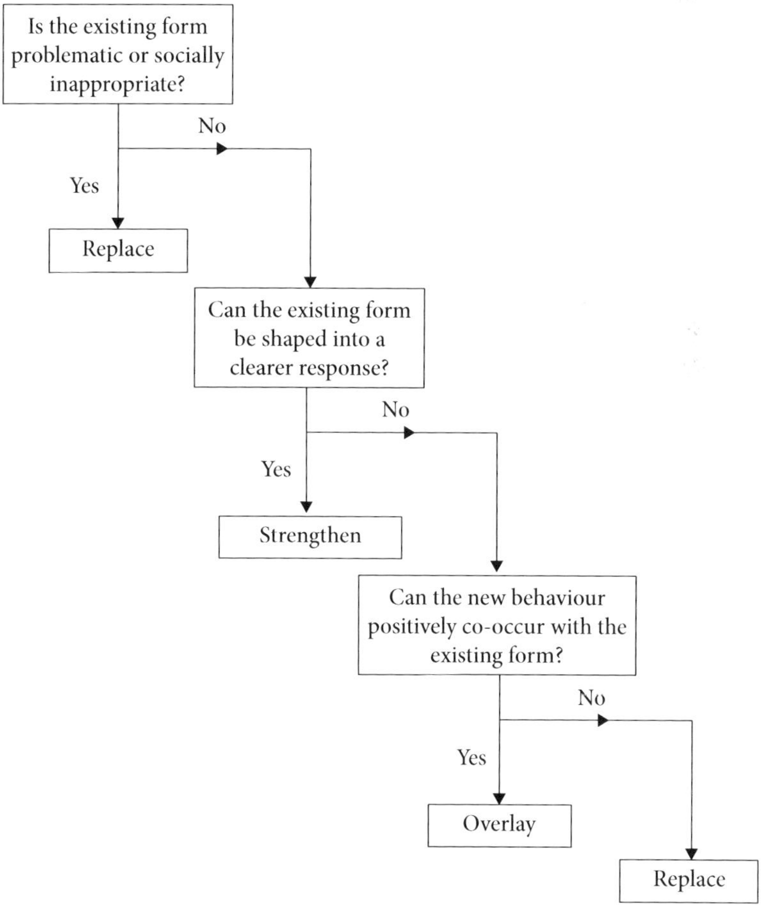

Figure 1. Decision rules for guiding choice of intervention between replacing, overlaying and strengthening (reproduced with permission from Keen 2001)

forms, some existing forms may be appropriate but ineffective because they may easily be overlooked or misunderstood, leading to communication breakdowns.

Under these circumstances, intervention may concentrate on either shaping the existing form into a stronger and clearer form or pairing the existing behaviour with another, complimentary behaviour. Consider the example of a child who, according to parent interview and observation, sometimes greets others by looking at them. Looking is an appropriate form of greeting and is not a behaviour that should usually be replaced or extinguished. Teaching the child to look at the person he is greeting more consistently would generally be considered to be a more appropriate intervention. However, if the child is reluctant to make eye contact, it may be difficult to teach him to look consistently as a form of greeting. In situations such as this, adding an additional greeting behaviour such as a wave could make his greeting easier to recognise and lead to greeting behaviour that could be clearer and more consistent. In this case, waving would be reinforced and would be the focus of the intervention, not looking.

A prelinguistic behaviour may persist, however, if it co-occurs with a replacement behaviour that is reinforced (Drasgow, Halle & Ostrosky 1998). In the study by Keen et al. (2001), this situation occurred and the looking behaviour did persist during intervention at the same level as it had occurred at baseline, while the waving behaviour increased during intervention. A slight modification to this intervention approach involves reinforcement of the existing and new behaviour simultaneously and is referred to in Figure 1 as 'overlay'. In the example above, looking was reinforced coincidentally. Using the overlay approach to intervention, both looking and waving would be targeted and explicitly reinforced.

The framework presented above highlights the importance of using assessment data to inform intervention decisions for children with unconventional and idiosyncratic communicative forms. Existing behaviours that may have a communicative message have the potential, through intervention, to be shaped into more conventional forms or augmented with forms that can be more easily observed and understood by communication partners. Some forms, however, may be inappropriate or problematic and could interfere with the acquisition of more appropriate forms of communication.

Summary and conclusion

This chapter has considered the potential communicative acts of children with autism from both a developmental and environmental perspective. Developmentally, some children with autism struggle to progress beyond the prelinguistic stage and continue to rely on primitive, idiosyncratic and unconventional forms of communication. While caregivers and teachers may interpret the child's potential communicative acts (PCAs) as forms of communication, the unconventional and idiosyncratic nature of these forms makes it difficult for those less familiar with the child to understand the child's message. While their typically developing peers progress through this phase, acquiring joint attention skills and more symbolic means of communication, these children exhibit joint attention deficits and may fail to show the behavioural indicators usually associated with intentional communication.

These impairments give rise to frustrations for the child and caregivers when attempting to communicate, and lead to frequent communication breakdowns and occurrences of problem behaviour. Skills to repair communication breakdowns are often limited and it is hypothesised that at times these children may use problematic forms of communication as a type of repair strategy. It appears that these children can be influenced to use different communicative forms in response to different contexts and communicative partners, which has implications for how we might assess their communicative forms. Three approaches to assessment were discussed and a combination of at least two of these is recommended to ensure a comprehensive knowledge of the child's communicative forms and functions.

A primary goal for parents and professionals is to help these children progress toward the use of communicative forms that can assist the child to effectively convey his/her message to others. As depicted in Figure 1, this means either shaping existing forms, learning new forms that can replace existing but inappropriate forms, or augmenting those that are appropriate but unclear. This should be undertaken in the context of an intervention that considers the development of joint attention skills and the implementation of a comprehensive augmentative and alternative communication system.

References

Adamson, L., & Chance, S. (1998). Coordinating attention to people, object and language. In A. Wetherby, S. Warren & J. Reichle (Eds.), *Transitions in Prelinguistic Communication* (pp. 15–37). Baltimore, MD: Paul H. Brookes.

Alexander, D., Wetherby, A., & Prizant, B. (1997). The emergence of repair strategies in infants and toddlers. *Seminars in Speech and Language, 18*, 197–212.

Bates, E., Camaioni, L., & Volterra, V. (1975). The acquisition of performatives prior to speech. *Merrill-Palmer Quarterly, 21*, 205–226.

Beukelman, D.R., & Mirenda, P. (2005). *Augmentative and Alternative Communication: Management of Severe Communication Disorders in Children and Adults* (3rd ed.). Baltimore, MD: Paul H. Brookes.

Brady, N.C., McLean, J.E., McLean, L.K., & Johnston, S. (1995). Initiation and repair of intentional communication acts by adults with severe to profound cognitive disabilities. *Journal of Speech and Hearing Research, 38*, 1334–1348.

Butterfield, N. (1991). Assessment of preverbal communicative abilities in students with severe intellectual disability. *Australia and New Zealand Journal of Developmental Disabilities, 17*, 347–364.

Charman, T. (1998). Specifying the nature and course of the joint attention impairment in autism in the preschool years. *Autism: The International Journal of Research and Practice, 2*, 61–79.

Cirrin, F., & Rowland, C. (1985). Communicative assessment of nonverbal youths with severe/profound mental retardation. *Mental Retardation, 23*, 52–62.

Coggins, T., & Carpenter, R. (1981). The communicative intention inventory: A system for observing and coding children's early intentional communication. *Applied Psycholinguistics, 2*, 235–251.

Dore, J. (1975). Holophrases, speech acts and language universals. *Journal of Child Language, 2*, 21–40.

Drasgow, E., Halle, J.W., & Ostrosky, M. (1998). Effects of differential reinforcement on the generalization of a replacement mand in three children with severe language delays. *Journal of Applied Behaviour Analysis, 31*, 357–374.

Durand, V.M. (1993). Functional communication training using assistive devices: Effects on challenging behavior and affect. *Augmentative and Alternative Communication, 9*, 168–176.

Durand, V.M., & Carr, E.G. (1991). Functional communication training to reduce challenging behavior: Maintenance and application in new settings. *Journal of Applied Behavior Analysis, 24*, 251–264.

Golinkoff, R.M. (1986). "I beg your pardon?": The preverbal negotiation of failed messages. *Journal of Child Language, 13*, 455–476.

Granlund, M., & Olsson, C. (1999). Efficacy of communication intervention for presymbolic communicators. *Augmentative and Alternative Communication, 15*, 25–37.

Halle, J.W. (1993). Innovative assessment measures and practices designed with the goal of achieving functional communication and integration. In Lisa Kuper (Ed.), *The Second National Symposium on Effective Communication for Children and Youth with Severe Disabilties: Topic Papers, Reader's Guide & Videotape* (pp. 201–251). McLean, Virginia.

Halle, J.W., Brady, N., & Drasgow, E. (2004). Enhancing socially adaptive communicative repairs of beginning communicators with disabilities. *American Journal of Speech-Language Pathology, 13*, 43–54.

Halliday, M. (1975). Learning how to mean. In E. Lenneberg & E. Lenneberg (Eds.), *Foundations of Language Development: A Multi-disciplinary Approach* (Vol. 1). New York, NY: Academic Press.

Harris, S., Kasari, C., & Sigman, M.D. (1996). Joint attention and language gains in children with Down syndrome. *American Journal on Mental Retardation, 100*, 608–619.

Iacono, T., Carter, M., & Hook, J. (1998). Identification of intentional communication in students with severe and multiple disabilities. *Augmentative and Alternative Communication, 14*, 102–114.

Iacono, T., Waring, R., & Chan, J.M. (1996). Sampling communicative behaviours in children with intellectual disability in structured and unstructured situations. *European Journal of Disorders of Communication, 31*, 106–120.

Kasari, C., Gulsrud, A.C., Wong, C., Kwon, S., & Locke, J. (2010). Randomized controlled caregiver mediated joint engagement intervention for toddlers with autism. *Journal of Autism and Developmental Disorders, 40*, 1045–1056.

Keen, D. (2001). *Analysis and Enhancement of Communication Behaviour in Children with Autism*. Brisbane: University of Queensland.

Keen, D. (2003). Communicative repair strategies and problem behaviours of children with autism. *International Journal of Disability, Development and Education, 50*, 53–64.

Keen, D. (2005). The use of non-verbal repair strategies by children with autism. *Research in Developmental Disabilities, 26*, 243–254.

Keen, D., Sigafoos, J., & Woodyatt, G. (2001). Replacing prelinguistic behaviors with functional communication. *Journal of Autism and Developmental Disorders, 31*, 385–398.

Keen, D., Sigafoos, J., & Woodyatt, G. (2005). Teacher responses to the communicative attempts of children with autism. *Journal of Developmental and Physical Disabilities, 17*, 19–33.

Luyster, R.J., Kadlec, M.B., Carter, A.S., & Tager-Flusberg, H. (2008). Language assessment and development in toddlers with autism spectrum disorders. *Journal of Autism and Developmental Disorders, 38*, 1426–1438.

McLean, J., & Snyder-McLean, L. (1987). Form and function of communicative behaviour among persons with severe developmental disabilities. *Australia and New Zealand Journal of Developmental Disabilities, 13*, 83–98.

McArthur, D, & Adamson, L. (1996). Joint attention in preverbal children: Autism and developmental language disorder. *Journal of Autism and Developmental Disorders, 26*, 481–496.

Meadan, H., Halle, J.W., Watkins, R.V., & Chadsey, J.G. (2006). Examining communication repairs of 2 young children with autism spectrum disorder: The influence of the environment. *American Journal of Speech-Language Pathology, 15*, 57–71.

Mirenda, P., Iacono, T., & Light, J. (Eds.). (2009). *AAC and autism*. Baltimore, MD: Paul H. Brookes.

Mundy, P., & Crowson, M. (1997). Joint attention and early social communication: Implications for research on intervention with autism. *Journal of Autism and Developmental Disorders, 27*, 653–676.

Mundy, P., Gwaltney, M., & Henderson, H. (2010). Self-referenced processing, neurodevelopment and joint attention in autism. *Autism, 14*, 408–429.

Reichle, J., Beukelman, D., & Light, J. (Eds.). (2002). *Implementing an Augmentative Communication System: Exemplary Strategies for Beginning Communicators*. Baltimore, MD: Paul H. Brookes.

Schuler, A., Peck, C., Willard, C., & Theimer, K. (1989). Assessment of communicative means and functions through interview: Assessing the communicative capabilities of individuals with limited language. *Seminars in Speech and Language, 10*, 51–62.

Sigafoos, J., Arthur-Kelly, M., & Butterfield, N. (2006). *Enhancing Everyday Communication for Children with Disabilities*. Baltimore, MD: Paul H. Brookes.

Sigafoos, J., Woodyatt, G., Keen, D., Tait, K., Tucker, M., Roberts-Pennell, D., et al. (2000). Identifying potential communicative acts in children with developmental and physical disabilities. *Communication Disorders Quarterly, 21*(2), 77–86.

Siller, M., & Sigman, M. (2002). The behaviors of parents of children with autism predict the subsequent development of their children's communication. *Journal of Autism and Developmental Disorders, 32*, 77–89.

Tomasello, M. (1995). Joint attention as social cognition. In C. Moore & P. Dunham (Eds.), *Joint Attention: Its Origins and Role in Development* (pp. 103–130). Hillsdale, NJ: Lawrence Erlbaum Associates.

Tomasello, M., Conti-Ramsden, G., & Ewert, B. (1990). Young children's conversations with their mothers and fathers: Differences in breakdown and repair. *Journal of Child Language, 17*, 115–130.

Warren, S., Yoder, P., Gazdag, G., Kim, K., & Jones, H. (1993). Facilitating prelinguistic communication skills in young children with developmental delay. *Journal of Speech and Hearing Research, 36*, 83–97.

Wetherby, A., Alexander, D., & Prizant, B. (1998). The ontogeny and role of repair strategies. In A. Wetherby, S.F. Warren & J. Reichle (Eds.), *Transitions in Prelinguistic Communication* (Vol. 7, pp. 135–159). Baltimore, MD: Paul H. Brookes.

Wetherby, A., & Prizant, B. (1989). The expression of communicative intent: Assessment guidelines. *Seminars in Speech and Language, 10*, 77–90.

Wetherby, A., & Prizant, B. (1992). Facilitating language and communication development in autism: Assessment and intervention guidelines. In D. Berkell (Ed.), *Autism: Identification, Education and Treatment* (pp. 107–134). Hillsdale, NJ: Lawrence Erlbaum Associates.

Wetherby, A., & Prizant, B. (1993). *Communication and Symbolic Behavior Scales*. Chicago, IL: Applied Symbolix.

Wetherby, A., & Prizant, B. (2002). *Communication and Symbolic Behavior Scales Developmental Profile*. Baltimore, MD: Paul H. Brookes.

Wetherby, A., & Prutting, C. (1984). Profiles of communicative and cognitive-social abilities in autistic children. *Journal of Speech and Hearing Research, 27*, 364–377.

Wetherby, A., Watt, N., Morgan, L., & Shumway, S. (2007). Social communication profiles of children with autism spectrum disorders in the second year of life. *Journal of Autism and Developmental Disorders, 37*, 960–975.

Wetherby, A., Yonclas, D., & Bryan, A. (1989). Communicative profiles of preschool children with handicaps: Implications for early identification. *Journal of Speech and Hearing Disorders, 54*, 148–158.

Whalen, C., & Schreibman, L. (2003). Joint attention training for children with autism using behavior modification procedures. *Journal of Child Psychology and Psychiatry and Allied Disciplines, 44*, 4556–4468.

Yoder, P., Warren, S.F., Kim, K., & Gazdag, G. (1994). Facilitating prelinguistic communication skills in young children with developmental delay II: Systematic replication and extension. *Journal of Speech and Hearing Research, 37*, 841–851.

Yoder, P., Warren, S.F., McCathren, R., & Leew, S. (1998). Does adult responsivity to child behavior facilitate communication development? In A. Wetherby, S.F. Warren & J. Reichle (Eds.), *Transitions in Prelinguistic Communication* (Vol. 7, pp. 39–58). Baltimore, MD: Paul H. Brookes.

CHAPTER 2

Facilitating emergent verbal repertoires in individuals with autism spectrum disorders and other developmental disorders

Insights from behaviour analysis

Richard J. May[1,2] & Simon Dymond[1]
[1]Swansea University / [2]University of South Wales

Applied behaviour analysis (ABA) is the science that underpins several evidence-based interventions currently undertaken with individuals with autism. With its grounding in learning theory, ABA has traditionally approached language instruction via the systematic application of operant conditioning principles (e.g. reinforcement, shaping, generalisation). However, recent advances in a research domain known as derived relational responding indicates that important language skills involving arbitrary stimulus relations may emerge in the absence of a direct training history. Available evidence suggests that the application of these procedures may enhance existing methods of teaching language skills to children with autism and other developmental disorders. The present article reviews the current status of the literature on facilitating emergent communication by relational responding. Studies involving procedures that have facilitated emergent verbal repertoires in individuals with autism and other developmental disabilities are described and evaluated, and further research challenges are discussed.

Applied behaviour analysis (ABA) is a "science in which tactics derived from the principles of behaviour are applied systematically to improve socially significant behaviour, and experimentation is used to identify the variables responsible for behaviour change" (Cooper, Heron & Heward 2007: p. 20). Put simply, the goal of ABA-based assessment and intervention is to establish meaningful differences in the behavioural repertoires of individuals through the application of behavioural principles and careful experimental analysis. Among many other accomplishments, ABA has recently helped to inform novel approaches to teaching functional language and communication skills to individuals with diagnoses of autism and other developmental disorders (LeBlanc, Dillon & Sautter 2009). Indeed, ABA methods now underpin several widely used evidence-based interventions that involve aspects of functional language learning, such as Early Intensive Behavioural Intervention (EIBI; Virués-Ortega 2010), the Picture Exchange Communication System (PECS; Frost & Bondy 1994), and Incidental Teaching (Hart & Risley 1975). These interventions each involve systematically targeting individual language skills and applying behavioural principles, such as shaping/fading, differential reinforcement, extinction, and stimulus control to the acquisition and maintenance of basic units of conversation and other communication skills (e.g. requesting, asking, and answering questions, etc.).

While this approach has resulted in a some promising outcomes (Eldevik, Hastings, Hughes, Jahr, Eikeseth & Cross 2010; Flippin, Reszka & Watson 2010; Reichow, Barton, Boyd & Hume 2011; Reichow & Wolery 2009), recent findings indicate that incorporating additional teaching elements may further enhance interventions. In particular, there is a growing body of research suggesting that language and communication skills can develop in the absence of a direct reinforcement history or explicit teaching. By planning instruction in particular ways, a range of novel, generative language skills have been shown to emerge in individuals with previously limited functional language.

Significant benefits may accrue from tailoring instruction to explicitly target emergent verbal behaviour in children with autism and other developmental disorders. In situations where curricula recommend the explicit teaching of all language forms, the sheer volume of teaching trials required to directly teach every component part of a minimal linguistic repertoire presents a serious practical challenge. For those using alternative and augmentative communication devices (AAC), the time-consuming nature of extensive teaching trials may be of particular concern. Alternative and augmentative communication devices are often utilised to provide learners with a functional means of communication in the absence of the typical speech development. Such systems generally consist of pictures, spoken and/or printed words that learners are taught to select, point to, or exchange with a communicative partner (e.g. PECS™: Frost & Bondy 1994; voice-output communication aids (VOCAs): Sigafoos et al. 2004). For instance, the PECS consists of a range of pictures or symbols that can be exchanged with a 'listener'. Exchanging a picture serves particular functions such as requesting an item or activity, or engaging in a conversational response. Learning to use the PECS involves a series of discrete steps aimed at ensuring that the child can discriminate between pictures of different objects or events, transfer a picture of the preferred object to a workbook, identify and locate a caregiver, and exchange the relevant picture for access to the preferred object (Frost & Bondy 1994).

At present, many AAC systems such as the PECS necessitate the direct teaching of each new communicative response. Although it may be desirable to teach particular requests via direct experience, an approach that involves directly training every request that a child may require is both time consuming and labour intensive. Ideally, therefore, language-training programs should seek to develop techniques that serve to establish appropriate communicative behaviour, like requesting, in the absence of explicit training.

Recent developments in the field of behaviour analysis may provide novel ways to both facilitate emergent language skills and re-conceptualize the behavioural approach to, and theories of, language. In particular, techniques, many of which originate in Skinner's (1957) analysis of verbal behaviour, have been elaborated and adapted to the challenge of developing economical teaching methods to establish appropriate language skills in the absence of extensive training. These methods present some exciting new possibilities for teaching language to children with autism and other developmental disorders (Carr & Felce 2000; Rehfeldt & Barnes-Holmes 2009). The aim of the current chapter is to provide an overview of this contemporary behaviour-analytic research domain.

Derived relational responding, stimulus equivalence, and the basic experiment

Psychologists have long been interested in the seemingly unique human capacity to classify and organise linguistic stimuli. Behaviour commonly defined as 'symbolic', such as categorization and concept formation, often cannot readily be traced to a history of direct learning. Over the past four decades, behaviour analysis has developed a productive approach to the study of symbolic behaviour, called derived relational responding. Derived relational responding has its foundations in the phenomenon of stimulus equivalence, whereby an organism treats one stimulus as being equivalent to another. Consideration of stimulus equivalence dates back to ancient Greece (Aristotle in *De Memoria et Reminiscentia*, 451b; 1941) and was the focus of research by experimental psychologists as early as the 1930s (e.g. Hull 1939). However, it was not until the 1970s that Murray Sidman began to devise a coherent set of experimental procedures with which to study it (Sidman 1994).

Sidman (1971) worked with an individual with intellectual disabilities who, before the study, could select a picture of a number of items when given their corresponding dictated names (e.g. "car"), name the various pictures and imitate vocally. This ability to select a picture given its name, which was repeated for many name-picture relations, is represented in Figure 1 with the letters A–B. Next, the participant was further taught to select printed words (e.g. CAR) when given its corresponding dictated name (e.g. "car"). This is represented in Figure 1 as A–C. Following this A–B and A–C training, the participant then went on to spontaneously (i.e. in the absence of feedback) select pictures given words (C–B), select words given pictures (B–C; Figure 1), and name all of the words. Sidman's (1971) findings were subsequently replicated and extended by Sidman and Cresson

(1973). They worked with a participant less proficient on name-picture matching and picture naming, but who subsequently demonstrated picture-word matching and word naming at up to 90% accuracy (see also, Green 1990; Sidman, Cresson & Willson-Morris 1974; Sidman & Tailby 1982; Smeets & Barnes-Holmes 2005).

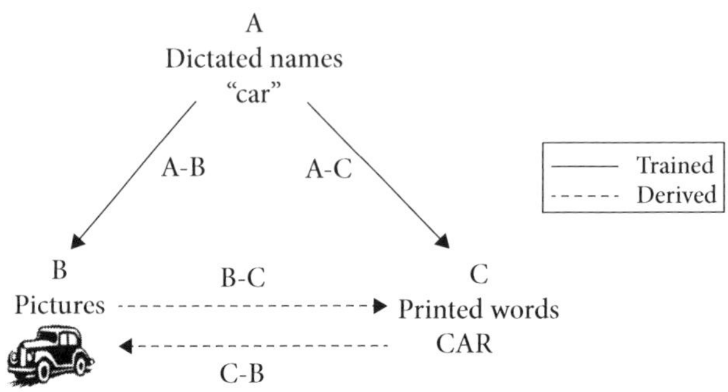

Figure 1. A schematic procedural summary of Sidman (1971)

These untrained 'derived stimulus relations' have since become the most widely studied topic in the experimental analysis of human behaviour (Dymond & Critchfield 2002). They are of considerable theoretical significance precisely because they are not readily explained by traditional behavioural principles (Hayes, Barnes-Holmes & Roche 2001; Sidman 1994). Neither B nor C, for instance, have a history of differential reinforcement with regard to each other, therefore, the presentation of one should not control the selection of the other. Also, the derived stimulus relations that emerge cannot be accounted for on the basis of generalization because the stimuli are all physically dissimilar. Other low-level associative processes also struggle to account for the reliable emergence of these auditory-visual and visual-visual stimulus relations (e.g. Hall 1996; Smyth, Barnes-Holmes & Barnes-Holmes 2008).

From the outset, however, research on derived relational responding has been of immediate relevance for attempts to facilitate novel communicative behaviour in individuals lacking such abilities. We will now review the existing research on derived relational responding, focusing on derived manding, derived intraverbals, derived textual behaviour, and derived tacting as examples of this contemporary approach.

Facilitating emergent verbal repertoires: Derived manding

Skinner (1957) described a mand as verbal behaviour by a speaker which results in a specific consequence being provided by a listener. Mands occur due to the particular state of deprivation or aversive stimulation of the speaker. For example, a mand may include uttering "water" where (a) the water is not present; (b) the utterance is made in the presence of a listener who mediates the delivery of the reinforcer (water); and (c) the response occurs as a result of the state of deprivation (thirst) of the speaker. The mand is the only form of verbal behaviour that is not under the control of a particular prior or antecedent stimulus (e.g. the water is not present); control is exerted by deprivation state of the speaker and the particular functional outcome (e.g. receiving the water) that follows its emission.

A *derived* mand occurs when a speaker requests an item, action or event that has not previously been provided for such a request (Barnes-Holmes et al. 2000; Rosales & Rehfeldt 2009). More specifically, derived manding may be said to have occurred when an object is requested that "(a) has never reinforced the mand in the past, (b) has never reinforced a different mand that might induce the current mand (i.e. response induction), (c) does not physically resemble an object that previously reinforced the mand (i.e. primary stimulus generalization), and (d) has never been paired with an object that previously reinforced the mand (i.e. respondent conditioning)" (Barnes-Holmes et al. 2000: p. 72).

For instance, if a child with autism learns to request juice using a picture of juice from the PECS, he or she may then be taught to relate the picture to its dictated name (Name ["juice"]-Picture [from PECS]: A–B), and to relate the dictated name to its corresponding written text (Name ["juice"]-Text [JUICE]: A–C). If the child subsequently requests juice using the written text (i.e. text exchange) – a behaviour that was never directly taught – then derived requesting has occurred (see Figure 2). Given this history, a person is also likely to speak the word "juice" both on being presented with a picture of juice (B–A) and the printed word (C–A), as well as pointing to pictures given the printed words (C–B) and vice versa (B–C), without any further training (Rehfeldt & Barnes-Holmes 2009; Sidman 1994).

Derived manding occurs under the control of both the individual's current motivational state and a history of derived relational responding; it is the presence of a history of derived relational responding that distinguishes derived mands from non-derived, directly learned mands. Emergent requesting repertoires of this kind have particular utility for learners with limited language repertoires since they result in generative communicative behaviour. Indeed, maximizing emergent forms of requesting may be particularly important for individuals who demonstrate behavioural and communicative rigidity that is often seen with children with autism (Rosales & Rehfeldt 2009).

To date, a number of studies have established derived manding skills in individuals with limited language repertoires with and without autism. Halvey and Rehfeldt (2005) sought to facilitate a derived manding repertoire in three adults with severe developmental disabilities by examining whether a derived vocal 'category' requesting response would emerge following a history of relational

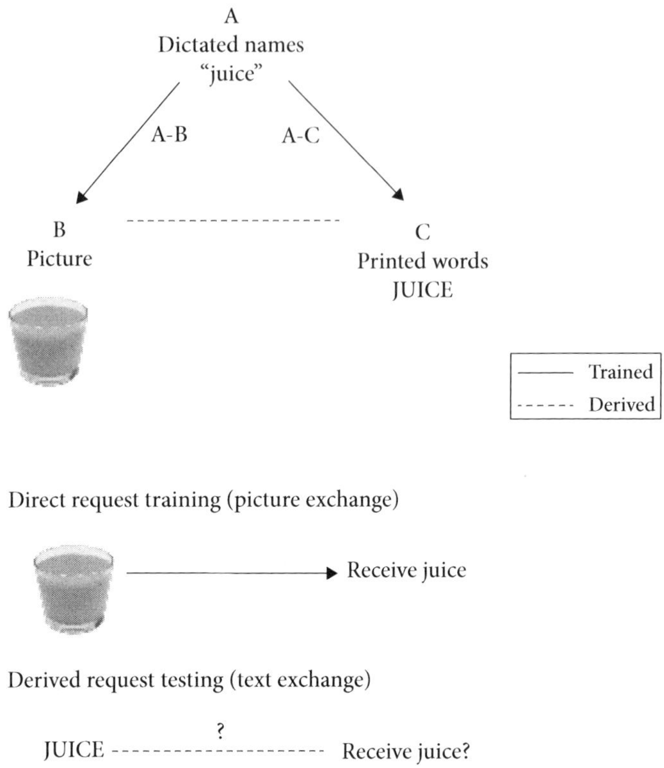

Figure 2. Schematic representation of trained and tested relations involved in establishing derived manding with text-exchange

responding with members of that category. Initially, three items from each of three distinct categories were selected as preferred items for each individual learner via a formalized preference assessment (DeLeon & Iwata 1996). Each participant was then given training to request one of the items from each category with the respective category name (e.g. training to request an apple by using the mand, "fruit"). Once participants demonstrated this mand repertoire, they were given conditional discrimination training to relate the category member with the two other members of the same category. That is, when presented with a picture of the item trained as a category vocal request, and three comparison stimuli consisting of three distinct categories, they were taught to select the picture of the preferred item from the same category. This training was repeated for both of the remaining category members. Finally, post-test probes indicated that participants reliably used the category name to request those items not previously used during mand training. Halvey and Rehfeldt's findings showed how a history of relational responding results in the emergence of derived vocal requests for related category members.

Rehfeldt and Root (2005) further examined the extent to which a derived manding repertoire could be facilitated by relational training. Rather than establishing a derived vocal category mand, the authors sought to establish novel mands with text exchange, following initial training with the PECS (Frost & Bondy 1994). Participants were three adults with severe mental retardation, described as having either rudimentary or no functional communication skills (formal language assessments were not conducted). Prior to the intervention, three items for each participant were selected as preferred items, and participants were pre-tested on a number of existing relations between the items and experimental materials. Relations between the dictated names of items (A) and the corresponding pictures (B), and between the dictated names (A) and the corresponding text (C) were pre-tested, as well as the extent to which participants would exchange a picture of an item for the corresponding item or match the text to the item. Following this pre-test phase, using a multiple probe across participants design (Kennedy 2005) the authors implemented PECS training for each of the three items. This was followed by a sequence of relational training involving pictures, text and the corresponding dictated names. Specifically, participants were trained to select the correct picture from an array given the dictated name of the item (A–B training), and to select the correct text given the name of the item (A–C training). Following this, the emergence of a derived manding repertoire was demonstrated by all three participants who reliably exchanged the correct text for the preferred items despite having no history of receiving the items for such an exchange in the past.

Rosales and Rehfeldt (2007) provided a partial replication and extension of the study described above. These authors also utilized the PECS to explicitly train a manding repertoire with two adults with developmental disabilities and limited language repertoires. However, as part of this mand training, and unlike the previous studies above, the authors ensured that the target items were not present when the mands occurred. This more closely approximates manding in the real world, since the reinforcer manded is usually not present when the mand response is made (Skinner 1957). To replicate such conditions, Rosales and Rehfeldt taught participants to request missing items needed to complete a chained task (e.g. Schuster, Gast, Wolery & Guiltinan 1988). For example, participants provided with a CD player and CD were taught to exchange a picture to request headphones (which were not present). The authors also assessed the extent to which participants exchanged text for the required items prior to any mand or relational training. Following these pretests, relational training was implemented whereby participants selected a picture from an array upon hearing the spoken words (A–B training) and selected text from an array upon hearing the spoken words (A–C training). The results indicated that both participants used text to mand for items following the relational training, despite this repertoire not being explicitly trained. The authors noted, however, that one month later, the derived mands were not maintained. Rather, the participants used vocal mands, a repertoire that neither of the individuals had demonstrated prior to or during the study. The authors speculated that vocal manding may have emerged as a result of the earlier relational training procedures establishing the spoken word, pictures, text and items as functionally substitutable for one another.

The research of Rehfeldt and colleagues described above entail many benefits in the economy of teaching functional communication skills to language-impaired individuals. For each item, the name, picture and text were established as functionally substitutable for one another, which led to new communicative behaviour which had never been explicitly taught. There are potential advantages for a communicative exchange involving text, not least of which is the fact that the request is more readily understood by a wider audience of 'listeners'. Transfering text rather than pictures may also be a favourable outcome where community integration and inclusion for adults with limited language repertoires are valued treatment goals.

Further research on derived manding

Murphy, Barnes-Holmes and Barnes-Holmes (2005) have further described methods of relational training to establish derived manding repertoires in children with autism. In their first study, Murphy et al. taught three children to request two different cardboard tokens (X1 and X2) in order to complete a token board and subsequently receive a reinforcer. Participants were taught to request the tokens by presenting A1 and A2 stimulus cards (nonsense syllables) respectively. Once these directly trained requests were established, the participants were given relational training (A–B: in the presence of A1[A2], picking B1[B2] was reinforced; and B–C: in the presence of B1[B2], picking C1[C2] was reinforced). Following this, tests for derived manding assessed the extent to which the children requested the X1 and X2 tokens with the C1 and C2 stimulus cards. For two of the three participants, the derived manding repertoire emerged immediately and without further training. The remaining participant required remedial training in the form of corrective feedback during derived mand tests following relational training with a number of new stimulus sets. Training with multiple exemplars has been found to facilitate derived relational responding where absent (e.g. Barnes-Holmes, Barnes-Holmes, Roche & Smeets 2001; Berens & Hayes 2007). Consistent with predictions, when presented with a novel stimulus set, the participant demonstrated derived manding.

Murphy and Barnes-Holmes (2009) further evaluated the emergence of derived manding in four children with autism. Participants first played a game in which the goal was to maintain a particular number of smiley-face tokens on a token board. Participants were given training to mand for *more* tokens by presenting stimulus card D1 (an arbitrary symbol) to the experimenter and to receive *less* tokens by presenting D2. Following mastery of this more/less manding procedure, participants were then given training with two further stimulus cards, A1 and A2. In the presence of A1 and two lines of smiley-faces of differing lengths, participants were taught to select the longer of the two lines; and in the presence of A2, participants were taught to select the shorter of the two lines. This ensured that functions of more-than and less-than were attached to the A1 and A2 stimuli, respectively. As in the Murphy et al. (2005) study, children were then given A–B and B–C relational training: they were required to select B1[B2] in the presence of A1[A2], and C1[C2] in the presence of B1[B2]. Following this training, all children passed the tests for derived manding by selecting C1 as a request for more smiley-faces and C2 as a request for fewer smiley-faces, over repeated trials.

Murphy and Barnes-Holmes (2010a) directly extended these findings by increasing from two to five the number of stimulus cards available to exchange as mands. Three adolescents with autism were taught to mand for either for 2, 1, 0, −1 or −2 tokens in order to maintain a particular number of tokens on the board. If they were able to achieve the required number of tokens by manding for the addition or removal of the correct amount of tokens, the participants were rewarded with points that could be later exchanged for prizes. Participants were taught to mand for the specific quantities by presenting one of a number of stimulus cards (A1, A2, A3, A4, or A5) in order to have to either have 2, 1, 0, −1 or −2 tokens delivered or removed respectively. Following this direct mand training, A–B and B–C relational training was undertaken in which, for example, in the presence of A1, selecting B1 was reinforced, and in the presence of B1, selecting C1 was reinforced. When all of the relations had been trained (A1–B1, A2–B2, A3–B3, A4–B4, A5–B5, B1–C1, B2–C2, B3–C3, B4–C4, and B5–C5), derived mand tests revealed that, for two participants, mand functions transferred to the equivalent C stimuli, in line with the relational training employed. Multiple exemplar training across a number of stimulus sets resulted in emergence of derived manding in the final participant.

Derived comparative relations and derived manding

The relational training procedures implemented by the studies described thus far have sought to establish stimulus relations where all of the stimuli serve a functionally identical purpose. In other words, if a learner is taught that the spoken word "juice" is the same as a picture of juice and the spoken word "juice" is also the same as the text 'JUICE', the learner may then substitute either the spoken word or the text as part of a novel request (Figure 2).

A prominent behavioural theory of language and cognition, relational frame theory (RFT; Hayes et al. 2001), proposes that equivalence is one type of a number of possible derived stimulus relations (Dymond & Roche 2013; Hayes et al. 2001; Törneke 2010). For instance, a substantial literature has amassed on comparative relations, such as more-than and less-than, which are by definition not functionally equivalent (Dymond, May, Munnelly & Hoon 2010; Munnelly, Dymond & Hinton 2010). To illustrate, consider a child who has a history of receiving 10 sweets in return for a blue token. If the child is subsequently told that a yellow token is worth *more than* the blue token, the child is likely to select the yellow token when given a choice between the two, despite having never experienced any consequences for exchanging yellow tokens. If she is subsequently told that the yellow token is now worth *less than* the blue token she is now likely to select the blue token. In this example, the functional properties of the tokens are transformed on the basis of the specified relation of more-than or less-than, rather than as a result of any physical properties of the tokens or history of having received differential consequences for using the tokens in the past.

In a further study, Murphy and Barnes-Holmes (2010b) directly examined the emergence of derived mands involving comparative relations of more-than/less-than in four children with autism and three typically developing children. Participants were given mand training with five stimulus cards (arbitrary symbols) representing five specific token values ranging from −2 to 2. Participants were then given relational training to pick the longer of two lines of tokens in the presence of X and to pick the shorter of two lines in the presence of Y, over various presentations of lines differing in length. Having established a 'more-than' function for X, and a 'less-than' function for Y, these two stimuli were used to train a comparative relational network consisting of printed nonsense words (labeled, for the purposes of clarity, A, B, C, D, and E). Blocks of trials were administered in which pairs of stimuli were presented (e.g. A and B). For each pair presented, participants' selection of one stimulus (e.g. A) was reinforced in the presence of the 'more than' cue (X) and selection of the other stimulus (e.g. B) was reinforced in the presence of the 'less than' cue (Y). By systematically presenting four pairs of stimuli, the following relational network was trained: A>B>C>D>E (i.e. A is more than B, B is more than C, C is more than D, D is more than E).

Following the training of the comparative relational network, participants were then re-presented with the mand game, however, this time they were presented with the nonsense syllables with which to request the addition or removal of tokens, rather than the directly trained cards. The final phase revealed that all but two of the seven participants manded for specific quantities of +2, +1, 0, −1 and −2 with the

A, B, C, D, and E stimuli. In other words, participants correctly manded with a member of the newly trained relational network in order to increase or decrease the number of tokens needed (in the absence of any consequences). Crucially, the functions of each of the stimuli of 'more' or 'less' had been transformed in accordance with the comparative relational network. For the participants for whom derived manding did not immediately emerge, multiple exemplar training was implemented. Corrective feedback provided during derived mand tests with two sets of stimuli, led to the emergence of derived manding in accordance with the comparative relations on a further set (Murphy & Barnes-Holmes 2010b).

These findings provide further evidence that relational responding can be utilized to engender emergent verbal repertoires. In addition, this novel behaviour may be determined by relational training involving comparative relations. While the nature of the particular tasks involved in the studies described above may seem somewhat arbitrary, facilitating relational repertoires may have important generalized effects in terms of verbal flexibility. Proponents of relational frame theory argue that an essential element of what can be considered 'verbal' behaviour is the ability to place stimuli in relation with one another and respond to the stimuli accordingly (Törneke 2010). Furthermore, it is the ability to respond to stimuli, not on the basis of a nonarbitrary relation between stimuli (e.g. physical dissimilarity), but on the basis of specific arbitrarily applicable contextual cues that have been established in a person's behavioural history. In the example given above, for example, a child may choose the yellow token over the blue token in accordance with the contextual cue of more-than and less-than, rather than on the basis of the nonarbitrary features of the stimuli involved (i.e. relative size of the tokens, colour etc.) It is proposed that responding relationally in accordance with contextual cues that are established and arranged via social convention (such as relations of 'equivalence' or 'comparison' described here) is a key feature of language and may be a crucial factor in establishing and maintaining flexible verbal behaviour (Hayes et al. 2001).

Facilitating emergent verbal repertoires: Derived intraverbals

Skinner defined an intraverbal as an instance of verbal behaviour emitted by a speaker in response to another verbal stimulus. For example, when a child answers "four" as a response to the question, "what is two plus two?" intraverbal responding is shown. In contrast to the mand, in which a particular reinforcer is specified by the speaker, the consequences mediated by a listener following an intraverbal response are more general, usually social, in nature. For example, a teacher saying "correct!", and other related forms of approval are examples of commonly used generalized conditioned reinforcers. In addition, the intraverbal response emitted, be it spoken, written or signed, bears no formal correspondence to the prior verbal stimulus (Skinner 1957). In natural language, conversational responses can generally be categorized as intraverbal behaviour (Stromer & Vogt 2009; Sundberg & Michael 2001).

Derived intraverbals are distinct in that they are established via a history of relational responding, rather than having been acquired through a direct history of reinforcement for using such a response in the past. For instance, a child who has been directly taught to respond to the stimulus "count to three", but can also respond appropriately to "count backwards from three" or "what comes between one and three?" in the absence of any further teaching, is emitting a derived intraverbal (Barnes-Holmes et al. 2000). For these responses to emerge, "the individual words *one*, *two*, and *three* participate in derived comparative relations such that the intraverbal counting response "one, two, three" entails "three and two after one" or entails "one before two, and three after two" (Barnes-Holmes et al. 2000: p. 75). Such procedures may be important in fostering flexible and complex verbal repertoires in individuals with language and communication difficulties, particularly in situations which can lead to favourable and inclusive social consequences, such as conversational competency (Stromer & Vogt 2009).

Perez-Gonzalez, Herszlikowicz and Williams (2008) provide an empirical demonstration of how directly taught intraverbals may be combined via relational training to facilitate novel spoken language. Typically developing children aged between 5 and 6 years old were taught to respond to four questions involving countries, cities and parks (see Figure 3). When the experimenter presented the statement, "Name the city of Argentina", participants were taught to say, "Buenos Aires", and when the statement, "Name the park of Buenos Aires" was given, participants were trained to say, "El Botanico". Participants were also trained to respond to two similar statements, "Name the city of Uruguay" ("Montevideo") and "Name the park of Montevideo" ("El Lecoc"), respectively. This training may be represented as A–B (where A1 is 'Argentina', A2 is 'Uruguay', B1 is 'Buenos Aires', and B2 is 'Montevideo') and B–C relational training (where C1 is 'El Botanico' and C2 is 'El Lecoc'). In the next phase of the study, Perez-Gonzalez et al. assessed the emergence of all possible derived intraverbals. For example, they probed the emergence of: "Name the country of Buenos Aires" (B–A), "Name the city of El Botanico" (C–B), "Name the country of El Botanico" (C–A), and "Name the park of Argentina" (A–C), this was repeated for both stimulus sets. However, test probes revealed that derived intraverbals emerged with only one of the six participants.

Perez-Gonzalez et al. then adapted the procedures with a naive group of participants. Prior to relational training, participants were instructed to identify, when presented with one of the stimuli, whether it was a city, country or park

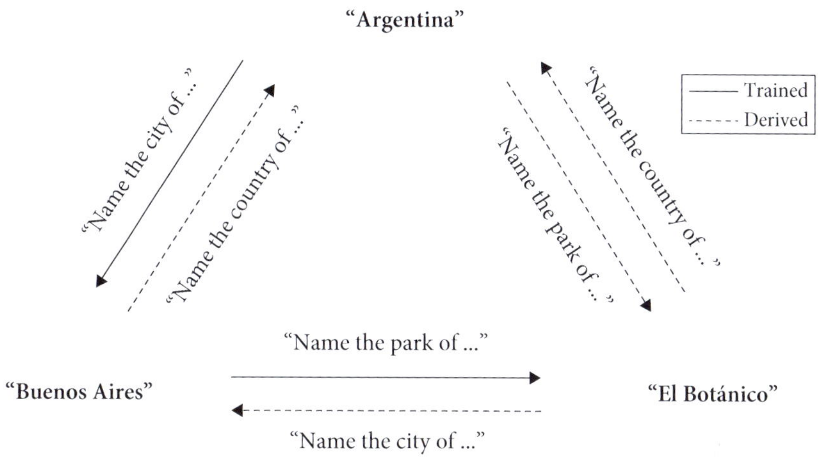

Figure 3. Schematic representation of Perez-Gonzalez et al.'s (2008) study

and, conversely, to vocalise the names of the cities, countries or parks. Intraverbal A–B and B–C training was then administered again, followed by test probes to evaluate emergent intraverbals. The preceding city, country and park training had a marked effect: all participants demonstrated emergence of all eight untrained target intraverbals. Furthermore, when the same participants were presented with novel stimulus sets, the authors observed that untrained emergence with the new stimuli was demonstrated more rapidly than with the earlier stimulus sets (Perez-Gonzalez et al. 2008).

Further studies investigating the emergence of derived interverbals have also been conducted with individuals with a diagnosis of autism (Grannan & Rehfeldt 2012; May, Hawkins & Dymond 2013). May et al. (2013) sought to facilitate emergence of derived intraverbals in three adolescents with autism and language delays. Each participant was directly taught to name pictures of fictional monsters (e.g. "What is the name of this monster?" ["Simon"]"), and to name a food preferred by each monster when presented with the monster picture (e.g. "What is the food that this monster eats?" ["Chips"]). The format of this training can be represented as A–B, A–C training, where A is the picture, B is the monster name, and C is the food name. Emergence of derived intraverbals was evaluated under test conditions (in the absence of feedback) whereby participants were asked questions concerning the names of the monsters and their food preferences, in the absence of the picture stimuli: "What food does Simon eat?" (B–C test) and "Which monster eats Chips?" (C–B test). The test phase indicated that intraverbal responses emerged for all three participants immediately following the relational training and in accordance with the multiple baseline design.

A novel means of facilitating the emergence of untrained intraverbal responses in children diagnosed with Pervasive Developmental Disorder (PDD) was reported by Perez-Gonzalez, Garcia-Asenjo, Williams and Carnerero (2007). Two children, aged 6 and 8 years old, were trained to respond to a number of statements involving an opposite relation. For example, when presented with the question "Name the opposite of hot?" (original relation), the children were given intraverbal training to vocally respond, "cold". Following training in a number of examples, emergence of the untrained reversed relation was tested (e.g. "Tell me the opposite of cold?") across the trained relations. Over a number of successive probes, neither participant demonstrated emergence of the untrained opposition relation. Once this repertoire had been established as absent, the first participant was given explicit intraverbal training to respond correctly to both the original and the reversed relations. As this training progressed over successive sets for the first participant, test probes revealed that emergence of the reversed relation began to occur without any explicit training. Identical training was then implemented for the second participant and the same effects of gradual untrained emergence were observed.

Additional studies with typically developing children have demonstrated variable effects of relational training on the emergence of spoken derived intraverbals. Petursdottir and colleagues (Petursdottir & Haflidadottir 2009; Petursdottir, Olafsdottir & Aradottir 2008) report the emergence of untrained intraverbals following training in a small foreign language vocabulary. In the study by Petursdottir et al. (2008), one group of children were trained to select an object given a foreign language name, and other group were taught to label an object with a foreign language name. Subsequently, when asked to respond to the foreign language words with their own native language and vice-versa (i.e. intraverbal tasks), some untrained intraverbals emerged. This emergence, however, was not consistent across all participants.

Petursdottir and Haflidadottir (2009) taught two young Icelandic-speaking children foreign language (Italian) relations in four different conditions. Across different sets of words, foreign-native intraverbal relations (e.g. "Tell me what [*foreign word*] is in Icelandic") and native-foreign intraverbal relations (e.g. "Tell me what [*native-language word*] is in Italian") were trained. In addition, the children were taught picture labelling with foreign words (e.g. "What is this *[shows object]*in Italian"), and taught to identify pictures when given the foreign words (e.g. "Point to [*foreign word*]"). Untrained relations were examined by testing each set of words trained in one condition, with the tasks from all the other conditions. For example, any word targeted in the labelling condition, was then probed in each of the other three conditions (identifying the picture when given the word, foreign-native intraverbal, and native-foreign intraverbal). The tests revealed that, although emergence did occur for some of the derived intraverbals, again, the facilitation of emergent responding in the novel language forms was inconsistent across participants.

Studies on the effects of the emergence of untrained intraverbal responding following other relational training have, to date, produced mixed results. Indeed, two further studies have indicated that intraverbal categorization skills do not readily emerge following training in other relations (Miguel, Petursdottir & Carr 2005; Petursdottir, Carr, Lechago & Almason 2008). In considering the range of findings reported here on intraverbal emergence, it is important to note that most of the studies that have demonstrated a consistent emergence of novel spoken intraverbals have included additional training components (Grannan & Rehfeldt 2012; Perez-Gonzalez et al. 2007, 2008). These training interventions, firstly, facilitated the emergence of intraverbals that initially failed to occur and, secondly, had apparent effects on the ease with which intraverbal emergence occurred with novel sets. Future research might look to both extend and refine such procedures and examine the relative efficacy of such interventions with individuals with impaired language repertoires.

Although much of the research described has been undertaken with young, typically developing populations without language impairment, developing new procedures may prove fruitful in establishing emergent intraverbal repertoires in individuals with communication difficulties. What follows is an illustrative example of how such an approach may have direct clinical utility for developing flexible early language repertoires. Consider a child who has been directly taught that a fire fighter (A) drives an engine (B) and uses a ladder (C). Given the explicit intraverbal training, "What does a fire fighter drive?" ("An engine"; A–B training) and "What might you find on an engine?" ("A ladder"; B–C training), by facilitating intraverbal emergence, we may be able to foster a range of untrained responses to such questions as, "Who drives an engine?", "On what would you find a ladder?", "What does a fire fighter use?" and, "Who uses a ladder?" Current educational curricula that recommend explicit and direct teaching of all such language tasks may ultimately benefit from incorporating procedures that plan for the direct teaching of two relations, with a further four emerging "for free".

Facilitating emergent verbal repertoires: Derived textual behaviour

Textual behaviour as described by Skinner (1957) is defined by three characteristic properties. First, textual behaviour is controlled by a verbal stimulus (usually written). Second, the stimulus and the response bear point-to-point correspondence with each other but, third, there is no formal similarity between the stimulus and the response product. Michael describes such a relationship as "where one stimulus is said to stand for another that it does not resemble" (1982: p. 2). In everyday language, reading aloud may be seen as an instance of textual behaviour. The verbal stimulus (the text) controls the response (speaking), which despite being symbolic for each other (point to point correspondence), they are still formally dissimilar (e.g. printed vs. auditory). *Derived* textual behaviour may occur when the vocal response occurs as a result of a history of relational responding. There are currently no formal, empirical demonstrations of derived textual behaviour, although prior research on relational training with auditory and visual stimuli may be relevant. For instance, in the first published study on stimulus equivalence by Sidman (1971), discussed above, oral reading was observed as an emergent skill following training to identify printed text when given the spoken name.

A recent study by Miguel, Yang, Finn and Ahearn (2009) sought to facilitate a variation of derived textual responding in two 6-year-old children with autism. The purpose of the procedure was to teach participants to use written words as alternatives to pictures as part of an independent activity schedule (MacDuff, Krantz & McClannahan 1993). Pretests assessed participants' ability to match pictures given printed words, match printed words given pictures, and demonstrate oral reading of the printed words. The children were systematically taught to select the correct picture when given a dictated word and select the correct text when given the dictated word. Following mastery of these trained relations, testing revealed the emergence of all untrained relations. That is, the children responded by correctly selecting the pictures given text, selecting text given pictures, and were able to read the text aloud, without further training. In the context of the independent schedule, the children now responded in the same way when provided with text as they had when given pictures.

The findings of Miguel et al. (2009) are encouraging, yet further research will be necessary to distinguish between the relative contributions of operant and respondent processes to the emergence of derived textual behaviour. Moreover, the development of preparations that unambiguously demonstrate derived and non-derived textual behaviour in language-impaired populations warrants further empirical attention.

Facilitating emergent verbal repertoires: Derived tacting

According to Skinner (1957), tacting is said to concern the "world of things and events which a speaker is said to 'talk about'" (p. 81). Tacts are learned when, for instance, a vocal response such as "apple" is reinforced in the presence of actual apples. In *derived* tacting, the tacted stimulus participates in derived relations with other objects and events. For instance, consider a child who learns to tact "apple" to actual apples, and later learns that apples are sometimes called "pomme" in French. Later, he or she may be presented with an apple and produce a derived verbal tact by saying "pomme" instead of the directly reinforced tact (i.e. "apple").

Few published studies have investigated the emergence of derived tacting in typically or atypically developing populations. This is perhaps unsurprising given that derived tacting probably occurs rarely in the natural environment and that the majority of tacts have some history of reinforcement. Nevertheless, as Barnes-Holmes et al. (2000) highlight, distinguishing between derived and non-derived tacting allows researchers to make "a clear functional distinction between formally similar responses that arise from very different behavioural histories" (p. 75). The existing studies that have examined the emergence of tact-like responding in either typically or atypically developing populations have tended to examine the effects on emergent expressive skills following simultaneous presentation of trained relations from auditory and visual modalities (Horne & Lowe 1996). For example, Groskreutz, Karsina, Miguel and Groskreutz (2010) describe a procedure that resulted in emergent tact and textual responding in children with autism. The three children involved in the study were given pre-tests for existing skills in selecting pictures (B) given dictated words (A), (A–B relations), selecting printed words (C) when given the dictated words (A), (A–C relations), and selecting pictures when given the printed words, (C–B relations). They were also given tests on their existing skills of oral labelling or tacting (B–D relations) and oral reading or textual responding (C–D relations). Next, training to select printed words from an array of three words when given a complex sample consisting of the dictated word and presentation of the picture (AB-C) was conducted. Following mastery of the trained relations phase, each participant was again tested with all possible relations (as they had during the pre-test). Each of the three children demonstrated emergence of all untrained relations following the training procedure, indicating that language training involving complex visual-auditory samples may result in a number of generative responses involving the individual components of the sample.

A further study carried out by LeBlanc, Miguel, Cummings, Goldsmith and Carr (2003) with two children diagnosed with autism, highlighted the emergence of vocal tact-like and intraverbal-like responding following a series of trained relations involving maps of US states, printed state names and printed capital names. During all trial presentations, vocal labelling of the stimuli by the experimenter was presented concurrently with presentation of the visual stimuli in the form of task related questions. An oral geography quiz was given prior to, and following, the relational training. The findings indicated that, despite vocal relations not explicitly being targeted during the training, one of the participants demonstrated reliable emergence during the post-tests.

Future research challenges

The research on synthesizing derived relational responding and verbal behaviour analysis is growing, yet there are many untapped avenues of investigation. Examining the utility of training 'expanded' relational networks, for example, is an important translational research challenge. In many of the examples given above, such as the research on derived manding by Rehfeldt and colleagues, the relational network typically consisted of three members: a picture, spoken word and item. Recall that in tests for emergent responding, Rehfeldt et al.'s findings indicated that each of the stimuli in these three-member relational networks became functionally equivalent for one another. There is an abundance of research showing that relational networks can extend beyond three members in young children (e.g. Smeets & Barnes-Holmes 2005) and it is here that the potential for improvements in efficiency of teaching practices may be realized. A three-member relational network involving two trained relations (A–B and A–C) entails that four relations, in addition to those trained, will be derived (B–A, C–A, C–B, and B–C). As has been described throughout, these relations emerge in the absence of further instruction. A four-member relational network requires only one additional taught relation (e.g. A–D) and yet by adding this single relation, a further *five* derived relations would be predicted to emerge (D–A, B–D, D–B, C–D, D–C). This occurs because the additonal stimulus (D) added to the network participates in relations with all the existing members.

These benefits can be further illustrated by way of a practical example. Figure 4 depicts a hypothetical relational network involving five members. Suppose a child had learned through explicit training to request one of the candy items with the text exchange (indicated by the open arrow). Having established this communicative exchange through direct training, a relational network could then be established through training to relate all the members of the candy to each other. It would be predicted that the child would then request all items included in the network using the text 'CANDY', despite having only been trained to use this text word to request one of the exemplar members. Such outcomes would confer significant benefits in the extended communicative repertoire of the learner. The learner would be able to utilise category words to mand for a range of items without any prior training to request for those specific items (Barnes-Holmes et al. 2000). In this way, future research should seek to demonstrate the functional and educational utility

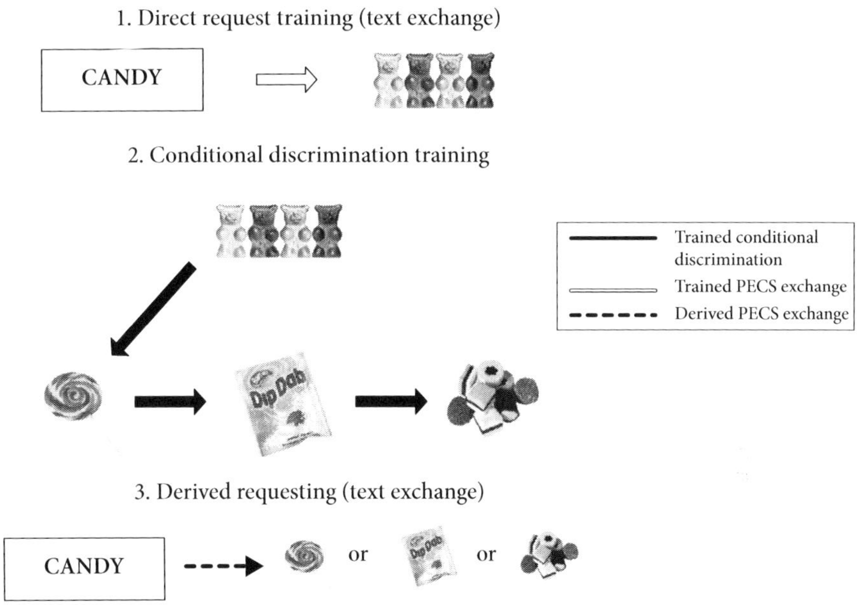

Figure 4. Schematic representation of 5-member relational network for training and testing derived manding using text-exchange. Solid arrows indicate trained relations, dashed lines indicate predicted derived manding, and open arrow indicates trained PECS

of training expanded networks of relations in boosting the verbal repertoires of learners with limited language.

Conclusion

Emergent verbal repertoires may be facilitated by a history of derived relational responding in which relations are established between pictures, spoken/written words, and other physically dissimilar stimuli. Targeting relational responding has been shown to facilitate the generalization and maintenance of skills usually only acquired after extensive periods of direct training. The boost in independent communicative episodes that result from a research synthesis of Skinner's (1957) verbal taxonomy with procedures and concepts from derived relational responding is still in its early stages but suggests that it has some potential to improve the lives of individuals with language impairment, such as children with autism. Researchers now need to move beyond merely demonstrating a role for derived relational responding and, instead, seek to develop innovative ways of incorporating a relational history into their language instruction and intervention strategies.

These challenges, combined with developments in other areas, such as the tremendous opportunities afforded by modern, low-cost portable computing solutions seem set to make this a central research topic for some time to come.

References

Aristotle. (1941). *De Memoria et Reminiscentia*, 415b, (J. I. Beare, trans). In R. McKeone (Ed.), *The Basic Works of Aristotle* (pp. 607–617). New York, NY: Random House.

Barnes-Holmes, D., Barnes-Holmes, Y., & Cullinan, V. (2000). Relational frame theory and Skinner's *Verbal Behavior*: A possible synthesis. *Behavior Analyst, 23*, 69–84.

Barnes-Holmes, Y., Barnes-Holmes, D., Roche, B., & Smeets, P.M. (2001). Exemplar training and a derived transformation of functions in accordance with symmetry: I. *The Psychological Record, 51*, 287–308.

Berens, N.M., & Hayes, S.C. (2007). Arbitrarily applicable comparative relations: Experimental evidence for a relational operant. *Journal of Applied Behavior Analysis, 40*, 45–71.

Carr, D., & Felce, D. (2000). Application of stimulus equivalence to language intervention for individuals with severe linguistic disabilities. *Journal of Intellectual and Developmental Disability, 25*, 181–205.

Cooper, J., Heron, T., & Heward, W. (2007). *Applied Behavior Analysis* (2nd ed.). Upper Saddle River, NJ: Pearson Merrill Prentice Hall.

DeLeon, I.G., & Iwata, B.A. (1996). Evaluation of a multiple-stimulus presentation format format for assessing reinforcer preferences. *Journal of Applied Behavior Analysis, 29*, 519–532.

Dymond, S., & Roche, B. (Eds.), (2013). *Advances in Relational Frame Theory: Research and Application*. Oakland, CA: New Harbinger.

Dymond, S., & Critchfield, T.S. (2002). A legacy of growth: Human operant research in *The Psychological Record* (1980–1999). *The Psychological Record, 52*, 99–106.

Dymond, S., May, R.J., Munnelly, A., & Hoon, A.E. (2010). Evaluating the evidence base for relational frame theory: A citation analysis. *The Behavior Analyst, 33*, 97–119.

Frost, L.A., & Bondy, A.S. (1994). *The Picture Exchange Communication System Training Manual*. Cherry Hill, NJ: Pyramid Educational Consultants.

Grannan, L., & Rehfeldt, R.A. (2012). Emergent intraverbal responses via tact and match-to-sample instruction. *Journal of Applied Behavior Analysis, 45*, 601–605.

Green, G. (1990). Differences in development of visual and auditory-visual equivalence relations. *American Journal on Mental Retardation, 95*, 260–270.

Groskreutz, N.C., Karsina, A., Miguel, C.F., & Groskreutz, M.P. (2010). Using complex auditory-visual samples to produce emergent relations in children with autism. *Journal of Applied Behavior Analysis, 43*, 131–136.

Hall, G. (1996). Learning about associatively activated stimulus representations: Implications for acquired equivalence and perceptual learning. *Animal Learning and Behavior, 24*, 233–255.

Halvey, C., & Rehfeldt, R.A. (2005). Expanding vocal requesting repertoires via relational responding in adults with severe developmental disabilities. *The Analysis of Verbal Behavior, 21*, 13–25.

Hart, B., & Risley, T. (1975). Incidental teaching of language in the preschool. *Journal of Applied Behavior Analysis, 8*, 411–420.

Eldevik, S., Hastings, R.P., Hughes, J.C., Jahr, E., Eikeseth, S., & Cross, S. (2010). Using participant data to extend the evidence base for intensive behavioral intervention for children with Autism. *American Journal on Intellectual and Developmental Disabilities, 115*, 381–405.

Flippin, M., Reszka, S., & Watson, L.R. (2010). Effectiveness of the Picture Exchange Communication System (PECS) on communication and speech for children with autism spectrum disorders: A meta-analysis. *American Journal of Speech and Language Pathology, 19*, 178–195.

Hayes, S.C., Barnes-Holmes, D., & Roche, B. (2001). *Relational Frame Theory. A Post- Skinnerian Account of Human Language and Cognition*. New York, NY: Kluwer Academic/Plenum.

Horne, P.J., & Lowe, C.F. (1996). On the origins of naming and other symbolic behavior. *Journal of the Experimental Analysis of Behavior, 65*, 185–241.

Hull, C.L. (1939). The problem of stimulus equivalence in behavior theory. *Psychological Review, 46*, 9–30.

Kennedy, C. (2005). *Single-case Designs for Educational Research*. Boston, MA: Allyn & Bacon.

LeBlanc, L.A., Dillon, C.M., & Sautter, R.A. (2009). Establishing mand and tact repertoires. In R.A. Rehfeldt & Y. Barnes-Holmes (Eds.), *Derived Relational Responding: Applications for Learners with Autism and other Developmental Disabilities* (pp. 79–108). Oakland, CA: New Harbinger.

LeBlanc, L.A., Miguel, C.F., Cummings, A.R., Goldsmith, T.R., & Carr, J.E. (2003). The effects of three stimulus equivalence testing conditions on emergent US Geography relations of children diagnosed with autism. *Behavioral Interventions, 18*, 279–289.

MacDuff, G.S., Krantz, P.J., & McClannahan, L.E. (1993). Teaching children with autism to use photographic activity schedules: Maintenance and generalization of complex response chains. *Journal of Applied Behavior Analysis, 26*, 89–97.

May, R.J., Hawkins, E., & Dymond, S. (2013). Effects of tact training on emergent intraverbal vocal responses in adolescents with autism. *Journal of Autism and Developmental Disorders, 43*, 996–1004.

Michael. J. (1982). Skinner's elementary verbal relations: Some new categories. *The Analysis of Verbal Behavior, 1*, 1–3.

Miguel, C.F., Petursdottir, A.I., & Carr, J.E. (2005). The effects of multiple-tact and receptive-discrimination training on the acquisition of intraverbal behavior. *The Analysis of Verbal Behavior, 21*, 27–41.

Miguel, C.F., Yang, H.G., Finn, H.E. & Ahearn, W.H. (2009). Establishing derived textual control in activity schedules with children with autism. *Journal of Applied Behavior Analysis, 42*, 703–709.

Munnelly, A., Dymond, S., & Hinton, E.C. (2010). Relational reasoning with derived comparative relations: A novel model of transitive inference. *Behavioural Procesess, 85*, 8–17.

Murphy, C., & Barnes-Holmes, D. (2009). Derived more/less relational mands with children diagnosed with autism. *Journal of Applied Behavior Analysis, 42*, 252–268.

Murphy, C., & Barnes-Holmes, D. (2010a). Establishing five derived mands in three adolescent boys with autism. *Journal of Applied Behavior Analysis, 43*, 537–543.

Murphy, C., & Barnes-Holmes, D. (2010b). Establishing complex derived manding with children with and without a diagnosis of autism. *The Psychological Record, 60*, 489–504.

Murphy, C., Barnes-Holmes, D., & Barnes-Holmes, Y. (2005). Derived manding with seven children diagnosed with autism: Synthesizing Skinner's *Verbal Behavior* with Relational Frame Theory. *Journal of Applied Behavior Analysis, 38*, 445–462.

Perez-Gonzalez, L.A., Garcıa-Asenjo, L., Williams, G., & Carnerero, J.J. (2007). Emergence on intraverbal antonyms in children with pervasive developmental disorder. *Journal of Applied Behavior Analysis, 40*, 697–701.
Perez-Gonzalez, L.A., Herszlikowicz, K., & Williams, G. (2008). Stimulus relations analysis and the emergence of novel intraverbals. *The Psychological Record, 58*, 95–129.
Petursdottir, A.I., & Haflidadottir, R.D. (2009). A comparison of four strategies for teaching a small foreign language vocabulary. *Journal of Applied Behavior Analysis, 42*, 497–745.
Petursdottir, A.I., Carr, J.E., Lechago, S.A., & Almason, S.M. (2008). An evaluation of intraverbal training and listener training for teaching categorization skills. *Journal of Applied Behavior Analysis, 41*, 53–68.
Petursdottir, A.I., Olafsdottir, A.R., & Aradottir, B. (2008). The effects of tact and listener training on the emergence of bi-directional intraverbal relations. *Journal of Applied Behavior Analysis, 41*, 411–415.
Rehfeldt, R.A., & Barnes-Holmes, Y. (Eds.). (2009). *Derived Relational Responding Applications for Learners with Autism and Other Developmental Disabilities.* Oakland, CA: New Harbinger.
Rehfeldt, R.A. & Root, S.L. (2005). Establishing derived requesting skills in adults with severe developmental disabilities. *Journal of Applied Behavior Analysis, 38*, 101–105.
Reichow, B., Barton, E.E., Boyd, B.A., & Hume, K. (2011). Early intensive behavioral intervention for increasing functional behaviors and skills for young children with autism spectrum disorders. *Cochrane Database of Systematic Reviews*, CD009260. DOI: 10.1002/14651858
Reichow, B., & Wolery, M. (2009). Comprehensive synthesis of early intensive behavioral interventions for young children with autism based on the UCLA Young Autism Project model. *Journal of Autism and Developmental Disorders, 39*, 23–41.
Rosales, R., & Rehfeldt, R.A. (2007). Contriving transitive conditioned establishing operations to establish derived manding skills in adults with severe developmental disabilities. *Journal of Applied Behavior Analysis, 40*, 105–121.
Rosales, R., & Rehfeldt, R.A. (2009). Extending functional communication through relational framing. In R.A. Rehfeldt & Y. Barnes-Holmes (Eds.) *Derived Relational Responding Applications for Learners with Autism and Other Developmental Disabilities.* Oakland, CA: New Harbinger.
Schuster, J.W., Gast, D.L., Wolery, M., & Guiltinan, S. (1988). The effectiveness of a constant time-delay procedure to teach chained responses to adolescentswith mental retardation. *Journal of Applied Behavior Analysis, 21*, 169–178.
Sidman, M. (1971). Reading and auditory-visual equivalences. *Journal of Speech and Hearing Research, 14*, 5–13.
Sidman, M. (1994). *Equivalence Relations and Behavior: A Research Story.* Boston, MA: Authors Cooperative.
Sidman, M., & Cresson, O. (1973). Reading and crossmodal transfer of stimulus equivalences in severe retardation. *American Journal of Mental Deficiency, 77*, 515–523.
Sidman, M., Cresson, O., & Willson-Morris, M. (1974). Acquisition of matching to sample via mediated transfer. *Journal of the Experimental Analysis of Behavior, 22*, 261–273.
Sidman, M., & Tailby, W. (1982). Conditional discrimination versus matching to sample: An expansion of the testing paradigm. *Journal of the Experimental Analysis of Behavior, 37*, 5–22.

Sigafoos, J., Drasgow, E., Halle, J.W., O'Reilly, M., Seely-York, S., Edrisinha, C., & Andrews, A. (2004). Teaching VOCA use as a communicative repair strategy. *Journal of Autism and Developmental Disorders, 34*, 411–422.

Skinner, B.F. (1957). *Verbal Behavior.* Acton, MA: Copley.

Smeets, P.M., & Barnes-Holmes, D. (2005). Auditory-visual and visual-visual equivalence relations in children. *The Psychological Record, 55*, 483–503.

Smyth, S., Barnes-Holmes, D., & Barnes-Holmes, Y. (2008). Acquired equivalence in human discrimination learning: The role of propositional knowledge. *Journal of Experimental Psychology: Animal Behavior Processes, 34*(1), 167–177.

Stromer, R., & Vogt, R. (2009). The formation and elaboration of stimulus classes. In A. Fitzer & P. Sturmey (Eds.), *Language and Autism: Applied Behavior Analysis, Evidence, and Practice* (pp. 218–249). Austin, TX: Pro-Ed.

Sundberg, M.L., & Michael, J. (2001). The benefits of Skinner's analysis of verbal behavior for children with autism. *Behavior Modification, 25*, 692–724.

Törneke, N. (2010). *Learning RFT: An Introduction to Relational Frame Theory and its Clinical Applications.* Oakland, CA: New Harbinger Publications.

Virués-Ortega, J. (2010). Applied behavior analytic intervention for autism in early childhood: Meta-analysis, meta-regression and dose-response meta-analysis of multiple outcomes. *Clinical Psychology Review, 30*, 387–399.

SECTION 2

Oral language

CHAPTER 3

Echolalia and language development in children with autism

Jacqueline M.A. Roberts
Griffith University

Echolalia, the immediate or delayed repetition of the speech of another, is associated with autism. Echolalia is usually described as a non-functional self-stimulatory or stereotypical behaviour, despite research and theory suggesting echolalia has several functions for people with autism and may also be important in language development. Reduction or elimination of echolalia is often cited as a therapeutic goal and is generally considered to be a positive intervention outcome. In this chapter, the relationship between echolalia and imitation in typical and disordered language development is discussed. The relationship between developing receptive language competence (Reynell Developmental Language Scales) and the amount of echolalia (language sample) in speech is examined in a group (n = 26) of children with Autistic Disorder compared to a group of children (n = 23) of children with Specific Language Impairment (SLI). The receptive language and the amount of echolalia in speech were assessed in both groups annually for three years. An inverse association between the amount of echolalia in speech and receptive language ability in children with autism was noted. Like imitation in typical development, echolalia may be exact or modified in some way (mitigated). These modifications can be classified into several types. The amount and type of mitigated echolalia in speech and its relationship to the receptive language ability of children with autism is described. The findings of this study are consistent with the view that echolalia plays an important role in the language development of children with autism. Implications for assessment and management of echolalia in children with autism are discussed.

Introduction

> 'That tongue of yours by which I have been tricked, shall have its power curtailed and enjoy the briefest use of speech.'
>
> Hera, Queen of Greek mythology, deprives the nymph Echo of spontaneous speech and reduces her to echoing the words of others.

Echolalia is defined as the rote and literal repetition of the speech of others (Kanner 1946). It may occur immediately, or after some time has passed, (delayed) and may be exact or altered slightly in specific ways (mitigated). While not exclusive to autism, echolalia is frequently noted in the speech of verbal children with autism and is considered to be characteristic of the disorder (Rutter & Lockyer 1967). Children with autism may have no speech at all (nonverbal) or be highly verbal, or anywhere in between these extremes. However, if people with autism spectrum disorders speak, it is likely that they will exhibit echolalia in their speech at some point (Lovaas 1981).

Echolalia remains a frequently misunderstood and, consequently, mismanaged characteristic of autism. Researchers have established that echolalia has functions for people with autism (Prizant & Duchan 1981, Prizant & Rydell 1984) and is important in the development of language in children with autism (Prizant 1987); however, this has not been studied systematically from a developmental perspective.

The current study examined longitudinally the changes in amount and type of echolalia in speech of children with autism and children with Specific Language Impairment (SLI). The aims of the study were (a) to examine the amount and type of echolalia in the language of young children with autism over time; (b) to determine how the amount and type of echolalia might relate to their language development, in particular the development of receptive language; and (c) to determine the extent to which echolalia is specific to autism by comparison with children with SLI. This study in important because it increases our understanding of this very common characteristic of autism, its potential role in language development for children with autism, and potentially improves management as a result.

Why echolalia?

Echolalia has been reported in the literature since 1825, when Itard wrote about his clinical observations of verbal echoing (echolalia) in an abandoned child found living wild in the woods. It has been noted in association with disabilities such as dementia senilis and some types of acquired aphasia (Pick 1924). The repetition of previously heard speech, either immediately or after a significant interval, has also been reported in the speech of children with communication disability and those with intellectual disability (Bishop 1989; Cantwell & Baker 1978; Darley 1964). Rydell and Mirenda (1991) found that verbal repetition, or echolalia, occurred in the speech of non-autistic individuals at times of high cognitive work load: for example, when there was a lack of shared event knowledge or conversational themes.

Historically, in relation to autism, echolalia has been explained and treated in various ways depending on the prevailing theoretical framework of the time. When autism was first described in the 1940s by Kanner (1943, 1946) and Asperger (1944), psychoanalysis was the dominant theoretical framework for all manner of physical and psychological conditions. As a result, echolalia was considered to be a hostile behaviour (Carluccio, Sours & Kalb 1964) indicative of a failure of ego development (Bettelheim 1967). With the application of behaviourist theory to autism, echolalia was considered to be a self-stimulatory behaviour (Griffith & Ritvo 1967) interfering with learning (Lovaas 1966). Recommended management involved extinguishing echolalia (usually by punishment) so learning could start (Lovaas Schriebman & Koegel 1974). Unfortunately, the preferred strategy for training speech in behavioural programs of the time was by rewarding the child for imitating a model, which must have been confusing for everyone.

There was one researcher who questioned both the psychoanalytic and behaviourist explanations of echolalia and autism current at that time. Warren Fay (1967, 1969) suggested that while some might not consider a child's attempts to participate vocally as a typically social behaviour, for children with autism, echolalia was, at the least, an attempt on the part of the child to take a conversational turn when he did not understand the speech of others.

"Thus if a doubt remains as to whether echolalia reflects the last failure of human connections or a struggle to maintain them, the child deserves the benefit of that doubt. A return to mutism, either by well meaning clinical intervention intent only upon echo abatement, marks the last failure" (Fay 1973: 487).

In the 1980s and 90s echolalia was considered to be a linguistic strategy used for a variety of communicative purposes, including cognitive and social functions (Prizant & Duchan 1981; Prizant & Rydell 1984; Rydell & Mirenda 1991). Potential functions of echolalia for a child with autism include (a) as a coping strategy in the face of high cognitive work load (Rydell & Mirenda 1991); (b) as a means of initiating or maintaining social contact (conversational turn taking) (Hurtig, Ensrud & Tomblin 1982); and (c) as a language acquisition strategy resulting in the eventual development of a more flexible rule-governed system (Kirchner & Prutting 1987). While there was some research into the likely communicative functions of echolalia for individuals with autism (Prizant & Duchan 1981; Prizant & Rydell 1984), there was little understanding of the dynamics that underlie echolalia, its neurological basis, or the role it plays in the development of communication skills (Rydell & Mirenda 1991).

Types of echolalia

There are different types of echolalia described in the autism literature. According to Prizant (1987), immediate echolalia can be an exact imitation or modified in some way (mitigated). Mitigated (or modified) echolalia is a term which has been used to refer to echolalia with structural change in the form of substitution, addition or reduction of elements in the echoed utterance or changes to the intonation, stress or other paralinguistic features (Bebko 1990; Prizant 1987; Roberts 1989). It has been differentiated from non-mitigated immediate echolalia in its structural uniqueness or supplementation of the model (Fay 1967). The term delayed echolalia refers to utterances repeated at a significantly later time than the model utterance (Kanner 1943; Prizant & Rydell 1984) and may also be exact or mitigated (Shapiro 1977). The definition of delayed echolalia has presented the most difficulty to researchers, since it relies on knowledge of the child and past context and is therefore difficult to operationally define and differentiate from spontaneous speech. It is possible that a child with autism produces language somewhere along a continuum of exactness, ranging from automatic echoes unrelated to the context to utterances that have only a slightly rote quality (Prizant & Rydell 1984). It is noteworthy that types of echolalia are similar to types of imitation.

Exact echolalia

Fay and Coleman (1977:396) described a child with the most automatic form of echolalia, extremely rapid accurate repetition, as "a human sound transducer". This child showed no sign of comprehension of the words she echoed. Fay and Coleman proposed that this behaviour indicated processing restricted to transduction from ear to articulation, divorced completely from syntactic, semantic and cognitive functions of the brain. They further argued that this kind of automatic echolalia has limited function. Exact echolalia produced without evident function has also been described as a form of pre-categorical imitation (Malvy et al. 1999). Exact echolalia may also be used for a range of functions such as requesting and rejecting by the person with autism (Prizant & Duchan 1981) or to mark a conversational turn (Fay 1967).

Mitigated echolalia

Modified echolalia, that is speech of others that is imitated and altered slightly, is referred to as mitigated echolalia. The term was first used by Pick (1924) to describe the slightly modified echolalic utterances produced by aphasic patients. Stengel (1947) described echolalic behaviour in the speech of children developing language and in people learning another language as mitigated echolalia. Stengel noticed two characteristic modifications: (a) the introduction of the first person singular into the repeated sentence, and (b) adding an answer to the echoed question or order. He considered these characteristics to be evidence of development in comprehension and expression.

Mitigations involving structural change through the use of substitution, addition or reduction of elements of the model utterance have been documented in the speech of children and adults with autism (Prizant 1987; Roberts 1989). Mitigated echolalia was operationally defined by Fay (1967). He described mitigated echoic patterns as echolalia that is either structurally unique from or a supplement to a pure echoic response. Fay observed three types of syntactic modifications in the speech of echolalic children: (a) Type I included a pure echoic segment, with the exception of pronominal reciprocation (e.g. 'Where did you sleep' is echoed as 'I sleep', 'What is this thing?' is echoed as 'That thing'); (b) Type II included a pure echoic segment preceded by or followed by affirmation or negation, or by reply, remark, or query (e.g. 'I'll show you how it works' is echoed as 'How it works, okay'); and (c) Type III included combinations of Types I and II or miscellaneous grammatical conversions or syntactical supplements to the pure echoic segment ('You have a dog, don't you?' is echoed as 'Yeah I have a dog don't I?'). Examples cited are from Fay (1967: 308).

Roberts (1989) used Fay's operational definitions of mitigated echolalia in her study of the relationship between receptive language ability and echolalia in the spontaneous speech of a group of 10 subjects with autism aged 4 to 17 years. She found that high levels of immediate echolalia were associated with low scores on receptive language tests. In addition, subjects with low levels of echolalia and high levels of receptive language ability tended to have the most mitigation. The mitigations observed in this study were all of Type II or III, indicating that none of the 10 participants used pronominal reciprocation. Most used mitigations indicating affirmation or negation, and some combined Type II with other grammatical conversions or syntactical supplements.

Pronoun reversal

Pronoun reversal is often cited as a particular characteristic of autistic language. In the light of explanations of echolalia, it seems likely that, for example, use of the pronoun 'you' for 'I' is the result of accurate echoing, either immediately or after a period of time, of phrases heard, rather than of the actual reversal of a pronoun. Kanner (1946) himself described pronoun reversal as an artifact of delayed echolalia. Fay (1969) stated that if a child with autism has only the speech of others at his disposal and cannot edit linguistically, the result is the non-conversion of pronouns in both immediate and delayed echolalia. It is unlikely that children understand pronouns separately from the total utterance, which they reproduce as a whole unit. True pronoun reversal, in the context of language development in children with autism, occurs when the child changes the pronoun in the echoed phrase and substitutes either a proper name or a more appropriate pronoun. This strategy would seem to indicate recognition of the function of pronouns and the beginning of attempts to use them appropriately.

There does, however, remain a tendency for able individuals with autism who have demonstrated control over personal pronouns to continue to use them in an odd and inconsistent manner (Lee, Hobson & Chiat 1994). Several authors (e.g. Hobson 1990; Lee et al. 1994) have suggested that this continued error is due to a limitation in self-other differentiation and/or self-concept, which is related to the theory of mind in autism: that is, the difficulty individuals with autism have imagining others as distinct from themselves with different thoughts and feelings. It is, therefore, not clear whether pronoun reversal is always an artifact of echolalia, although several investigators suggest that this seems the most likely explanation for the majority of occurrences (Bebko 1990; Fay 1969; Roberts 1989).

While there have been suggestions in the research literature that echolalia is a language acquisition strategy for children with autism resulting in the eventual development of a more flexible rule-governed system (Kirchner & Prutting 1987) and that mitigation of the echoed utterance marks movement towards expressive and receptive competence (Stengel 1947), there has been no systematic longitudinal examination of language development, exact echolalia and mitigated echolalia in children with autism. Evidence that the amount of exact immediate echolalia decreases in speech as language competence increases would support the suggestion that children with autism become less reliant on imitation and more linguistically competent as they develop. Increasing mitigation in the echoed utterances as receptive language competence grows would provide evidence of the nature of the language development process in autism, in particular if this is compared to children with Specific Language Impairment.

The current study

This study set out to; describe the amount and type of echolalia in the speech of children with autism longitudinally over a period of three years; to determine how the amount and type of echolalia might relate to their development of receptive language; and determine the extent to which echolalia is specific to autism by comparison with children with SLI. Children with SLI were chosen for comparison with the Autistic Disorder group because both groups have a significant developmental language disorder; however children with SLI do not meet the social and behavioural criteria required for a diagnosis of Autism.

Method

Participants

A total of 49 participants were recruited (26 with AD, 23 with SLI). All participants met the following criteria: spontaneous spoken language production sufficient to generate a minimum 100 utterance language sample; no gross medical, neurological or sensory disorders (in particular hearing and vision reported as within normal limits); no evidence of a motor speech disorder; and English as the first language. The mean chronological age at the start of the study for the autism group was 47 months (range = 37–54), for the SLI group mean was 45 months (range = 33–44). There was a marked gender bias in both groups (male: female, AD 22:4, SLI 19:4). All participants lived at home with their families and none was taking medication at any time throughout the data collection period.

Criteria for participant selection for the autism group were a diagnosis of Autistic Disorder (as per DSM III-R, 1987) with significant language disorder and performance IQ within the typical range (i.e. 70+; excluding children with a significant intellectual disability). The diagnosis of children with Autistic Disorder (AD) was done independently of the study by medical practitioners experienced in the assessment of children with autism using DSM-III at referring child development clinics in major Sydney hospitals. Children with autism also scored a minimum of 1 SD below the mean on the Reynell Developmental Language Scales (RDLS) (Reynell 1977) for receptive and/or expressive language. Participants in the autism group received one or more of a variety of interventions over their three years of participation in the study, ranging from weekly speech therapy sessions to full time enrolment in a special school for children with autism. None of the participants had intervention specifically designed to modify echolalia.

For the SLI group, criteria were: a minimum of 1 SD below the mean on a standardised language assessment, the absence of sufficient characteristics of autism for a diagnosis of AD and performance IQ within the typical range (i.e. 70+; excluding children with a significant intellectual disability).

Procedures

Data were collected between 1990 and 1995. The following variables were measured at three annual assessments: the amount of immediate echolalia in speech, the proportion of the immediate echolalia that was mitigated, and receptive language scores (standardised measure). All assessments were carried out by two clinically qualified and experienced speech pathologists (the author, and a research assistant). Assessments were conducted in familiar, non-clinical settings (in most cases in the home) with a familiar person (usually the child's mother) to ensure that the language sample was representative of the participant's communication ability (Bernard-Opitz 1982; Tager-Flusberg et al. 1990).

Language testing

Raw scores for expressive and receptive language scales were obtained for the Reynell Developmental Language Scales (RLDS) (Reynell 1977). Receptive language score was chosen as a measure of language ability because it has been argued to be more accurate over time for children with language disability than are measures of expressive language only, or measures combining both expressive and receptive language scores (Cole, Schwartz, Notai, Dale & Mills 1995). In addition it is likely that, in highly echolalic children, expressive language may not necessarily reflect competence in the sense usually understood in language development; i.e. because the utterances may be produced from memory rather than by application of linguistic rules.

Language Sample

A language sample was elicited using a consistent set of toys. The samples were collected and video recorded during interactions between the child and one of the clinicians and then with a familiar other, usually the mother. A total corpus of a minimum of 100 utterances was recorded for all participants at each assessment. Language samples were analysed to determine the amount of immediate echolalia, exact and mitigated, in the first 100 utterances of the language sample. In order to determine measures of echolalia and mitigated echolalia, all examples of immediate echolalia (including mitigated) were noted. Immediate echolalia was defined as the repetition of all or part of another's utterance (not self) within one conversational turn (Phillips & Dyer 1977). Responses to requests for repetition were not considered to be echolalic, nor were responses to direct questions offering a choice (e.g. Do you want to play with the cars or the playdoh?), unless the whole utterance was repeated. It was not possible to control for delayed echolalia, hence, in this study the term echolalia refers to immediate echolalia only. An echolalic utterance was further classified as mitigated if the model utterance was changed or modified (Prizant 1987). The operational definition of mitigated echolalia used in this study was based on descriptions of types of mitigated echolalia by Stengel (1947), Fay (1967), Shapiro Roberts and Fish (1970), and types of imitation noted in the speech of young children by Clark (1977), and Kirchner and Prutting (1987). Types of mitigated echolalia and examples, taken from participants' language samples, are shown in Table 1.

In order to demonstrate the amount of mitigated echolalia relative to the total amount of echolalia in language samples at each assessment, the percentage of total echolalia that was mitigated in relation to the total was calculated.

Design and statistical considerations

A longitudinal follow-up design was used. Pearson's correlations were computed to examine the relationship between the raw scores on the receptive language test and each of the other two variables – number of echolalic utterances in

Table 1. Types of mitigated echolalia

Type		Description	Example
Type 1	Syntactic Edit	Pronoun editing including substitution of pronouns or proper names.	R. I got it C. You got it
		Other syntactic editing including substitution of words in the same class, eg articles 'a' & 'the'	R. That was funny C. It was funny
Type 2	Expansion	Indication of affirmation or negation	R. Making big ball C. No more big ball
		Response to a question	R. What's she bringing, bringing breakfast C. Bringing breakfast, pizza
		Other	R. In here C. In here boys
Type 3	Reduction	Telegraphic; omitting grammatical morphemes.	R. And he jumped C. Jump
		Other (If child echoed the last word(s) of the preceding utterance this was not considered to be reduction.)	R. What is coming out from the fire hose. Lots of water. C. The fire hose
Type 4	Combinations of Types 1, 2, & 3.	Reduction and expansion	R. What are you doing? C. You know what doing
		Syntactic editing + reduction	R. Has he got any eyes? C. His eyes.
		Syntactic editing + expansion	R. Is that all right ? C. Yes, it can be all right.
		Syntactic editing + reduction + expansion	R. Can you see? C. I see them all.

Note: Type 4 examples of echolalia, the closest type to spontaneous speech, were rare (< 1% total mitigated echolalia) in the language samples

100 utterance language sample (percent echolalia), and percentage of echolalic utterances containing mitigated echolalia, at each assessment time for each of the AD and SLI groups. High negative correlations between receptive language and echolalia plus positive correlations between receptive language and percent mitigated echolalia were expected for the AD group. Two 2-tailed tests were used although the direction of correlations was predicted. Regression analysis was used for both groups at each assessment time to examine the relationship between receptive language (raw score) and the amount of echolalia and the percentage mitigated echolalia.

Reliability

The reliability of the transcription and analysis of the language samples was established by the re-transcription and re-analysis of 10% of all data by an independent speech pathologist who was blind to the diagnosis of the participants. The overall mean agreement on the amount of echolalia in the language samples and the classification of the echolalia as mitigated or non-mitigated was 97%, with a range of 96% to 98% across the re-analysed samples.

Results

The percent of participants in the AD group with significant amounts of echolalia (10% or more) (Wetherby & Gaines 1982) in their speech at each assessment was as follows: assessment one 100%, assessment two 89%, assessment three 54%. For the SLI group participants, percentages were as follows: assessment one 61%, assessment two 22%, assessment three 0%.

In Table 2, the means and standard deviations for receptive language, echolalia and percent mitigated echolalia are shown for the AD and SLI groups at each assessment. In both groups, receptive language scores increased over time. It is also of note that the mean receptive scores for the AD and SLI groups show that the AD group had, on average, a greater receptive language deficit at each point in time. For echolalia, the mean for the AD group at assessment 1 was double that of the SLI group suggesting that echolalia is characteristic of children with autism but not exclusive to this population. The level of echolalia in the speech of the SLI group was at negligible levels at Times 2 and 3 (less than10%). In the autism group the trend for the echolalia to become increasingly mitigated was very marked over the assessment period.

Table 2. Means and standard deviations for raw scores on the receptive language test, percentage of utterances containing echolalia, and percentage of echolalic utterances containing mitigated echolalia for the AD and SLI groups at each assessment

Assessment	Receptive language		% Utterances echolalic		% Echolalia mitigated	
	AD	SLI	AD	SLI	AD	SLI
1	19.1 (12.2)	34.1 (8.3)	35.6 (17.9)	17.7 (15.9)	39.4 (19.6)	55.3 (26.7)
2	35.5 (9.8)	47.4 (7.1)	23.1 (13.7)	6.3 (4.0)	54.5 (19.5)	70.8 (33.8)
3	45.2 (10.7)	56.6 (9.2)	12.3 (9.2)	4.6 (2.6)	72.2 (19.8)	71.6 (33.2)

In Table 3 Pearson's correlation coefficients are shown for the AD and SLI groups at each assessment for receptive language and echolalia, and for receptive language and percentage mitigated echolalia. The results of corresponding regression analyses are shown in Figure 1.

Table 3. Pearson's correlation coefficients between raw scores on the receptive language test and either percentage of utterances containing echolalia (% Echolalic) or percentage of echolalic utterances containing mitigated echolalia (% Mitigated), for the AD and SLI groups at each assessment

Assessment time	AD		SLI	
	% Echolalic	% Mitigated	% Echolalic	% Mitigated
1	–0.49*	0.53**	–0.51*	0.29
2	–0.50**	0.45*	–0.53**	–0.05
3	–0.69**	0.56**	–0.10	0.04

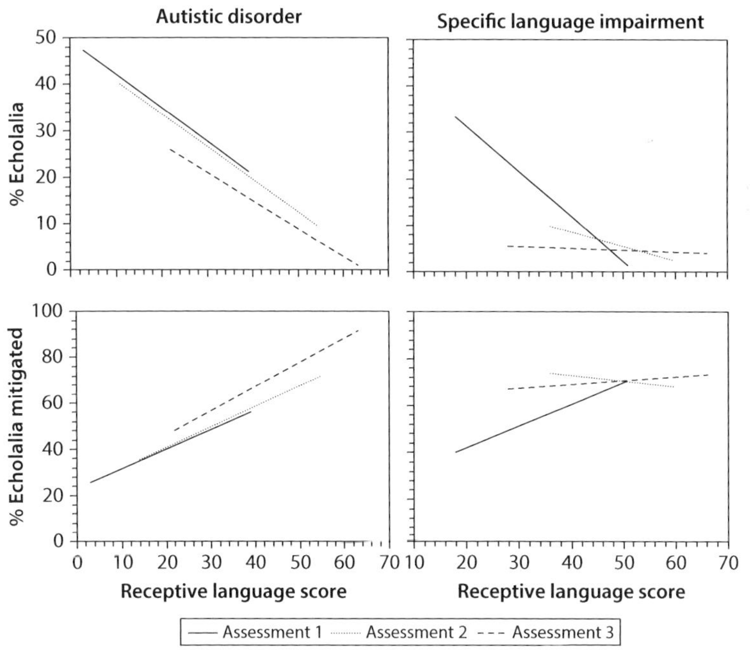

Figure 1. Regression fits for percentage of utterances containing echolalia (% Echolalic) or percentage of echolalic utterances containing mitigated echolalia (% Mitigated), as a function of receptive language score

For the AD group, there was a significant negative correlation between receptive language and echolalia at all three time points. That is, the lower the receptive language score, the higher the level of immediate echolalia in speech. There was also a positive correlation between receptive language scores and the percentage of echolalia that was mitigated, that is, the higher the receptive language score, the greater proportion of echolalia that was mitigated.

For the SLI group at Times 1 and 2 there was a significant negative correlation between receptive language and echolalia, which was no longer present at Time 3. There was no significant correlation between receptive language and proportion of mitigated echolalia in the SLI group. It can be seen from Table 2 that the mean amount of echolalia in speech of the SLI group at Times 2 and 3 was negligible. As a result correlation data is not informative.

Discussion

The first finding of the study relates to the extent echolalia is found in autism. In the present study, 100% of the AD group had 10% or more echolalia in their speech at the time of their first assessment (age range 37–54 months, mean 47 months). Together with Rutter and Lockyer's (1967) report that 75% of verbal children with autism go through a period of marked echolalia, our results indicate that echolalia may be characteristic of *v*erbal children with Autistic Disorder, at least in the early stages of their language development. Please note these findings do not apply to Aspergers Syndrome, which was not a formal diagnostic category at the time the data for this study was collected. In addition all the participants in this study had a clinically significant language delay which technically precludes a diagnosis of Aspergers Syndrome. Neither do the findings of this study apply to nonverbal children with autism, or children with significant intellectual disability and autism.

The second finding relates to whether echolalia is exclusive to autism. In the present study, 14 children in the SLI group of 23 met the criteria (10% or more in language sample) for echolalia in the first year of assessment. The results of this study suggest that language delay in Autistic Disorder is invariably associated with echolalia in the early stages of language development but it is not exclusive to autism and may be observed in the speech of young children with language disorder. However data from this study suggests that echolalia is not as pervasive or persistent in the SLI population as it is in the AD population.

The third and main finding of the study relates to the relationship between language skill development and immediate echolalia, both exact and mitigated. The correlations indicated that there was a strong and consistent negative association between receptive language ability and the amount of echolalia in speech for children in the AD group at each of the three annual assessments. In addition, low levels of echolalia tended to be increasingly highly mitigated over time. The results of the present study support the findings of Roberts (1989) that low receptive language scores are associated with high levels of immediate echolalia, of which little is mitigated. These results also provide support for Fay and Butler's (1968) statement that 'mitigated echoers' have higher receptive language scores; this was particularly apparent at times 2 and 3 for the autism group. In the SLI group at Time 1 the same pattern prevailed as for the autism group: lower receptive language scores were associated with higher levels of echolalia. However, the amount of echolalia in speech at times 2 and 3 was negligible.

The results suggest that the trends that were evident when group means for receptive language score, amount of echolalia and proportion of mitigated echolalia were examined at any one point in time, held true over time for individual participants in the autistic group. If receptive language, echolalia and mitigated echolalia are related to each other, it is likely that they are sensitive to some common underlying mechanism (Bates, Bretherton & Snyder 1988). The problem then becomes the identification of this mechanism and the developmental process for language particular to verbal children with Autistic Disorder.

Echolalia and imitation of speech

In the literature, it has been suggested that some typically developing children pass through a marked imitative period at a younger age than did the participants in the present study (Bloom 1991; Clark 1977; Rees 1975). High levels of imitation are not uncommon in the speech of children up to the age of 30 months (Bloom 1991). If imitation persists after this age, it is generally associated with communication disability, and particularly with autism (Howlin 1982; Rutter & Lockyer 1967; Zipf 1965).

There are parallels evident between the definition of imitation in the typical population and the classification of echolalia and mitigated echolalia in the present study. The classification system for mitigations developed for the present study was based on the work of investigators such as Clark (1977), who described the imitation of typically developing children, and Kirchner and Prutting (1987), who described imitation in children with language disability. Exact, immediate imitation was considered by Clark (1977) to require less communicative competence on the part of the typical child than does the production of variations, such as substitutions and additions, which, she suggested, are likely to be evidence of the child's emerging linguistic competence. Similarly, examination of the levels of exact and mitigated echolalia in the language samples of the participants in the present study and the association between receptive language scores and levels of mitigation suggest that, for young verbal children with autism, the production of mitigations is also evidence of developing linguistic competence.

For children developing language typically, Kirchner and Prutting (1987) suggested that imitation is a process that allows temporary storage and rehearsal of linguistic units, while mechanisms for linguistic rule extraction are developing. It is apparent from the present and other studies (e.g. Fay 1969; Prizant 1987; Roberts 1989) that many children with language disability, particularly those with autism, use echolalia more extensively and over a longer period than typical children use imitation. It is likely that, for verbal children with autism, the ability to extract linguistic rules from heard speech is deficient, resulting in the need for a longer than usual period of temporary storage and rehearsal of linguistic units (Kirchner & Prutting 1987). For less able verbal children with autism, echolalia may not be a transitional phase in that they continue to have difficulty with linguistic rules and use echolalia as a communicative strategy throughout their lives (Prizant 1987). As suggested by Prizant (1983), the participants' reproduction of chunks of language they have just heard may be a strategy for retaining information in short term memory. In the early stages of language development, the utterance is heard, retained in short term memory and then produced without understanding, possibly in response to a need to keep the conversation going in the absence of the means to generate a novel utterance (Prizant 1983). In the case of immediate exact echolalia, it cannot be assumed that the participants in the present study understood the rules that govern the generation of the utterances they produced (Fay 1973). It is likely that the echolalia observed in the speech of participants was indicative of difficulty generating novel utterances, which was likely to be the result of failure to develop adequate control over the rules that govern language production (Schuler & Prizant 1985). It is proposed that this difficulty, in turn, results in prolonged (past the age of 30 months) dependence on imitation, described as echolalia.

In summary, according to the literature, it appears that the distinction between echolalia and imitation is primarily a matter of timing. It is suggested that the mechanism available to typical children to analyse language and derive rules for the generation of utterances is impaired in the language-disabled population, and to the greatest extent in children with autism. As a result, children with autism rely on verbal imitation as the primary means of language acquisition for longer than do echolalic children with SLI, while both groups utilise it with greater frequency and over a more extended period than do children with typical language development.

Mitigated echolalia

Children utilising a predominantly imitative style need to develop analytic skills for the development of spontaneous, generative, multi-word language (de Villiers & de Villiers 1987). The increased amount of mitigation observed over time, in the speech of children in the autism group in particular, suggested that they were developing some ability to process speech and, possibly, to derive the rules that govern language production (Prizant 1987). As children with autism develop linguistically, it is likely that they acquire the ability to retain a heard utterance in short term memory, then to process it at a higher level, resulting in a mitigated echolalic utterance. The appearance of this ability marks an important developmental stage. It indicates some ability to retain and then process the heard utterance in a way that demonstrates understanding of at least some of the utterance and some understanding of the rules governing the production of utterances (Prizant 1987). It indicates that the child is able to change the echoed utterance in a *systematic* way requiring the use of some sort of linguistic processing. In the present study, the increased use of mitigations was associated with a reduction in the total amount of echolalia (i.e. less echolalia was produced over time and what was produced became increasingly mitigated) and improved receptive language scores. Further research exploring the nature of mitigated echolalia is warranted to address, in more detail, the issue of the precise nature of the relationship between the increased use of mitigations and developing linguistic competence.

There has been some evidence in the literature that could be interpreted to suggest that children with SLI also rely on imitative learning strategies to develop language. Connell (1987) demonstrated that these children learned new language structures most efficiently when imitative teaching strategies were used (i.e. when the child was required to imitate a model, in contrast to being given a model without being required to imitate). In contrast, Connell found that, in a typically developing group, using imitation in addition to modeling to teach a language structure did not improve learning. Connell suggested that this difference is related to the respective learning styles of children in the two groups. He proposed that children with SLI have greater difficulty recognising critical characteristics of models than do typical children, and that imitation assists them in this process because their learning style is different. Connell concluded that children respond best to those strategies that reflect their predominant learning style.

Implications for assessment and management

The measurement of the amount and type of echolalia in speech and the assessment of receptive language ability over time is likely to provide useful information about the development of language competence in young children with high levels of echolalia. The increasing presence of mitigated echolalia in the speech of echolalic children with autism or SLI is likely to be a positive prognostic indicator. It is suggested, therefore, that the measurement of receptive language ability, levels of echolalia and the relative amount of mitigation in speech are likely to be useful indicators of a child's progress towards the development of spontaneous functional language.

A process of language development in young cognitively able children with Autistic Disorder that differs from that observed in the typically developing population was suggested in the present study. Rather than developing intervention programs for echolalic children based on models of typical development, it may be more productive to base them on the process that has been observed in this population. In the case of children with autism a combination of modeling and imitation is likely to be the most effective learning strategy. The facilitation of language development in children with autism may be best achieved by further examining developmental patterns characteristic of this group and repeating, promoting and extending these strategies. While much work remains to be done to better understand the process of language acquisition in children with Autism Spectrum Disorder without intellectual disability, in developing intervention programs it is possible to begin to consider the use of echolalia and mitigated echolalia as tools to facilitate language development.

Limitations of the study

Participants with Autistic Disorder and performance IQ in the typical range represent a subgroup on the autism spectrum. Caution is warranted in making assumptions that imply that echolalia is a stage through which all verbal children with autism move in the development of spontaneous functional speech. Although all but four of the echolalic participants in the present study had ceased to echo significantly by the end of this study, less able verbal children with autism may present with a different pattern. For example, when Landry and Loveland (1988) compared a group of verbal participants with autism with a SLI and a typical group, they found that the children with autism had high levels of echolalia in their speech at a much later chronological age (M = 8;9) than the participants in the present study. Their results suggested that, for less able children with autism, significant echolalia is likely to continue to be a feature of their language throughout their lives. All the participants in this study had delayed language development, that is, children meeting criteria for Aspergers Disorder were not included.

The applicability of the findings to different groups on the autism spectrum warrants further investigation, particularly for those with more severely impaired cognitive and language skills and those with superior cognitive and language development.

Further research

Several issues for further research arise from the present study. First is the need for further analysis of mitigated echolalia. The identification of echolalia as mitigated or non-mitigated had high inter-rater reliability (97%) and, as a result, the identification of echolalia and its description as mitigated or non-mitigated was considered to be reliable. Further research is warranted to develop the classification system for mitigated echolalia to enable the prevalence of different types of echolalia to be analysed.

Second, further research is warranted into the effects of age and intellectual development on language acquisition in able children with autism and children with SLI to assess outcomes in late childhood. Outcomes could be compared for (a) the amount of echolalia and mitigated echolalia, if any, remaining in speech; (b) the relationship between echolalia, if any, and receptive/expressive language competence; (c) the relationship between the amount of echolalia in speech and psychological stress, including that resulting from receptive communication problems (Rydell & Mirenda 1991); and long term follow-up to assess the effect of maturation on the diagnosis and classification of participants is warranted.

Conclusion

It is likely that for verbal children with Autistic Disorder and some with language disability, echolalia is, in part, a language acquisition strategy. The nature of the echolalia observed in the language samples changed over time as participants increasingly utilised mitigated echolalia. This change was associated with increased language competence and suggests that changes in the amount and type of echolalia may also be evidence of developmental progression. Thus, the amount and type of echolalia in the speech of able children with autism is potentially a marker of the development of language competence, which may be useful in the assessment of these children. The most effective intervention is likely to be one that utilises these strengths. The challenge for researchers and practitioners is to better understand this process and to develop interventions that are relevant to facilitate language development of these children.

References

American Psychiatric Association (1987). *Diagnostic and Statistical Manual, 3rd edition, revised (DSM III-R)*. Washington, DC: American Psychiatric Association.

American Psychiatric Association (1994). *Diagnostic and Statistical Manual, 4th edition, (DSM-IV)*. Washington, DC: American Psychiatric Association.

Asperger, H. (1944). Die Autistichen Psychopathen im Kindesalter. *Archive fur Psychiatrie und Nervenkrankheiten 117*, 76–136.

Bates, E., Bretherton, I., & Snyder, L. (1988). *From First Words to Grammar*. Cambridge: CUP.

Bebko, J.M. (1990). Echolalia, mitigation and autism: Indicators from child characteristics for the use of sign language and other augmentative language systems. *Sign-Language Studies, 66*, 61–78.

Bernard-Opitz, V. (1982). Pragmatic analysis of the communicative behaviour of an autistic child. *Journal of Speech and Hearing Disorders, 47*, 99–109.

Bettelheim, B. (1967). *The Empty Fortress*. New York, NY: Free Press.

Bishop, D.V.M. (1989). Autism, Asperger's Syndrome and Semantic-Pragmatic Disorder: Where are the boundaries? *British Journal of Disorders of Communication, 24*, 107–121.

Bloom, L. (1991). *Language Development from Two to Three*. Cambridge: CUP.

Cantwell, D.P., & Baker, L. (1978). Imitations and echoes in autistic and dysphasic children. *Journal of the American Academy of Child Psychiatry, 17*, 604–613.

Carluccio, C., Sours, J.A., & Kalb, L.C. (1964). Psychodynamics of echo-reactions. *Archives General Psychiatry, 10*, 623–629.

Clark, R. (1977). What's the use of imitation? *Journal of Child Language, 4*, 341–358.

Cole, K.N., Schwartz, I.S., Notati, A.R., Dale, P.S. & Mills, P.E. (1995). Examination of the stability of two methods of defining specific language impairment. *Applied Psycholinguistics, 16*, 103–123.

Connell, P.J. (1987). An effect of modelling and imitation teaching procedures on children with and without specific language impairment. *Journal of Speech and Hearing Research, 30*, 105–113.

Darley, F.L. (1964). *Diagnosis and Appraisal of Communication Disorders*. Englewood Cliffs, NJ: Prentice-Hall.

de Villiers, P.A. & de Villiers, J.G. (1987). Commentary on language and autism. In D.J. Cohen & A.M. Donnellan (Eds.), *Handbook of Autism and Pervasive Developmental Disorders*. New York, NY: John Wiley & Sons.

Fay, W.H. (1967). Mitigated echolalia of children. *Journal of Speech and Hearing Research, 10*, 305–310.

Fay, W.H. (1969). On the basis of autistic echolalia. *Journal of Communication Disorders, 2*, 37–47.

Fay, W.H. (1973). On the echolalia of the blind and of the autistic child. *Journal of Speech and Hearing Disorders, 38*, 478–489.

Fay W.H. & Butler B.V. (1968). Echolalia, IQ, and the developmental dichotomy of speech and language systems. *Journal of Speech and Hearing Research, 11*, 358–364.

Fay, W.H. & Coleman, R.O. (1977). A human sound transducer: Temporal capabilities of a profoundly echolalic child. *Brain and Language, 4*, 396–402.

Griffith, R. & Ritvo, E. (1967). Echolalia: Concerning the dynamics of the syndrome. *Journal of the American Academy of Child Psychiatry, 6*, 184–193.

Hobson, R.P. (1990). Beyond cognition: A theory of autism. In G. Dawson (Ed.) *Autism: New Perspectives on Diagnosis, Nature and Treatment*. New York, NY: Guilford.

Howlin, P. (1982). Echolalia and spontaneous phrase speech in autistic children. *Journal of Child Psychology and Psychiatry, 23*(3), 281–293.

Hurtig, R., Ensrud, S. & Tomblin, J. (1982). The communicative function of question production in autistic children. *Journal of Autism and Developmental Disorders, 12*, 57–69.

Kanner, L. (1943). Autistic disturbances of affective contact. *Nervous Child, 2*, 217–250.

Kanner, L. (1946). Irrelevant and metaphorical language in early infantile autism. *American Journal of Psychiatry, 103*, 242–246.

Kirchner, D.M. & Prutting, C.A. (1987). Spontaneous verbal repetition: A performance-based strategy for language acquisition. *Clinical Linguistics & Phonetics, 1*, 147–169.

Landry, S.H. & Loveland, K.A. (1988). Communication behaviours in autism and developmental language delay. *Journal of Child Psychology and Psychiatry, 5*, 621–634.

Lee, A., Hobson, R.P., Chiat, S. (1994). I you, me, and autism: An experimental study. *Journal of Autism and Developmental Disorders, 24,* 15–176.
Lovaas, O.I. (1966). A program for the establishment of speech in psychotic children. In J.K. Wing (Ed.), *Early Childhood Autism.* Oxford: Pergamon.
Lovaas, O. 1981. *Teaching Developmentally Disabled Children: The Me Book.* Austin, TX: Pro-Ed.
Lovaas, O.I., Schriebman, L., & Koegel, R.L. (1974). A behavioural modification approach to the treatment of autistic children. *Journal of Autism and Childhood Schizophrenia, 4,* 111–129.
Malvy, J., Roux, S., Zakian, A., Debuly, S., Sauvage, D., & Barthélémy, C. (1999). A brief clinical scale for the early evaluation of imitation disorders in autism. *Autism, 3,* 357–369.
Phillips, G.M., & Dyer, C. (1977). Late onset echolalia in autism and allied disorders. *British Journal of Disorders of Communication, 12,* 47–59.
Pick, A. (1924). On the pathology of echographia. *Brain, 47,* 417–429.
Prizant, B.M. (1983). Language acquisition and communicative behaviour in autism; toward an understanding of the 'whole' of it. *Journal of Speech and Hearing Disorders, 48,* 296–307.
Prizant, B.M. (1987). Theoretical and clinical implications of echolalic behaviour in autism. In T. Layton (Ed.), *Language and Treatment of Autistic and Developmentally Disordered Children.* Springfield, IL: Charles Thomas.
Prizant, B.M. & Duchan, J.F. (1981). The functions of immediate echolalia in autistic children. *Journal of Speech and Hearing Disorders, 46,* 241–249.
Prizant, B.M. & Rydell, P. (1984). An analysis of the functions of delayed echolalia in autistic children. *Journal of Speech Hearing Research, 46,* 183–192.
Rees, N.S. (1975). Imitation and language development issues and clinical implications. *Journal of Speech and Hearing Disorders, 40,* 339–350.
Reynell, J.K. (1977). *Reynell Developmental Language Scales.* Windsor: NFER Publishing.
Roberts, J.M.A. (1989). Echolalia and comprehension in autistic children. *Journal of Autism and Developmental Disabilities, 19,* 271–281.
Rutter, M. & Lockyer, L. (1967). A five to fifteen year follow up study of infantile psychosis II: Social and Behavioural outcome. *British Journal of Psychiatry, 113,* 1183–1199.
Rydell, P.J. & Mirenda, P. (1991). The effects of two levels of linguistic constraint on echolalia and generative language production in children with autism. *Journal of Autism and Developmental Disorders, 21,* 151–157.
Schuler A.L. & Prizant B.M. (1985). Echolalia. In E. Schopler & G.B. Mesibov (Eds.), *Communication Problems in Autism,* 163–184. New York, NY: Plenum Press.
Shapiro, T. (1977). The quest for a linguistic model to study the speech of autistic children. *Journal of the American Academy of Child Psychiatry, 16,* 608–619.
Shapiro, T., Roberts, A. & Fish, B. (1970). Imitation and echoing in young schizophrenic children. *Journal of the American Academy of Child Psychiatry, 9,* 548–567.
Stengel, E. (1947). A clinical and psychological study of echo-reactions. *Journal of Mental Science, 18,* 598–612.
Tager-Flusberg, H., Calkins, S., Nolin, T., Baumberger, T., Anderson, M., Chadwick-Dias, A. (1990). A longitudinal study of language acquisition in autistic and Down Syndrome children. *Journal of Autism and Developmental Disorders, 20,* 1–21
Wetherby, A.M. & Gaines, B.H. (1982). Cognition and language Development in Autism. *Journal of Speech and Hearing Disorders, 47,* 63–70.
Wechsler Pre School and Primary Scale of Intelligence (1976). New York, NY: The Psychological Corporation.
Zipf, G.K. (1965). *Human Behaviour and the Principle of Least Effort.* New York, NY: Hafner.

CHAPTER 4

Do autism spectrum disorders and specific language impairment have a shared aetiology?

A review of the evidence

Lauren J. Taylor, Murray T. Maybery & Andrew J.O. Whitehouse
University of Western Australia

There has been considerable debate in the literature regarding the aetiological relationship between Autism Spectrum Disorder (ASD) and Specific Language Impairment (SLI). While some authors have suggested that similarities in the language phenotypes of the conditions represent a theoretically significant aetiological overlap, others argue that the overlap is superficial and not reflective of shared causes. This chapter reviews the published literature with regard to the hypothesised aetiological relationship between ASD and SLI. Specifically, we review studies investigating behavioural and linguistic overlap between ASD and SLI, before considering results of neurological and molecular genetic studies. While several studies have highlighted phenotypic similarities between ASD and SLI, there is a considerable degree of inconsistency throughout the literature and current evidence does not support aetiological overlap. Important avenues for future research are investigating whether there are shared neurological and genetic pathways contributing to ASD and SLI.

Introduction

While language impairment is accepted as a defining feature of Autism Spectrum Disorder (ASD), there is debate as to whether characteristics of this impairment are unique to ASD or are shared with other childhood communication disorders. Language delay, a slower trajectory of language acquisition, is often the first indicator to parents that their child may not be developing in a typical fashion. Clinically speaking, language delay is also frequently parents' primary concern when seeking intervention. However, the language phenotype of ASD is complex and variable, as some children fail to develop language and others acquire prolific vocabularies, but have difficulty with the social use of language.

Language difficulties are components of a number of other developmental disorders, most notably Specific Language Impairment (SLI). SLI is diagnosed when children experience a clinically significant delay in language development despite having adequate hearing, nonverbal intelligence and educational opportunities (Bishop 2003). The structural language impairments (i.e. in phonology, morphology, syntax) of children with SLI contrast with the pragmatic language impairments (i.e. in social communication) and broader developmental difficulties of children with ASD. On the basis of these distinctions, ASD and SLI have traditionally been considered distinct disorders, with different aetiologies.

Several researchers (Lewis, Murdoch & Woodyatt 2007; Rapin & Allen 1983; Rapin & Dunn 2003; Rapin, Dunn, Allen, Stevens & Fein 2009) have attempted to subcategorise children on the autism spectrum according to their structural language ability. One subgroup of children with ASD that has been described by several authors is characterised by mixed expressive and receptive language impairments. In a series of studies, Rapin and colleagues found that a substantial proportion of children with ASD (59% in one study, 63% in another) presented with impaired phonological and syntactical skills (Rapin & Dunn 2003; Tuchman, Rapin & Shinnar 1991). Results of a longitudinal study similarly highlighted distinct clusters of language ability in children with ASD (Lewis et al. 2007), as did more recent results of a cluster analysis (Rapin et al. 2009). In each of these studies, one cluster of children with ASD was characterised by impaired expressive phonological skill (Lewis et al. 2007; Rapin & Dunn 2003; Rapin et al. 2009). These results highlight that a substantial proportion of children with ASD present with deficits in phonology and syntax in addition to their pragmatic impairments and broader autistic symptomatology.

A further study conducted by Kjelgaard and Tager-Flusberg (2001) subdivided children with ASD into 'normal' (ALN; standard scores greater than 85), 'borderline' (standard scores between 70 and 84), and 'impaired' (ALI; standard scores less than 70) language groups based on their performance on the Peabody Picture Vocabulary Test-III and Clinical Evaluation of Language Fundamentals (CELF; Wiig, Secord & Semel 1992) preschool, or III. The language 'impaired' subgroup of children with ASD (ALI) performed poorly on tests of phonological processing, vocabulary, and higher-order grammatical and semantic skills; a pattern of performance that is reminiscent of children with SLI. Kjelgaard and Tager-Flusberg (2001) proposed that this subgroup of children with ASD may share similar genetic risk factors with children with SLI. However, Williams, Botting and Boucher (2008) argued that Kjelgaard and Tager-Flusberg's (2001) interpretation of their results was only partly justified, as articulatory phonological impairments are a common feature of language profiles in SLI, but were not seen in children with ASD. Nonetheless, the research has stimulated significant interest into the aetiological relationship between ASD and SLI. One position is that the phenotypic similarities between ASD and SLI reflect of shared underlying causes (Kjelgaard & Tager-Flusberg 2001; Tager-Flusberg 2006). A contrasting position is that phenotypic similarities between ASD and SLI are merely superficial and do not reflect a common aetiology (Whitehouse, Barry & Bishop 2007, 2008). Substantive conclusions from this debate have not yet been reached.

The current chapter includes a comprehensive review of the literature pertaining to the hypothesised aetiological relationship between ASD and SLI. Specifically, we review the literature that has examined linguistic characteristics of SLI (namely poor nonword and sentence repetition, tense-marking errors) in children with ASD. In addition, we summarise evidence highlighting the 'blurring' of diagnostic boundaries between ASD and SLI. Neurobiological links between ASD and SLI, such as atypical lateralisation for language and volumetric abnormalities in the cerebral cortex are also discussed. Finally, we consider genetic links between ASD and SLI, specifically focusing on family and molecular genetic studies. Thus, our overall aim is to review evidence from behavioural, neurological and molecular genetic levels in light of the hypothesised aetiological relationship between ASD and SLI. Understanding the relationship between these two conditions has important implications for diagnostic and intervention purposes. Moreover, understanding the aetiological relationship between ASD and SLI will advance theoretical conceptualisations of the disorders and facilitate investigations of genetic influences shared by the two conditions.

Linguistic and cognitive links between ASD and SLI

Comparisons between the language phenotypes of ASD and SLI offer an important contribution to the debate about aetiological overlap between the two conditions. Much of the early research investigating language in children with ASD included heterogeneous samples of children who had varying degrees of language impairment. More recent studies have included subgroups of children with ASD based on research highlighting distinct clusters of language ability across the autism spectrum (Lewis et al. 2007; Rapin & Dunn 2003; Rapin et al. 2009). One crucial comparison is between children with ALI (i.e. autism with an additional structural language impairment) and SLI. ALI is defined as impaired performance (i.e. more than 1.5SD below the mean) on standardised measures of expressive and receptive language (e.g. Kjelgaard & Tager-Flusberg 2001). Studies comparing the language phenotypes of ALI and SLI have provided important insights into the debate about shared aetiologies.

Evidence for phenotypic overlap between ASD and SLI comes from a recent study that reported no significant differences between children with ALI and those with SLI on receptive, expressive and total language scores on the CELF-III (Lindgren, Folstein, Tomblin & Tager-Flusberg 2009). In contrast, Lloyd, Paintin and Botting (2006) found that children with SLI performed significantly worse than children with ASD and also significantly worse than children with shared symptoms (children who displayed some features of both SLI and ASD) on expressive and total language scores of the CELF-III. The group of children with shared symptoms could arguably be defined as ALI; however, children were allocated to the 'shared group' based on teaching needs rather than clinical features. Importantly, Lloyd et al. (2006) found the language profile of children with shared symptoms more closely resembled the ASD than the SLI group. In addition, while children with shared symptoms demonstrated poorer receptive than expressive skills, the opposite was observed for children with SLI. Further support for contrasting patterns of expressive and receptive abilities between children with ALI and children with SLI comes from Loucas et al. (2008), who found a discrepancy in the profile of expressive and receptive abilities for children with SLI relative to children with ALI. While children with SLI had stronger receptive than expressive language, the levels of receptive and expressive language difficulties were comparable in children with ALI.

Few other investigations have directly compared the language abilities of children with ALI and those with SLI. The following sections review studies which have examined the language abilities of the two conditions independently.

Phonology

Phonological impairments are a defining feature of SLI (Bartak et al. 1975; Conti-Ramsden & Crutchley 1997). Children with SLI exhibit deficits on phonological discrimination (Briscoe, Bishop & Norbury 2001), phonological awareness (Briscoe et al. 2001) and expressive phonology tasks (Briscoe et al. 2001), and several studies have found that these difficulties often last well into early adulthood (Clegg, Hollis, Mawhood & Rutter 2005). In contrast, phonology skills are relatively unimpaired in the vast majority of children with ASD (Bartolucci & Pierce 1977; Boucher 1976; Kjelgaard & Tager-Flusberg 2001; Rapin & Dunn 2003; Rapin et al. 2009). For example, Rapin et al. (2009) found that only 24% of their sample of 118 children with ASD had phonological difficulties as indexed by the Photo Articulation Test (PAT; Pendergast, Dickey, Selmar & Soder 1984). Cleland, Gibbon, Peppé, O'Hare and Rutherford (2010) reported similar findings, with only 11.5% of their sample of 69 children with ASD scoring at least one standard deviation below the normal mean on the Goldman Fristoe Test of

Articulation (GFTA-2; Goldman & Fristow 2000). Studies have found that phonological errors, when they occur in children with ASD, are predominantly in gliding, cluster reduction, final consonant deletion and phoneme substitution (Bartolucci, Pierce, Steiner & Eppel 1976; Cleland et al. 2010). While less frequent in ASD, these phonological errors are similar to those observed in children with SLI, who make errors in the production of vowel sounds, accuracy of stops and nasals, phoneme substitutions, cluster reduction and initial and final consonant deletion (Aguilar-Mediavilla, Sanz-Torrent & Serra-Raventos 2002; Bortolini & Leonard 2000; Leonard 1982; Orsolini, Sechi, Maronato, Bonvino & Corcelli 2001).

Morphosyntax

Like phonological difficulties, morphosyntactic deficits are a defining characteristic of SLI (Botting 2002; Conti-Ramsden & Crutchley 1997; Hewitt, Hammer Yont & Tomblin 2005; Rice 1997). Children with SLI can be distinguished from typically developing (TD) children based on shorter and less grammatically-complex utterances (Johnston & Kahmi 1984). Experimental studies have also found that children with SLI make more grammatical errors in case marking, use of possessive and plural *-s*, and past tense inflections compared to younger TD children matched on mean length of utterance (Bedore & Leonard 1998; Bishop 1994; Bishop & Adams 1990). In addition, studies of the narrative abilities of children with SLI have highlighted deficits in sentence and story length, story organisation and tense-marking (Botting 2002).

Morphosyntactic deficits are less common among children with ASD (Rapin & Allen 1983; Rapin & Dunn 2003; Rapin et al. 2009), and for those children who do exhibit morphosyntactic difficulties, findings have been inconsistent. Early studies found that children with ASD had delayed morphosyntactic development (Bartolucci, Pierce & Steiner 1980; Pierce & Bartolucci 1977; Waterhouse & Fein 1982). More recent studies have also documented difficulties among children with ALI, particularly with higher-order grammatical (e.g. number of morphological errors) and syntactic (e.g. number of coordinate clauses, verb complements) skills (Capps, Losh & Thurber 2000; Kjelgaard & Tager-Flusberg 2001). However, Tager-Flusberg (1995) found no differences between children with ASD and TD children on measures of complexity (mean length of utterance, number of different words used).

Studies that have directly compared ASD and SLI groups on morphosyntactic aspects of language are also inconsistent in outcome. One early study found that ASD and SLI groups could not be distinguished in their use of morphological rules, transformational rules, or phrase structure rules (Cantwell et al. 1978).

Norbury Nash, Baird and Bishop (2004) investigated linguistic characteristics of subgroups of children with communication disorders using the Children's Communication Checklist – Second Edition (CCC-2). The Children's Communication Checklist (CCC) and its revision, the CCC-2, are parent-report measures designed to distinguish between structural and pragmatic language impairments in populations of children known to have delayed language development (Bishop 1998). Norbury et al. (2004) found that while children with ASD and those with SLI had syntax scores below the normal mean, the syntactic difficulties were significantly worse for children with SLI relative to the ASD children. However, in a separate study, Norbury and Bishop (2003) investigated the narrative abilities of children with ASD and those with SLI, and found no group differences in understanding the global structure of a story, or on morphosyntactic measures such as sentence complexity (e.g. number of subordinate clauses, complement clauses, verb complements and passive constructions) and frequency of tense-marking errors.

Semantics

Several studies have found that semantic impairments are common in children with SLI and those with ASD. For example, Norbury et al. (2004) reported similar levels of parent-reported semantic difficulties (CCC-2) among SLI and ASD children.

Norbury and Bishop also conducted an extensive direct investigation of the semantic abilities of children with SLI and ASD (Norbury & Bishop 2002; Norbury 2005). In the first study, children listened to a series of stories about familiar topics (e.g. a birthday party) and were required to answer literal and inferential questions related to the story (Norbury & Bishop 2002). While both clinical groups had more difficulty answering both types of questions than did their age-matched TD peers, children with ASD tended to perform worse than the SLI group on questions requiring inferences. Furthermore, five of the ten (50%) ASD children were found to have a story comprehension deficit, compared with four of the 16 (25%) SLI children.

More recently, Norbury (2005) examined lexical ambiguity resolution in children with ALN, ALI, SLI, and their TD peers. Children were presented with ambiguous words (i.e. words with multiple meanings, such as bank) along with a picture that represented one of the possible interpretations of the word. Participants were required to respond "yes" or "no" depending on whether they thought the picture represented one of the word meanings. Children with ALI and children with SLI made significantly more errors than children with ALN and TD children on pictures that represented the less frequent of the two interpretations of each word, indicating that the language impaired children might be unfamiliar with less frequent, alternative word meanings. In a subsequent study, children saw a visual presentation (i.e. on a computer screen) of a sentence, followed by a coloured picture, and were required to indicate whether the picture was consistent with the overall meaning of the sentence. Children with ALI and those with SLI made more errors on ambiguous sentences (i.e. sentences that ended with an ambiguous word) than the ALN and TD groups, indicating that they derived less facilitation from the sentence context in interpreting the final word. Thus, results of this study provide evidence for phenotypic overlap between ALI and SLI.

Pragmatic language

Extensive research has found that pragmatic language difficulties are a pervasive feature of ASD. Pragmatic language encompasses the social conventions and rules governing language use (Boucher 2003). In ASD, pragmatic impairments include: failure to follow conversational rules; failure to use language appropriate for the context; frequent interrupting; overly pedantic and long-winded speech; and stereotyped language (Baltaxe 1977; Eales 1993; Eisenmajer et al. 1998; Ramberg, Ehlers, Nydén, Johansson & Gillberg 1996). Atypicalities in nonverbal pragmatics (such as gesture) and aspects of prosody (such as pitch, loudness, vocal quality and speech flow) have also been reported among individuals with ASD (Fine, Bartolucci, Ginsberg & Szatmari 1991; McCann, Peppé, Gibbon, O'Hare & Rutherford 2007; Peppé, McCann, Gibbon, O'Hare & Rutherford 2007; Rapin & Allen 1983; Shriberg et al. 2001).

Pragmatic language can be measured using parent-report questionnaires (such as the CCC or CCC-2) and standardised language assessments. A pragmatic composite score on the CCC and CCC-2 is calculated by summing scores on subscales assessing inappropriate initiation, coherence, stereotyped language, use of context and rapport. Children with ASD typically fall significantly below (1.5–2 SD) the normative mean on the pragmatic composite score of the CCC and CCC-2 (Bishop & Baird 2001; Philofsky, Fidler & Hepburn 2007).

The pragmatic language difficulties of individuals with ASD are also evident in their poor performance on the Test of Pragmatic Language (TOPL). In this assessment, children are presented with pictures of commonly encountered communicative interactions. Items increase in difficulty, initially assessing behaviours such as polite greetings and progressing to assess attribution of mental states. For example, in one scenario, a child is presented with a picture of a boy at the doctor's office, who is holding his stomach and has a distressed facial expression. The child is asked what he/she thinks the boy would say to the doctor (Young, Diehl, Morris, Hyman & Bennetto 2005). Young et al. (2005) found that individuals with ASD performed significantly worse (1.5 SD lower) on the TOPL than a TD comparison group matched on chronological age, IQ, receptive language and expressive language. In a further study, Lewis, Woodyatt and Murdoch (2008) found that adults with ASD were less adept at understanding inference, appreciating humour and producing emphatic stress in comparison to adults with no history of developmental disorder.

Considerably less research has compared pragmatic abilities in SLI and ASD. Bartak and colleagues found that children with ASD differed from children with SLI in terms of more frequent use of echolalia, pronominal reversal, metaphorical language and inappropriate remarks (Bartak et al. 1975). From these findings, the authors concluded that while the language profile of SLI is characterised by language delay, the language phenotype of ASD is characterised by deviance (i.e. abnormal language use) as well as delay. Cantwell et al. (1978) also found that abnormal language use (such as echolalia and idiosyncratic language) was significantly more prevalent in children with ASD relative to children with SLI. Moreover, children with SLI showed greater spontaneity (i.e. greater frequency of non-prompted remarks) in their communication, whereas children with ASD tended to inflexibly adhere to specific topics of interest. However, in a follow-up study Eales (1993) found that children with ASD and those with SLI were equally likely to make inappropriate utterances arising from a failure to execute communicative intent. Nevertheless, more recent research has tended to confirm the earlier observations. Schaeffer et al. (2005) investigated pragmatic and grammatical language in children with SLI and found that they did not exhibit pragmatic language impairments. Also, while Norbury et al. (2004), and more recently Loucas et al. (2010), reported that children with SLI exhibited mild pragmatic language difficulties as measured by the CCC-2, these difficulties were less severe than those observed in children with ASD.

SLI markers in ASD

Three purported psycholinguistic markers for SLI (at least in English-speaking individuals) are impaired nonword repetition, poor oral motor (oromotor) skills (Barry, Yasin & Bishop 2007) and deficits in the acquisition and use of tense-marking morphemes (e.g. the addition of *-ed* to indicate past tense; Rice & Wexler 1996; Tager-Flusberg & Joseph 2003). Evidence supporting the hypothesised aetiological overlap between ASD and SLI would come from studies finding that children with ALI also have difficulty with these skills.

In nonword repetition tasks, meaningless phoneme sequences are aurally presented to participants, who are then required to repeat these 'nonwords' verbatim (Gathercole, Willis, Baddeley & Emslie 1994). Nonword repetition is thought to index phonological short-term memory, a proposed core cognitive deficit in SLI (Gathercole & Baddeley 1990). Extensive research indicates that children with ALI perform comparably to children with SLI, and significantly worse than TD children on tests of nonword and sentence repetition (Kjelgaard & Tager-Flusberg 2001; Lindgren et al. 2009; Loucas et al. 2010; Riches, Loucas, Baird, Charman & Siminoff 2010; Riches, Loucas, Baird, Charman & Simonoff 2011; Tager-Flusberg 1996, 2006; Whitehouse et al. 2008a). However, Botting and Conti-Ramsden (2003) found that while children with ASD and children with SLI performed more than 1 SD below the normative mean on the nonword repetition task, the latter group performed significantly worse than the ASD group. Furthermore, several authors have found contrasting patterns of errors on nonword and sentence repetition tasks between ALI and SLI groups. For instance, children with SLI tend to make significantly more errors than children with ALI on longer nonwords relative to shorter nonwords (Riches et al. 2010; Riches et al. 2011; Whitehouse et al. 2008a). The discrepant error patterns between children with ALI and children with SLI on psycholinguistic markers for SLI may be indicative of different underlying cognitive impairments.

Comparably less research has examined oromotor skills and tense-marking in children with autism. Botting and Conti-Ramsden (2003) found no differences between an undifferentiated group of children with ASD and children with SLI on a tense-marking task. More recently, Roberts, Rice and Tager-Flusberg (2004) examined tense-marking in subgroups of children with ASD and found that children with ALI made significantly more errors than children with ALN. Roberts et al. (2004) also reported significant correlations between tense-marking and nonword repetition performance for children with ALI, and drew comparisons with the language abilities observed in SLI children. However, the types of errors made by the children with ALI were not strictly morphological in that these children were more likely than the children with ALN to not respond, or to provide echolalic responses. Other errors were likely to arise as a consequence of pragmatic language impairments in ASD, rather than structural language deficits (see Williams et al. 2008). Findings that differed from those of Roberts et al. (2004) were reported by Eigsti et al. (2007), who found that children with ALI used tense-marking morphemes appropriately. Importantly, Eigsti et al. (2007) measured tense-marking in a non-structured play situation, whereas Roberts et al. (2004) used a structured experimental task. Therefore, discrepancies in the reported use of tense-marking morphemes for children with ALI may reflect methodological differences between the studies rather than qualitative differences in tense-marking ability. Finally, Whitehouse et al. (2008a) found that children with ALI performed within normal limits (and significantly better than children with SLI) on a test of oromotor sequencing.

ASD markers in SLI

Several studies have used standardised diagnostic measures of ASD to assess autistic symptomatology in individuals with SLI. Bishop and Norbury (2002) found that a substantial minority of children with SLI met criteria for ASD or Pervasive Developmental Disorder-Not Otherwise Specified (PDD-NOS) on the ADI-R or the ADOS-G. Similarly, Leyfer, Tager-Flusberg, Dowd, Tomlin and Folstein (2008) found that 41% of a group of children with SLI met ASD cut-offs in the social and communication domains. Longitudinal data have also shown that some individuals diagnosed with SLI as children demonstrate behaviours reminiscent of ASD when reassessed in adolescence and adulthood (Howlin, Mawhood & Rutter 2000; Mawhood, Howlin & Rutter 2000). For example, Conti-Ramsden et al. (2006) reported that 3.9% of a sample of adolescents with a history of SLI exhibited sufficient behavioural characteristics of ASD to warrant an ASD diagnosis; a figure that is approximately four times current ASD prevalence estimates (Rice 2009). However, it has been argued that these findings may reflect 'diagnostic substitution', where recent broadening of ASD diagnostic boundaries may result in children who were previously diagnosed with SLI now meeting contemporary criteria for ASD (Bishop, Whitehouse, Watt & Line 2008).

Summary

This review of the linguistic and cognitive characteristics of ALI and SLI has revealed inconsistent findings. On the one hand, several studies have highlighted similarities in the language abilities of children with ALI and those with SLI, particularly with regard to the type of phonological errors demonstrated by these children (i.e. in phoneme substitution, cluster reduction and initial and final consonant deletion) (Aguilar-Mediavilla, Sanz-Torrent & Serra-Raventos 2002; Bortolini & Leonard 2000; Leonard 1982; Nettelbladt 1992; Orsolini, Sechi, Maronato, Bonvino & Corcelli 2001) as well as certain morphosyntactic and semantic errors (Bishop 2003; Cantwell et al. 1978; Kjelgaard & Tager-Flusberg 2001; Norbury 2005; Norbury et al. 2004). In addition, numerous studies have reported similar nonword and sentence repetition performance in children with ALI and those with SLI (Kjelgaard & Tager-Flusberg 2001; Lindgren et al. 2009; Loucas et al. 2010; Riches, Loucas, Baird, Charman & Siminoff 2010; Riches, Loucas, Baird, Charman & Simonoff 2011; Tager-Flusberg 1996, 2006; Whitehouse et al. 2008a). However, as Williams et al. (2008) argued, nonword repetition tasks may tap multiple underlying cognitive and linguistic processes. Therefore, deficits in nonword repetition for children with ALI and those with SLI could result from different underlying causes. This point seems to be particularly salient given that Whitehouse et al. (2008a) observed a different pattern of nonword repetition errors made by these two groups.

Important distinctions can also be made between ALI and SLI children. Articulation and phonological impairments are markedly less prevalent in ALI relative to SLI (Bartolucci & Pierce 1977; Boucher 1976; Kjelgaard & Tager-Flusberg 2001; Rapin & Dunn 2003; Rapin et al. 2009). In addition, pragmatic impairments, a defining feature of ASD, occur relatively infrequently in SLI (Bartak et al. 1975; Cantwell et al. 1978; Schaeffer et al. 2005; Loucas et al. 2010). Furthermore, while Roberts et al. (2004) provided evidence showing that children with ALI have tense-marking deficits, others have not replicated this finding (Eigsti et al. 2007; see also Botting & Conti-Ramsden 2003).

The empirical literature is limited by the paucity of studies that have directly compared the linguistic profiles of ALI and SLI. As such, it is difficult to determine whether or not the superficial similarities between the two conditions reflect common underlying cognitive and linguistic processes and overlapping aetiologies. Direct comparisons of ALI and SLI groups will be well-placed to inform future theories on the aetiological relationship between ASD and SLI.

Neurobiological links between ASD and Specific Language Impairment

The majority of individuals with typical language development have the most crucial cortical areas involved in language production lateralised to the left-hemisphere (Binder, Frost, Hammeke, Cox, Rao & Prieto 1997; Knecht, Deppé et al. 2000; Knecht et al. 1998; Knecht, Drãger et al. 2000). Cerebral dominance for language has been the focus of considerable research attention in both ASD and SLI and has been investigated using indirect measures (see Hollier, Maybery & Whitehouse this volume), as well as structural and functional neuroimaging techniques. These latter findings will be reviewed here.

Structural neuroimaging studies

The primary language centres in the human brain (i.e. Broca's and Wernicke's areas) are centred around the perisylvian structures at the juncture of the temporal and frontal lobes (Binder et al. 1997; Ojemann 1991). There is increasing literature showing that children with SLI have atypical perisylvian asymmetries relative to TD individuals. Studies using Magnetic Resonance Imaging (MRI) in particular, have reported enlarged right perisylvian areas in children with SLI relative to the volumes for these areas in TD controls (Gauger, Lombardino & Leonard 1997; Plante, Swisher, Vance & Rapcsak 1991).

There is less consistent evidence for atypical laterality in ASD. Using MRI, Herbert et al. (2002) identified larger right frontal language areas for boys with ASD compared to TD boys. More recently, Knaus et al. (2010) examined associations between language lateralisation and anatomical characteristics in TD and ASD individuals using structural MRI. There were no significant differences in frontal and temporal grey matter volumes between TD and ASD groups. Interestingly, individuals with atypical language laterality (regardless of diagnostic classification) had significantly larger grey matter volumes in frontal and temporal language regions and there was a non-significant trend for these individuals to also have larger grey matter volumes in the posterior superior temporal gyrus and planum temporale (part of Wernicke's Area) than individuals with typical lateralisation. Diffusion tensor images also indicated higher fractional anisotropy of the regions that connect posterior receptive areas of the brain to the frontal cortex in individuals with typically lateralised language, relative to those with atypical language lateralisation. From these findings, Knaus et al. (2010) argued that differences in anatomical volumes in language areas are driven by differences in language laterality rather than by ASD diagnosis.

In two studies, Herbert and colleagues performed quantitative volumetric analyses on whole cortex MRI scans of children with ASD and children with SLI (Herbert, Ziegler, Deutsch et al. 2003; Herbert, Ziegler, Makris et al. 2003). Children with SLI had larger total brain volumes relative to TD children, and there was a non-significant trend for children with ASD to also have larger brain volumes relative to the TD group. With statistical control for total brain size, there was a trend for children with ASD and children with SLI to have larger cerebral white matter volumes and smaller cerebral cortex volumes relative to TD control participants (Herbert, Ziegler, Deutsch et al. 2003; Herbert, Ziegler, Makris et al. 2003).

In a further study, Herbert et al. (2004) provided a direct comparison of the morphological asymmetries in children with ASD and children with SLI using MRI. While TD boys showed significant left asymmetries in cerebral cortex and right asymmetries in caudate and cerebral white matter, these structures were not significantly asymmetrical in boys with SLI or boys with ASD. With regard to language-related regions, boys with SLI and boys with ASD exhibited less leftward asymmetry in subregions of Broca's area in the inferior frontal lobe, relative to TD boys. Further, compared to the TD group, both the ASD and SLI groups showed greater leftward asymmetry in the planum temporale and anterior supramarginal gyrus (part of the parietal lobe involved in language perception and processing) and greater rightward asymmetry in the posterior supramarginal gyrus. Overall, volumetric asymmetry in the SLI and ASD groups was closely similar and both groups differed significantly from the TD group.

Only one study has directly compared volumetric asymmetries between boys with ALI and boys with SLI. Using MRI, De Fossé et al. (2004) examined grey and white matter brain volumes in nine boys with SLI and 16 boys with ALI and found a similar pattern of reversed asymmetry in fronto-cortical language regions between groups. Both groups showed increased volumes in right compared to left frontal language areas, whereas boys with ALN and TD control participants showed the opposite volumetric differences. In contrast, no differences in asymmetry between the groups were observed in Wernicke's area.

Functional neuroimaging studies

Flagg and colleagues used magnetoencephalography (MEG) to record brain responses to vowel sounds and found opposing developmental trajectories between ALI and TD children; where TD children developed leftward lateralisation (i.e. left hemisphere dominance), children with ALI developed rightward lateralisation (Flagg, Cardy, Roberts & Roberts 2005). More recently, Redcay and Courchesne (2008) performed fMRI on toddlers with ASD, who were played speech sounds while they were sleeping. While TD children showed greater activations in left hemisphere frontal and temporal regions, children with ASD showed the opposite (i.e. greater activations in right hemisphere frontal and parietal regions). Further, there was a trend for children with ASD to show greater right than left hemisphere activation in frontal, temporal, occipital and parietal regions and the caudate nucleus. Conversely, TD children showed greater left than right hemisphere activations in frontal, temporal and parietal regions. Kleinhans et al. (2008) also observed weaker left-lateralised activation for individuals with ASD relative to control participants during a letter fluency task. Further, while all control participants exhibited leftward lateralisation, individuals with ASD were more likely to have right, bilateral, absent, or weak left-lateralised activation (measured using fMRI).

Using electroencephalography, Shafer and colleagues found reversed asymmetry (i.e. enhanced rightward activation) in perisylvian cortical regions of participants with SLI when processing auditory grammatical information (Shafer, Schwartz, Morr, Kessler & Kurtzberg 2000). Five of the seven SLI participants showed reduced positivity at the left temporal site and enhanced positivity at the right temporal site, relative to children with typical language development. Using functional Magnetic Resonance Imaging (fMRI), Hugdahl et al. (2004) also found differences between individuals with SLI and TD participants. fMRI was performed while participants heard individual phonemes, meaningless phonemic combinations, and words. While both groups demonstrated bilateral activations in the temporal lobes for all conditions, activations for the SLI participants were smaller and weaker than for the TD participants. In addition, TD participants exhibited greater activation in the left temporal lobe, whereas activations in the SLI group were more concentrated in upper and posterior pars of the superior temporal gyrus. Reduced activations in the superior temporal sulcus and medial temporal gyrus were also observed for the SLI group relative to the TD group.

One study has directly compared the functional lateralisation of language abilities in children with ASD and those with SLI (Whitehouse & Bishop 2008b). In this study, hemispheric dominance for language was indexed using functional transcranial Doppler ultrasonography (fTCD), which measures changes in blood flow velocity in the left and right middle cerebral arteries, while participants complete a word generation task (involving silently generating words beginning with a particular letter, then verbalising these words). Behavioural data revealed no significant differences in performance on the word generation task between individuals with ASD and those with SLI. However, the ASD and TD groups showed predominantly greater left than right hemisphere activation, whereas eight of the 11 adults with SLI had increased blood flow in the middle cerebral artery lateralised to the right hemisphere or blood flow was increased bilaterally.

Summary

Studies using indirect measures of cerebral dominance in children with SLI and those with ASD have yielded inconsistent results (see Hollier et al. this volume, for a review). Neuroimaging studies that have examined ASD and SLI in isolation have highlighted similarities between the conditions, particularly in enlarged cortical volumes for both conditions (Herbert, Ziegler, Deutsch et al. 2003; Herbert, Ziegler, Makris et al. 2003). However, direct comparisons of structural abnormalities in ASD and SLI are inconsistent; while Herbert et al. (2005) found comparable patterns of asymmetry in ASD and SLI, De Fossé et al. (2004) found reversed asymmetry in frontal language regions for boys with SLI and for boys with ALI, but not for boys with ALN. It is noteworthy to mention that De Fossé et al. (2004) compared volumetric abnormalities in children with ALI and SLI, whereas Herbert et al. (2005) compared asymmetry in ASD and SLI. It is possible that a considerable proportion of Herbert et al.'s (2005) ASD sample actually consisted of children with ALI, which could have led to the comparable patterns of asymmetry in ASD and SLI. Results of several functional imaging studies provide support for atypical cerebral lateralisation in ASD and SLI (Flagg et al. 2005; Hugdahl et al. 2004; Kleinhans et al. 2008; Knaus et al. 2010; Redcay & Courchesne 2008; Shafer et al. 2000). However, in the only direct comparison of functional activation between children with ASD and those with SLI, Whitehouse and Bishop (2008b) found opposing patterns of cerebral lateralisation for language between the two conditions.

There is a considerable body of evidence, particularly from findings of enlarged brain volumes and atypical lateralisation in ASD and SLI, which suggests overlapping neurological abnormalities. It is possible that the similarities are driven by language impairments in ASD (i.e. ALI), rather than ASD perse. Nonetheless, future research devoted to exploring the neurological mechanisms that underpin language in ASD and SLI will be well-placed to inform debate about the aetiological relationship between the two conditions.

Genetic links between ASD and Specific Language Impairment

Twin studies have found that ASD and SLI are both heritable conditions (Bailey et al. 1995; Bishop, North & Donlan 1996; Folstein & Rutter 1977a, 1977b; Rutter 2000). Results of family studies also indicate that relatives of individuals with ASD and SLI show milder variants of the respective phenotypes. With regard to potential overlap between SLI and ASD, twin, family and molecular genetic studies have sought to determine whether the two conditions share common heritable risk factors.

Twin studies

One twin study only has examined the purported overlap between ASD and SLI. Dworzynski et al. (2007, 2008) examined shared developmental pathways between early language development and specific impairments in the social, communication and behavioural domains of ASD. Results revealed a relationship between early language difficulties and later autistic traits, but the relationship was specific to social communication aspects of the autistic phenotype. In addition, the association between early language difficulties and higher levels of autistic-like traits was entirely mediated by shared genetic influences. These findings suggest that later pragmatic skills and early language competence may stem partly from the same cause.

Family studies

Family studies have provided mixed evidence regarding the hypothesised aetiological overlap between ASD and SLI. Early investigations found that family members of children with ASD have an elevated rate of history of language impairment (Bailey et al. 1998; Tomblin, Hafeman & O'Brien 2003). A further study reported similar language characteristics among parents of children with ASD and parents of children with SLI (Ruser et al. 2007).

However, there is an accumulating body of research that has found little evidence for phenotypic overlap among family members of ASD and SLI probands.

Pilowsky et al. (2003) found that the formal language abilities of siblings of children with ASD (assessed via the CELF) were within normal limits, and significantly better than the abilities shown by siblings of children with SLI. Furthermore, Whitehouse et al. (2007) found a 'double dissociation' between the performance of parents of children with ASD and parents of children with SLI on a range of language measures (such as reading efficiency, spelling accuracy, receptive grammatical knowledge, phonemic decoding, nonword repetition and oromotor sequences). While the parents of children with ASD had intact linguistic performance and impaired social communication skills, the parents of children with SLI exhibited impaired linguistic performance and intact social communication skills.

Further support for isolated impairments in pragmatic language for parents of children with ASD comes from family studies showing that lesser variants of ASD include communication impairments that are restricted to the pragmatic domain (Bolton et al. 1994; Folstein & Rosen-Sheidley 2001). In addition, Whitehouse et al. (2010) reported that parents of a child with ASD were more likely to score poorly on a single domain of the Communication Checklist – Adult (CC-A) (i.e. language structure, pragmatics, or social engagement), rather than on multiple subscales. The predominant area of difficulty for parents of children with ASD was social engagement, which is consistent with an earlier report of weaknesses in social skills and communication in the parents of ASD children (Bishop et al. 2004). Together these studies suggest that impairments in social communication rather than language *per se* may be part of the heritable communication deficit in ASD. Further evidence for this view comes from the study by Lindgren et al. (2009), who found that relatives of children with ALI and of children with ALN performed at a similar level, and significantly better than relatives of children with SLI, on a range of linguistic measures, including nonword repetition, which is a purported marker for heritable linguistic impairment (Barry et al. 2007; Bishop, North & Donlan 1996; Conti-Ramsden, Botting & Faragher 2001).

Molecular genetic studies

In recent years, an increasing number of molecular genetic studies have sought to identify genes that may confer susceptibility to ASD and/or SLI. ASD, in particular, has received considerable research attention, and susceptibility loci have been identified on chromosomes 2, 4, 7, 13, 16, 17 and 19 (Barrett et al. 1999; Philippe, Martinez, Guilloud-Bataille, Gillberg, Rastam et al. 1999; The International Molecular Genetic Study of Autism Consortium 1998). While studies of SLI are fewer in number, it is notable that candidate regions have been identified on chromosomes 7q (O'Brien, Zhang, Nishimura, Tomblin & Murray 2003) and 16q (Monaco & The SLI Consortium 2007; The SLI Consortium 2002), which overlap with the findings from several ASD studies.

One locus of particular interest has been chromosome 7q35, which has been linked with ASD (Alarcón, Yonan, Gilliam, Cantor & Geschwind 2005; see also Badner & Gershon 2002 for a meta-analysis). A specific gene located on chromosome 7q35 that has garnered significant research interest is Contactin Associated Protein-Like 2 (CNTNAP2). CNTNAP2 encodes a member of the neurexin superfamily – neuronal transmembrane proteins involved in cell adhesion – and shows enriched expression in language-related circuits of the brain (Abrahams, Tentler, Perederiy, Oldham & Geschwind 2007). Moreover, this gene is directly regulated by FOXP2 a transcription factor mutated in rare monogenic forms of speech and language disorder (Fisher & Scharff 2009; Lai, Fisher, Hurst, Vargha-Khadems & Monaco 2001; MacDermot et al. 2005). Several researchers have found that polymorphisms in the CNTNAP2 gene were over-transmitted in multiple incidence ASD families, highlighting CNTNAP2 as a potential ASD-susceptibility gene (Alarcón et al. 2008; Arking et al. 2008; Bakkaloglu et al. 2008). Interestingly, in a study of children with SLI, Vernes et al. (2008) found statistically significant associations between CNTNAP2 polymorphisms and impaired nonword repetition, a known heritable risk factor for SLI. Genetic variants in the exon 13–15 region of CNTNAP2 have also been associated with language delay in ASD (Alarcón et al. 2008; Poot et al. 2010) and early language acquisition in typical development (Whitehouse, Bishop, Ang, Pennell & Fisher 2011). In addition, O'Brien and colleagues (2003) found a significant association between the language phenotype of SLI and genetic markers on chromosome 7q31, proximal to FOXP2 (O'Brien, Zhang, Nishimura, Tomblin & Murray 2003). Notably, markers on 7q have also been associated with language delay in ASD (Bradford et al. 2001).

Summary

The findings of studies investigating genetic overlap between ASD and SLI are inconsistent. On the one hand, there is evidence supporting genetic overlap: longitudinal twin studies have found relationships between early lexical development and later pragmatic skills (Dworzynski et al. 2008; Dworzynski et al. 2007) and molecular genetic studies have identified potential areas of overlap between ASD and SLI, most notably for a locus on chromosome 7q (Alarcón et al. 2008; Poot et al. 2010; Vernes et al. 2008). On the other hand, results of family studies provide evidence against aetiological overlap. For example, the relatively intact structural language skills observed in relatives of children with ASD points to distinct aetiologies for ASD and SLI (Whitehouse et al. 2007). Failure to find impaired nonword repetition in relatives of children with ALI (Lindgren et al. 2009) provides additional evidence against aetiological overlap between the two conditions. While current genetic evidence does not support aetiological overlap between ASD and SLI, this remains a promising area for future research.

General conclusions and directions for future research

ASD and SLI are characterised by communication difficulties. SLI represents a specific deficit in structural aspects of language, while ASD is a pervasive developmental disorder, with language impairment occurring within the context of broader social and behavioural difficulties. On the basis of these phenotypic differences, ASD and SLI have traditionally been considered as distinct disorders, with distinct aetiologies. However, in recent years, there has been debate as to whether ASD and SLI are aetiologically related disorders, or separate conditions with distinct causes.

Putative markers for SLI – including nonword repetition, oromotor skills and tense-marking – have been investigated in ALI. The contrasting error patterns on tests of nonword repetition and reported differences in oromotor skills and the use of tense-marking morphemes between children with ALI and SLI provide evidence that the language impairment in children with ALI and those with SLI may stem from different underlying cognitive mechanisms. One possible explanation is that language impairments in children with ASD are secondary to social communication impairments or restricted behaviours and interests that define autism (e.g. Whitehouse et al. 2007). However, the evidence here for this model is weak, with two recent studies finding no significant relationships between language impairment and severity of autistic symptoms (Loucas et al. 2008; Lindgren et al. 2009). Findings that autistic symptoms emerge in individuals with SLI over time have also been used to argue for aetiological overlap. However, some have argued that this could be explained by diagnostic substitution, where broadening diagnostic boundaries have resulted in individuals who were previously diagnosed with SLI meeting current diagnostic criteria for ASD (Bishop et al. 2008).

There are some discrepancies within the literature relating to whether similar neurological abnormalities underpin ASD and SLI. Several studies have reported shared characteristics of brain morphology in ASD and SLI (e.g. Herbert et al. 2004; De Fossé et al. 2004), which appear to be driven by similarities between ALI and SLI. Other functional imaging studies show contrasting patterns of cerebral lateralisation for language function in these conditions (Whitehouse & Bishop 2008b). Overall, there are indications that atypical language in ASD and SLI may have a common basis in structural and functional anomalies. However, research has not yet isolated specific neurological characteristics that are shared between ASD and SLI.

Results of several family studies show that subtle signs and cognitive markers for ASD and SLI are restricted primarily to the relatives of individuals with that particular disorder, and do not extend to relatives of the alternative disorder

(Lindgren et al. 2009; Whitehouse et al. 2007). However, there are contrasting reports showing an elevated risk of a clinical diagnosis of SLI in family members of ASD probands (Bailey et al. 1998; Tomblin et al. 2003). Further, studies have started to identify similar genetic variants conferring risk for ASD and SLI (Alarcón et al. 2008; Arking et al. 2008; Bakkaloglu et al. 2008; Poot et al. 2010; Vernes et al. 2008).

The current literature may be more consistent with an 'aetiological fractionation' account of ASD and SLI, whereby ASD is considered to involve multiple underlying impairments, each with one or more independent causes (Bishop 2003; Happé & Ronald 2008). While some children may inherit one component of the autistic triad (i.e. impaired social skills), other children will inherit the full constellation of autistic symptoms and thus present with the 'syndrome' of ASD. It is then possible that a risk factor for structural language impairments is also inherited by some children with ASD, resulting in ASD with associated language difficulties (Loucas et al. 2008; Ronald, Happé & Plomin 2005).

Future research should address the potential behavioural and genetic 'fractionation' of the autistic triad of impairments in relatives of children with ASD and also relatives of children with SLI. By comparing the performance of these two groups of relatives on heritable markers for SLI (e.g. nonword repetition) and aspects of the broader ASD phenotype (e.g. impaired social communication), we would be able to identify the extent to which these traits 'splinter' in these relatives. Evidence supporting aetiological fractionation would come from studies finding that (a) relatives of children with SLI show no raised incidence of the broader ASD phenotype when compared to relatives of TD children (but still show some evidence of structural language problems), whereas (b) relatives of children with ASD show the opposite, that is, elevated rates of the broader ASD phenotype compared to relatives of TD children, and no evidence of structural language difficulties.

Final remarks

Considerable research has sought to elucidate the phenotypic and aetiological relationship between ASD and SLI. While there are some linguistic similarities between individuals with ASD and SLI, it is unclear whether these represent a common aetiology. Future research efforts should be directed towards evaluating the independence of the two disorders through considering whether broader autism phenotype traits are significantly elevated in relatives of children with SLI and whether structural language difficulties are more prevalent in relatives of children with ASD. Advances in neurological and molecular genetic research may also isolate specific neurobiological and genetic markers of each of the conditions, thus elucidating potential shared aetiologies. Such investigations are important clinically, to improve assessment and diagnostic practices, and theoretically, to enhance understanding of the aetiology of these complex conditions.

References

Abrahams, B.S., Tentler, D., Perederiy, J.V., Oldham, M.C., & Geschwind, D.H. (2007). Genome-wide analyses of human perisylvian cerebral cortical patterning. *Proceedings of the National Academy of Sciences in the United States of America, 104*, 17849–17854.

Aguilar-Mediavilla., E., Sanz-Torrent, M., & Serra-Raventos, M. (2002). A comparative study of the phonology of pre-school children with specific language impairment (SLI), language delay (LD) and normal acquisition. *Clinical Linguistics and Phonetics, 16*, 573–596.

Alarcón, M., Abrahams, B.S., Stone, J.L., Duvall, J.A., Perederiy, J.V., Bomar, J., et al. (2008). Linkage, association, and gene-expression analyses identify CNTNAP2 as an autism susceptibility gene. *The American Journal of Human Genetics, 82*, 150–159.

Alarcón, M., Yonan, A., Gilliam, T., Cantor, R.M., & Geschwind, D.H. (2005). Quantitative genome scan and ordered-subtests analysis of autism endophenotypes support language QTLs. *Molecular Psychiatry, 10*, 747–757.

Arking, D.E., Cutler, D.J., Brune, C.W., Teslovich, T.M., West, K., Ikeda, M., et al. (2008). A common genetic variant in the neurexin superfamily member CNTNAP2 increases familial risk of autism. *The American Journal of Human Genetics, 82*, 160–164.

Badner, J.A., & Gershon, E.S. (2002). Regional meta-analysis of published data supports linkage of autism with markers on chromosome 7. *Molecular Psychiatry, 7*, 56–66.

Bailey, A., Le Couteur, A., Gottesman, I., Bolton, P., Siminoff, E., Yuzda, E., et al. (1995). Autism as a strongly genetic disorder: Evidence from a British twin study. *Psychological Medicine, 25*, 63–77.

Bailey, A., Palferman, S., Heavey, L., & Le Couteur, A. (1998). Autism: The phenotype in relatives. *Journal of Autism and Developmental Disorders, 28*(5), 369–389.

Bakkaloglu, B., O'Roak, B.J., Louvi, A., Gupta, A.R., Abelson, J.F., Morgan, T.M., et al. (2008). Molecular cytogenetic andaysis and resequencing of Contactin Associated Protein-Like 2 in autism spectrum disorders. *The American Journal of Human Genetics, 82*, 165–173.

Baltaxe, C.A.M. (1977). Pragmatic deficits in the language of autistic adolescents. *Journal of Pediatric Psychology, 2*, 176–180.

Barrett, S., Beck, J.C., Bernier, R., Bisson, E., Braun, T.A., Casavant, T.L., et al. (1999). An autosomal genomic screen for autism collaborative linkage study of autism. *American Journal of Medical Genetics, 88*, 609–615.

Barry, J.G., Yasin, I., & Bishop, D.V.M. (2007). Heritable risk factors associated with language impairments. *Genes, Brain and Behavior, 6*, 66–76.

Bartak, L., Rutter, M., & Cox, A. (1975). A comparative study of infantile autism and specific developmental receptive language disorder, I: The children. *British Journal of Psychiatry, 126*, 127–145.

Bartolucci, G., & Pierce, S.S. (1977). A preliminary comparison of phonological development in autistic, normal, and mentally retarded subjects. *International Journal of Language and Communication Disorders, 12*, 137–147.

Bartolucci, G., Pierce, S.S., Streiner, D., & Eppel, P.T. (1976). Phonological investigation of verbal autistic and mentally retarded subjects. *Journal of Autism and Child Schizophrenia, 6,* 303–316.

Bartolucci, G., Pierce, S.S., Streiner, D. (1980). Cross-sectional studies of grammatical morphemes in autistic and mentally retarded children. *Journal of Autism and Developmental Disorders, 10,* 39–50.

Bedore, L.M, & Leonard, L.B. (1998). Specific language impairment and grammatical morphology: a discriminant function analysis. *Journal of Speech, Language, and Hearing Research, 41,* 1185–1192.

Binder, J.R., Frost, J.A., Hammeke, T.A., Cox, R.W., Rao, S.M., & Prieto, T. (1997). Human brain language areas identified by functional magnetic resonance imaging. *The Journal of Neuroscience, 17,* 353–362.

Bishop, D.V.M. (1998). Development of the Children's Communication Checklist (CCC): A method for assessing qualitative aspects of communicative impairment in children. *Journal of Child Psychology and Psychiatry, 39*(6), 879–891.

Bishop, D.V.M. (1994). Grammatical errors in specific language impairment: Competence or performance limitations? *Applied Psycholinguistics, 15,* 507–550.

Bishop, D.V.M. (2003). Autism and specific language impairment: Categorical distinction or continuum. *Autism: Neural Basis and Treatment Possibilities* (pp. 213–234). Chichester: Wiley.

Bishop, D.V.M., & Adams, C. (1990). A prospective study of the relationship between specific language impairment, phonological disorders and reading retardation. *Journal of Child Psychology and Psychiatry, 31,* 1027–1050.

Bishop, D.V.M., & Baird, G. (2001). Parent and teacher report of pragmatic aspects of communication: Use of the Children's Communication Checklist in a clinical setting. *Developmental Medicine and Child Neurology, 43,* 809–818.

Bishop, D.V.M., Maybery, M., Maley, A., Wong, D., Hill, W., & Hallmayer, J. (2004). Using self-report to identify the broad phenotype in parents of children with autism spectrum disorders: a study using the Autism Spectrum Quotient. *Journal of Child Psychology and Psychiatry, 45*(8), 1431–1436.

Bishop, D.V.M., & Norbury, C.F. (2002). Exploring the borderlands of autistic disorder and specific language impairment: a study using standardised diagnostic instruments. *Journal of Child Psychology and Psychiatry, 43*(7), 917–929.

Bishop, D.V.M., North, T., & Donlan, C. (1996). Nonword repetition as a behavioural marker for inherited language impairment: evidence from a twin study. *Journal of Child Psychology and Psychiatry, 37*(4), 391–403.

Bishop, D.V.M., Whitehouse, A.J.O., Watt, H.J., & Line, E.A. (2008). Autism and diagnostic substitution: Evidence from a study of adults with a history of developmental language disorder. *Developmental Medicine and Child Neurology, 50,* 341–345.

Bolton, P.F., MacDonald, H., Pickles, A., Rios, P., Goode, S., Crowson, M., et al. (1994). A case-control family history study of autism. *Journal of Child Psychology and Psychiatry, 35*(5), 877–900.

Bortolini, U. & Leonard, L.B. (2000). Phonology and children with specific language impairment: Status of structural constraints in two languages. *Journal of Communication Disorders, 33,* 131–150.

Botting, N. (2002). Narrative as a tool for the assessment of linguistic and pragmatic impairments. *Child Language Teaching and Therapy, 18,* 1–21.

Botting, N., & Conti-Ramsden, G. (2003). Autism, primary pragmatic difficulties, and specific language impairment: can we distinguish them using psycholinguistic markers? *Developmental Medicine and Child Neurology, 45,* 515–524.

Boucher, J. (1976). Articulation in early childhood autism. *Journal of Autism and Childhood Schizophrenia, 6,* 297–302.

Boucher, J. (2003). Language development in autism. *International Congress Series, 1254,* 247–253.

Bradford, Y., Haines, J., Hutcheson, H., Gardiner, M., Braun, T., et al. (2001). Incorporating language phenotypes strengthens evidence of linkage to autism. *American Journal of Medical Genetics, 105,* 539–547.

Briscoe, J., Bishop, D.V.M., & Norbury, C.F. (2001). Phonological processing, language, and literach: A comparison of children with mild-to-moderate sensorineural hearing loss and those with specific language impairment. *Journal of Child Psychology and Psychiatry, 42,* 329–340.

Cantwell, D., Baker, L., & Rutter, M. (1978). A comparative study of infantile autism and specific developmental receptive languge disorder – IV. Analysis of syntax and language function. *Journal of Child Psychology and Psychiatry, 19,* 351–362.

Capps, L., Losh, M., & Thurber, C. (2000). "The Frog ate the Bug and Made His Mouth Sad": Narrative competence in children with autism. *Journal of Abnormal Child Psychology, 28,* 193–204.

Clegg, J., Hollis, C., Mawhood, L., & Ruttern M. (2005). Developmental langauge disorders – a follow-up in later adult life. Cognitive, language and psychosocial outcomes. *Journal of Child Psychology and Psychiatry, 46,* 128–149.

Cleland, J., Gibbon, F.E., Peppé, S.J.E., O'Hare, A., & Rutherford, M. (2010). Phonetic and phonological errors in children with high functioning autism and Asperger Syndrome. *International Journal of Speech-Language Pathology, 12,* 69–76.

Collaborative Linkage Study of Autism. (1999). An autosomal genomic screen for autism. *American Journal of Medical Genetics, 88,* 609–615.

Conti-Ramsden, G., Botting, N., & Faragher, B. (2001). Psycholinguistic markers for specific language impairment. *Journal of Child Psychology and Psychiatry, 42*(6), 741–748.

Conti-Ramsden, G., & Crutchley, A. (1997). The extent to which psychometric tests differentiate subgroups of children with SLI. *Journal of Speech, Language and Hearing Research, 40,* 765–777.

De Fossé, L., Hodge, S.M., Makris, N., Kennedy, D.N., Caviness, V.S., McGrath, L., et al. (2004). Language-association cortex asymmetry in autism and specific language impairment. *Annals of Neurology, 56,* 757–766.

Dworzynski, K., Ronald, A., Hayiou-Thomas, M., McEwan, F., Happé, F., Bolton, P.F., et al. (2008). Developmental path between language and autistic-like impairments: A twin study. *Infant and Child Development, 17,* 121–136.

Dworzynski, K., Ronald, A., Hayiou-Thomas, M., Rijsdijk, F., Happé, F., Bolton, P.F., et al. (2007). Aetiological relationship between language performance and autistic-like traits in childhood: a twin study. *International Journal of Language & Communication Disorders, 42*(3), 273–292.

Eales, M.J. (1993). Pragmatic impairments in adults with childhood diagnoses of autism or developmental receptive language disorder. *Journal of Autism and Developmental Disorders, 23,* 593–617.

Eigsti, I.M., Bennetto, L., & Dadlani, M.B. (2007). Beyond pragmatics: Morphosyntactic development in autism. *Journal of Autism and Developmental Disorders, 37*, 1007–1023.

Eisenmajer, R., Prior, M., Leekam, S., Wing, L., Ong, B., Gould, J., et al. (1998). Delayed language onset as a predictor of clinical symptoms in pervasive developmental disorders. *Journal of Autism and Developmental Disorders, 28*, 527–533.

Fine, J., Bartolucci, G., Ginsberg, G., & Szatmari, P. (1991). The use of intonation to communicate in pervasive developmental disorders. *Journal of Child Psychology and Psychiatry, 32*, 771–782.

Fisher, S.E., & Scharff, C. (2009). FOXP2 as a molecular window into speech and language. *Trends in Genetics, 25*, 166–177.

Flagg, E.J., Cardy, J.E.O., Roberts, W., & Roberts, T.P.L. (2005). Language lateralisation development in children with autism: Insights from the late field magnetoencephalogram. *Neuroscience Letters, 386*, 82–87.

Folstein, S., & Rosen-Sheidley, B. (2001). Genetics of autism: complex aetiology for a heterogeneous disorder. *Nature, 2*, 943–955.

Folstein, S., & Rutter, M. (1977a). Genetic influences and infantile autism. *Nature, 265*, 726–728.

Folstein, S., & Rutter, M. (1977b). Infantile autism: a genetic study of 21 twin pairs. *Journal of Child Psychology and Psychiatry, 18*, 297–321.

Gathercole, S.E., & Baddeley, A. (1990). Phonological memory deficits in language disordered children: is there are causal connection? *Journal of Memory and Language, 29*, 336–360.

Gathercole, S.E., Willis, C.S., Baddeley, A., & Emslie, H. (1994). The children's test of nonword repetition: A test of phonological working memory. *Memory, 2*(2), 103–127.

Gauger, L.M., Lombardino, L.J., & Leonard, C.M. (1997). Brain morphology in children with specific language impairment. *Journal of Speech, Language and Hearing Research, 40*, 1272–1284.

Goldman, R., & Fristoe, M. (2000). *Goldman Fristoe 2 Test of Articulation*. Circle Pines, MN: American Guidance Service.

Happé, F., & Ronald, A. (2008). The 'fractionable autism triad': A review of evidence from behavioural, genetic, cognitive and neural research. *Neuropsychology Review, 18*, 287–304.

Herbert, M.R., Harris, G.J., Adrien, K.T., Ziegler, D.A., Makris, N., Kennedy, D.N., et al. (2002). Abnormal asymmetry in language association cortex in autism. *Annals of Neurology, 52*, 588–596.

Herbert, M.R., Ziegler, D.A., Deutsch, C.K., O'Brien, L.M., Kennedy, D.N., Filipek, P.A., et al. (2004). Brain asymmetries in autism and developmental language disorder: A nested whole-brain analysis. *Brain, 123*, 213–226.

Herbert, M.R., Ziegler, D.A., Deutsch, C.K., O'Brien, L.M., Kennedy, D.N., Filipek, P.A., et al. (2005). Brain asymmetries in autism and developmental language disorder: A nested whole-brain analysis. *Brain, 123*, 213–226.

Herbert, M.R., Ziegler, D.A., Deutsch, C.K., O'Brien, L.M., Lange, N., Bakardjiev, A., et al. (2003). Dissociations of cerebral cortex, subcortical and cerebral white matter volumes in autistic boys. *Brain, 126*, 1182–1192.

Herbert, M.R., Ziegler, D.A., Makris, N., Bakardjiev, A., Hodgson, J., Adiren, K.T., et al. (2003). Larger brain and white matter volumes in children with developmental language disorder. *Developmental Science, 6*, F11–F22.

Hewitt L.E., Hammer C.S., Yont K.M., Tomblin J.B. (2005). Language sampling for kindergarten children with and without SLI: mean length of utterance, IPSYN, and NDW. *Journal of Communication Disorders, 38*, 197–213.

Howlin, P., Mawhood, L., & Rutter, M. (2000). Autism and developmental receptive language disorder – a follow-up comparison in early adult life, II: Social, behavioural, and psychiatric outcomes. *Journal of Child Psychology and Psychiatry, 41*(5), 561–578.

Hugdahl, K., Gunderson, H., Brekke, C., Thomsen, T., Rimol, L.M., Ersland, L., et al. (2004). fMRI brain activation in a Finnish family with specific language impairment compared with a normal control group. *Journal of Speech, Language and Hearing Research, 47*, 162–172.

International Molecular Genetic Study of Autism Consortium. 1998. A full genome screen for autism with evidence for linkage to a region on chromosome 7q. *Human Molecular Genetics, 7*, 571–578.

Johnston, J.R., & Kahmi, A.G. (1984). Syntactic and semantic aspects of the utterances of language-impaired children: the same can be less. *Merrill-Palmer Quarterly, 30*, 65–86.

Kjelgaard, M.M., & Tager-Flusberg, H. (2001). An investigation of language impairment in autism: implications for genetic subgroups. *Language and Cognitive Processes, 16*(2/3), 287–308.

Kleinhans, N.M., Müller, R.-A., Cohen, D., & Courchesne, E. (2008). Atypical functional lateralisation of language in autism spectrum disorders. *Brain Research, 1221*, 115–125.

Knaus, T.A., Silver, A.M., Kennedy, M., Lindgren, K.A., Dominick, K.C., Siegel, J., et al. (2010). Language laterality in autism spectrum disorder and typical controls: A functional, colummetric, and diffusion tensor MRI study. *Brain and Language, 112*, 113–120.

Knecht, S., Deppe, M., Dräger, B., Bobe, L., Lohmann, H., Ringelsten, E.-B., et al. (2000). Language lateralization in healthy right-handers. *Brain, 123*, 74–81.

Knecht, S., Deppe, M., Ebner, A., Henningson, H., Huber, T., Jokeit, H., et al. (1998). Noninvasive determination of language lateralization by functional transcranial doppler sonography. *Stroke, 29*, 82–86.

Knecht, S., Dräger, B., Deppe, M., Bobe, L., Lohmann, H., Flöel, A., et al. (2000). Handedness and hemispheric language dominance in healthy humans. *Brain, 123*, 2512–2518.

Lai, C.S.L., Fisher, S.E., Hurst, J.A., Vargha-Khadem, F., & Monaco, A.P. (2001). A forkhead-domain gene is mutated in a severe speech and language disorder. *Nature, 413*, 519–523.

Leonard, L.B. (1982). Phonological deficits in children with developmental language impairment. *Brain and Language, 16*, 73–86.

Lewis, F.M., Murdoch, B.E., & Woodyatt, G.C. (2007). Linguistic abilities in children with autism spectrum disorder. *Research in Autism Spectrum Disorders, 1*, 85–100.

Lewis, F.M., Woodyatt, G.C., & Murdoch, B.E. (2008). Linguistic and pragmatic language skills in adults with autism spectrum disorder: A pilot study. *Research in Autism Spectrum Disorders, 2*, 176–187.

Leyfer, O.T., Tager-Flusberg, H., Dowd, M., Tomblin, J.B., & Folstein, S. (2008). Overlap between autism and specific language impairment: comparison of Autism Diagnostic Interview and Autism Diagnostic Observation Schedule scores. *Autism Research, 1*, 284–296.

Lindgren, K.A., Folstein, S., Tomblin, J.B., & Tager-Flusberg, H. (2009). Language and reading abilities of children with autism spectrum disorders and specific language impairment and their first-degree relatives. *Autism Research, 2*, 22–38.

Lloyd, H., Paintin, K., & Botting, N. (2006). Performance of children with different types of communication impairment on the Clinical Evaluation of Language Fundamentals (CELF). *Child Language Teaching and Therapy, 22*(1), 47–67.

Loucas, T., Charman, T., Pickles, A., Siminoff, E., Chandler, S., Meldrum, D., et al. (2008). Autistic symptomatology and language ability in autism spectrum disorder and specific language impairment. *Journal of Child Psychology and Psychiatry, 49*(11), 1184–1192.

Loucas, T., Riches, N.G., Charman, T., Pickles, A., Siminoff, E., Chandler, S., et al. (2010). Speech perception and phonological short-term memory capacity in language impairment: Preliminary evidence from adolescents with specific language impairment (SLI) and autism spectrum disorders (ASD). *International Journal of Language & Communication Disorders, 45*(3), 275–286.

MacDermot, K.D., Bonora, E., Sykes, N., Coupe, A.-M., Lai, C.S.L., Vernes, S.C., et al. (2005). Identification of FOXP2 truncation as a novel cause of developmental speech and language deficits. *The American Journal of Human Genetics, 76*, 1074–1080.

Mawhood, L., Howlin, P., & Rutter, M. (2000). Autism and developmental receptive language disorder – a comparative follow-up in early adult life, I: Cognitive and langauge outcomes. *Journal of Child Psychology and Psychiatry, 41*(5), 547–559.

McCann, J., Peppé, S., Gibbon, F.E., O'Hare, A., & Rutherford, M. (2007). Prosody and its relationship to language in school-aged children with high functioning autism. *International Journal of Language and Communication Disorders, 42*, 682–702.

Monaco, A.P., & The SLI Consortium. (2007). Multivariate linkage analysis of specific language impairment. *Annals of Human Genetics, 71*, 1–14.

Norbury, C.F. (2005). Barking up the wrong tree? Lexical ambiguity resolution in children with language impairments and autistic spectrum disorders. *Journal of Experimental Child Psychology, 90*, 142–171.

Norbury, C.F., & Bishop, D.V.M. (2002). Inferential processing and story recall in children with communicaiton problems: a comparison of specific language impairment, pragmatic language impairment and high-functioning autism. *International Journal of Language and Communication Disorders, 37*, 227–251.

Norbury, C.F., & Bishop, D.V.M. (2003). Narrative skills of children with communication impairments. *International Journal of Language and Communication Disorders, 38*, 287–313.

Norbury, C.F., Nash, M., Baird, G., & Bishop, D.V.M. (2004). Using a parental checklist to identify diagnostic groups in children with communication impairment: a validation of the Children's Commuication Checklist-2. *International Journal of Language and Communication Disorders, 39*, 345–364.

O'Brien, E.K., Zhang, X., Nishimura, C., Tomblin, J.B., & Murray, J.C. (2003). Association of specific language impairment to the region of 7q31. *The American Journal of Human Genetics, 72*, 1536–1543.

Ojemann, G.A. (1991). Cortical organization of language. *The Journal of Neuroscience, 11*, 2281–2287.

Orsolini, M., Sechi, E., Maronato, C., Bonvino, E. & Corcelli, A. (2001). Nature of phonological delay in children with specific language impairment. *International Journal of Language and Communication Disorders, 36*, 63–90.

Pendergast, K., Dickey, S.E., Selmar, J.W., & Soder, A.L. (1984). *Photo Articulation Test*. Chicago, IL: Stoelting.

Peppé, S., McCann, J., Gibbon, F.E., O'Hare, A., & Rutherford, M. (2007). Receptive and expressive prosodic ability in children with high-functioning autism. *Journal of Speech, Language and Hearing Research, 50*, 1015–1028.

Philippe, A., Martinez, M., Guilloud-Bataille, M., Gillberg, C., Råstam, M., et al. (1999). Genome-wide scan for autism susceptibility genes. *Human Molecular Genetics, 8*, 805–812.

Philofsky, A., Fidler, D.J., & Hepburn, S. (2007). Pragmatic language profiles of school-age children with autism spectrum disorders and Williams Syndrome. *American Journal of Speech-Language Pathology, 16*, 368–380.

Pierce, S., & Bartolucci, G. (1977). A syntactic investigation of verbal autistic, mentally retarded, and normal children. *Journal of Autism and Childhood Schizophrenia, 7*(2), 121–133.

Pilowsky, T., Yirmiya, N., Shalev, R.S., & Gross-Tsur, V. (2003). Language abilities of siblings of children with autism. *Journal of Child Psychology and Psychiatry, 44*(6), 914–925.

Plante, E., Swisher, L., Vance, R., & Rapcsak, S. (1991). MRI findings in boys with specific language impairment. *Brain and Language, 41*, 52–66.

Poot, M., Beyer, V., Schwaab, I., Damatova, N., van't Slot, R., Prothero, J., et al. (2010). Disruption of CNTNAP2 and additional structural genome changes in a boy with speech delay and autism spectrum disorder. *Neurogenetics, 11*, 81–89.

Ramberg, C., Ehlers, S., Nydén, A., Johansson, M., & Gillberg, C. (1996). Language and pragmatic functions in school-age children on the autism spectrum. *European Journal of Disorders of Communication, 31*, 387–414.

Rapin, I., & Allen, D.A. (1983). Developmental language disorders: nosologic considerations. In U. Kirk (Ed.), *Neuropsychology of Language, Reading, and Spelling*. New York, NY: Academic Press.

Rapin, I., & Dunn, M. (2003). Update on the language disorders of individuals on the autistic spectrum. *Brain and Development, 25*, 166–172.

Rapin, I., Dunn, M., Allen, D.A., Stevens, M.C., & Fein, D. (2009). Subtypes of language disorders in school-age children with autism. *Developmental Neuropsychology, 34*(1), 66–84.

Redcay, E., & Courchesne, E. (2008). Deviant functional magnetic resonance imaging patterns of brain activity to speech in 2-3-year-old children with autism spectrum disorder. *Biological Psychiatry, 64*, 589–598.

Rice, C. (2009). Prevalence of autism spectrum disorders – Autism and developmental disabilities monitoring network. *Morbidity and Mortality Weekly Report, 58*(SS-10), 1–20.

Rice, M.L. (1997). Specific language impairments: In search of diagnostic markers and genetic contributions. *Mental Retardation and Developmental Disabilities Research Reviews, 3*, 350–357.

Rice, M.L., & Wexler, K. (1996). Toward tense as a clinical marker of specific language impairment in English-speaking children. *Journal of Speech and Hearing Research, 39*, 1239–1257.

Riches, N.G., Loucas, T., Baird, G., Charman, T., & Siminoff, E. (2010). Sentence repetition in adolescents with specific language impairments and autism: an investigation of complex syntax. *International Journal of Language & Communication Disorders, 45*(1), 47–60.

Riches, N.G., Loucas, T., Baird, G., Charman, T., & Simonoff, E. (2011). Non-word repetition in adolescents with specific language impairment and autism plus language impairments; a qualitative analysis. *Journal of Communication Disorders, 44*, 23–36.

Roberts, J.A., Rice, M.L., & Tager-Flusberg, H. (2004). Tense marking in children with autism. *Applied Psycholinguistics, 25*, 429–448.

Ronald, A., Happé, F., & Plomin, R. (2005). The genetic relationship between individual differences in social and nonsocial behaviours characteristic of autism. *Developmental Science, 8*(5), 444–458.

Ruser, T.F., Arin, D., Dowd, M., Putnam, S., Winklosky, B., Rosen-Sheidley, B., et al. (2007). Communicative competence in parents of children with autism and parents of children with specific language impairment. *Journal of Autism and Developmental Disorders, 37*, 1323–1336.

Rutter, M. (2000). Genetic studies of autism: From the 1970s into the millenium. *Journal of Abnormal Child Psychology, 28*(1), 3–14.

Shafer, V.L., Schwartz, R.G., Morr, M.L., Kessler, K.L., & Kurtzberg, D. (2000). Deviant neurophysiological asymmetry in children with language impairment. *NeuroReport, 11*, 3715–3718.

Shriberg, L.D., Paul, R., McSweeny, J.L., Klin, A., Cohen, D.J., & Volkmar, F.R. (2001). Speech and prosody characteristics of adolescents and adults with high functioning autism and asperger syndrome. *Journal of Speech, Language and Hearing Research, 44*, 1097–1115.

Tager-Flusberg, H. (1995). 'Once upon a ribbit': Stories narrated by autistic children. *British Journal of Developmental Psychology, 13*, 45–59.

Tager-Flusberg, H. (1996). Brief Report: Current theory and research on language and communication in autism. *Journal of Autism and Developmental Disorders, 26*(2), 169–172.

Tager-Flusberg, H. (2006). Defining language phenotypes in autism. *Clinical Neuroscience Research, 6*, 219–224.

Tager-Flusberg, H., & Joseph, R.M. (2003). Identifying neurocognitive phenotypes in autism. *Philosophical Transactions of the Royal Society of London B, 358*, 303–314.

The Autism Genome Project Consortium. (2007). Mapping autism risk loci using genetic linkage and chromosomal rearrangements. *Nature Genetics, 39*, 319–328.

The SLI Consortium. (2002). A genomewide scan identifies two novel loci involved in specific language impairment. *The American Journal of Human Genetics, 70*, 384–398.

Tomblin, J.B., Hafeman, L.L., & O'Brien, M. (2003). Autism and autism risk on siblings of children with specific language impairment. *International Journal of Language & Communication Disorders, 38*(3), 235–250.

Tuchman, R.F., Rapin, I., & Shinnar, S. (1991). Autistic and dysphasic children, I: Clinical characteristics. *Pediatrics, 88*, 1211–1218.

Vernes, S.C., Newbury, D.F., Abrahams, B.S., Winchester, L., Nicod, J., Groszer, M., et al. (2008). A functional genetic link between distinct developmental language disorders. *The New England Journal of Medicine, 359*, 2337–2345.

Waterhouse, L., & Fein, D. (1982). Language skills in developmentally disabled children. *Brain and Language, 15*, 307–333.

Whitehouse, A.J.O., Barry, J.G., & Bishop, D.V.M. (2007). The broader language phenotype of autism: A comparison with specific language impairment. *Journal of Child Psychology and Psychiatry, 48*(8), 822–830.

Whitehouse, A.J.O., Barry, J.G., & Bishop, D.V.M. (2008a). Further defining the language impairment of autism: Is there a specific language impairment subtype? *Journal of Communication Disorders, 41*, 319–336.

Whitehouse, A.J.O., & Bishop, D.V.M. (2008b). Cerebral dominance for language function in adults with specific language impairment and autism. *Brain, 131*, 3193–3200.

Whitehouse, A.J.O., Bishop, D.V.M., Ang, Q.W., Pennell, C.E., & Fisher, S.E. (2011). CNTNAP2 variants affect early language development in the general population. *Genes, Brain and Behavior, 10*, 451–456.

Whitehouse, A.J.O., Coon, H., Miller, J., Salisbury, B., & Bishop, D.V.M. (2010). Narrowing the broader autism phenotype: A study using the Communication Checklist – Adult (CC-A). *Autism, 14*, 559–574.

Wiig, E.H., Secord, W.A., & Semel, E. (1992). *Clinical Evaluation of Language Fundamentals-Preschool.* San Diego, CA: The Psychological Corporation.

Williams, D., Botting, N., & Boucher, J. (2008). Language in autism and specific language impairment: where are the links? *Psychological Bulletin, 134*(6), 944–963.

Young, E.C., Diehl, J.J., Morris, D., Hyman, S.L., & Bennetto, L. (2005). The use of two language tests to identify pragmatic language problems in children with autism spectrum disorders. *Language, Speech, and Hearing Services in Schools, 36*, 62–72.

CHAPTER 5

Prosody and autism

Joanne Arciuli
University of Sydney

This chapter focuses on prosodic processing in individuals with autism spectrum disorders (ASD). An overview of key studies linking prosodic difficulties with ASD is provided. Methods reviewed include behavioural assessment, acoustic analyses, electrophysiological measures, and brain imaging. It is difficult to draw strong conclusions from previous research as there has been little consistency across studies in terms of the types of prosody that were examined, whether or not both comprehension and production of prosody were investigated, and the nature and size of the samples that were assessed. There is consensus that only some individuals with ASD experience problems with prosody. Importantly, different types of prosodic impairment have been observed across individuals with ASD and it seems likely that these are associated with different causal mechanisms. Some possible mechanisms underpinning prosodic impairment that have been put forward over the years include a cognitive deficit relating to Theory of Mind, motor speech impairment, lack of social motivation to align one's speech with others, atypical audio-vocal regulation, and deficient pitch encoding. Future research endeavours should include increased effort to pinpoint causal mechanisms and explore targeted remediation of prosodic difficulties in individuals with ASD.

Prosody plays a pivotal role in human interaction. All of the world's languages exhibit some kind of prosody, which operates across a range of linguistic and affective domains. Difficulty with prosodic processing is not an obscure phenomenon; it has been reported in apraxia of speech, hearing impairment, Parkinson's disease, aphasia, Down syndrome, esophageal speakers, and second language learning (e.g. those learning English). Yet, prosody has been described as the Cinderella of speech science remaining "in the cellar, with few visitors" (Crystal 2009: p. 257). Indeed, in comparison with other aspects of speech and language, research on prosody has only relatively recently begun to gain momentum.

This chapter focuses on prosodic processing in individuals with autism spectrum disorders (ASD). Aberrant prosody has long been associated with ASD, having been noted in the very earliest descriptions of the autistic syndrome (Kanner 1943). Broad descriptions of expressive prosody have included: "monotonic, sing-song-like, robotic, parroted, machine-like, odd, over-exaggerated, and/or stilted" (Jarvinen-Pasley, Peppé, King-Smith & Heaton 2008: p. 1328). Of the 70–80% of those with ASD that have functional spoken language (Rogers 2006), around half may demonstrate difficulties with prosody (Paul, Shriberg, McSweeney, Cicchetti, Klin & Volkmar 2005; Shriberg, Paul, McSweeny, Klin, Cohen & Volkmar 2001; Simmons & Baltaxe 1975). Prosodic atypicalities have been reported at all levels of ability in ASD, including high-functioning autism (Peppé, McCann, Gibbon, O'Hare & Rutherford 2007; Shriberg et al. 2001). The nature and degree of abnormal prosody appears to be variable across individuals. Interestingly, abnormal prosody is one of the earliest characteristics to appear (Paul, Fuerst, Ramsay, Chawarska & Klin 2011; Wetherby et al. 2004) and often persists in the face of improvements in other aspects of language function (e.g. DeMeyer et al. 1973; Simmons & Baltaxe 1975).

Most research in this area has centred on English prosody. Accordingly, this chapter focuses on studies that have examined English. The chapter begins with a brief definition of prosody and explanation of its importance for communication. An overview of key studies linking prosodic difficulties with ASD is provided along with discussion of some of the mechanisms which may underpin prosodic difficulties in individuals with autism. Areas in need of future research are outlined.

What is prosody?

Prosody is an umbrella term for the "rhythmic, dynamic and melodic features of language" (Samuelsson, Plejert, Nettelbladt & Anward 2011: p. 46). Perceptual correlates of prosody include pitch, loudness, and duration. Acoustically, prosody is realised through relative variation in fundamental frequency (measured in Hz), amplitude (measured in dB) and duration (Lehiste 1970, amongst many others). Pausing, vowel quality and other features such as spectral balance and spectral tilt may also play a role depending upon the language and the type of prosody in question (e.g. Fear et al. 1995; Van Kuijk & Boves 1999). Prosody can operate in different ways; for instance, in terms of the relative prominence of adjacent units (e.g. syllables within single words), and in terms of changes over time (e.g. the intonation contour of a sentence).

In English, prosody is important at a number of levels. For example, the alternation of strong and weak syllables assists with the identification of word boundaries in continuous speech (e.g. Jusczyk, Houston & Newsome 1999). The alternation of strong and weak syllables *within* single words is known as lexical stress; consider the minimal pair 'INcense' (a noun) versus 'inCENSE' (a verb).

In each of these disyllabic words one syllable is more prominent than the other. In the word 'INcense' the first syllable is given prominence through higher pitch, increased loudness and/or longer duration relative to the second syllable; whereas, in the word 'inCENSE' the second syllable is given prominence relative to the first. Emphatic stress, also known as contrastive stress, provides semantic focus at the utterance level; for example, consider 'The BOY is playing cards' versus 'The boy is playing CARDS' (the words denoted by capital letters may be of higher pitch, increased loudness and/or longer duration). Prosody can help differentiate sentence types such as questions versus statements (e.g. through rising or falling pitch contours). It is often modified according to social function (e.g. higher pitch in child-directed speech). Emotional aspects of communication tend to be marked by prosody (e.g. indicating whether a speaker is happy or angry). Prosody can also be involved in conveying more complex meaning and mood, such as that associated with irony.

Why is prosody important?

Prosody plays an important role in human interactions for a number of reasons. It is clearly beneficial to be able to identify and produce affective prosody in a suitable way during communication. It has been argued that vocal expressions of emotion are akin to facial expressions of emotion in that they contain invariant features "which are universally exploited by speakers and can be decoded across languages irrespective of the linguistic ability and experience of the listener" (Pell, Monetta, Paulmann & Kotz 2009: p. 116). It is assumed that the authors made this statement with regard to typically developing individuals.

Certain types of prosody are important because they are "properly linguistic" (Wilson & Wharton 2006: p. 1559). It is thought that early sensitivity to prosody in typically developing infants has a central role in language acquisition (e.g. the prosodic bootstrapping hypothesis: Morgan & Demuth 1996). Typically developing infants prefer the prosodic patterns of their native language (e.g. Mehler, Jusczyk, Lambertz, Halsted, Bertoncinic & Amiel-Tilson 1988; Jusczyk, Cutler & Redanz 1993). Prosody is also important for comprehension. It has been shown that lexical stress plays a role in spoken word recognition on the part of the listener (Arciuli & Slowiaczek 2007; Arciuli & Cupples 2003, 2004; Cooper et al. 2002). Slowiaczek (1990) demonstrated that mis-stressing English words (e.g. 'resCUE') impedes spoken word recognition. Studies using sentences presented via synthesised speech have revealed that when fundamental frequency is manipulated (to reduce prosodic variation), intelligibility is compromised (Laures & Weismer 1999; Wingfield, Lombardi & Sokol 1984). Thus, a speaker is less likely to be intelligible if prosody is compromised. Klopfenstein's (2009) review of the interaction between prosody and intelligibility provides a helpful review of research in relation to special populations where prosody is affected.

Prosody is also important because listeners may make judgements about a speaker based on prosody. Paul, Shriberg, McSweeny, Cicchetti, Klin, and Volkmar (2005) revealed a relationship between prosody-voice scores and ratings of socialisation and communicative abilities for 30 participants with ASD. In their study of 40 participants with intellectual impairment, Shriberg and Widder (1990) found that prosody-voice scores were associated with measures of independent living.

Previous studies of prosodic processing in ASD

This section provides an overview of key studies in this area. It begins with discussion of some of the formal tools that have been used to assess prosody in ASD; namely, the Prosody-Voice Screening Profile (Shriberg, Kwiatkowski & Rasmussen 1990) and the Profiling Elements of Prosody in Speech-Communication (Peppé & McCann 2003). The review paper by McCann and Peppé (2003) and follow up comprehensive study of receptive and expressive prosody undertaken by Paul, Augustyn, Klin and Volkmar (2005) are outlined. This is followed by a discussion of acoustic studies of prosody in ASD. The section concludes with a brief overview of previous research that has investigated complex prosody in ASD and some research on the relationship between prosody and other aspects of language in ASD. The aim is not to provide a systematic review of every study undertaken in this area but, rather, to showcase the kinds of research questions and methods which have attracted interest.

Formal assessment of prosody

There are strikingly few instruments available for the assessment of prosody. In this regard, prosody research has been described as being "decades behind" compared with research into other aspects of speech and language (Diehl & Paul 2009: p. 287).

In one of the few studies to utilise a formal prosody assessment tool to assess conversational speech production, the Prosody-Voice Screening Profile (PVSP: Shriberg, Kwiatkowski & Rasmussen 1990), Shriberg et al. (2001) examined 3 groups of male participants: speakers with High-Functioning Autism (HFA), speakers with Asperger syndrome (AS), and typically developing speakers. There were 15 participants in each of the first two groups (a total of 30 participants with ASD) and 53 participants in the control group. Shriberg and colleagues found few prosody-related differences between the HFA and AS groups; however, these groups were found to differ from the control group in terms of stress placement. For the most part, atypical productions in the HFA and AS groups were associated with the utterance level (in this case, use of contrastive stress) rather than word level (i.e. use of lexical stress). The paper contained discussion of a variety of mechanisms that may underpin their finding of impaired prosody production in ASD including perceptual, motor, and pragmatic difficulties as well as resource demands in a limited-capacity system. The researchers appeared to favour a pragmatic explanation arguing that contrastive stress requires explicit attention to the listeners' needs and, in this sense, may represent a form of social cognition. However, it seems possible that underlying mechanisms may be interrelated especially as the study did not incorporate any tests designed to probe this array of subskills (e.g. perceptual, motor, pragmatic abilities) directly. The study included a broad sample of participants ranging in age from 10–50 years but did not include exploration of age-related effects.

Peppé and McCann (2003) developed the Profiling Elements of Prosody in Speech-Communication (PEPS-C) as a means of collecting data on various aspects of prosody. It contains 12 subtasks which can be used to obtain measures of expressive and receptive prosody. In their study of 31 individuals with high-functioning autism (mean age of 9 years and 10 months) and a significantly younger group of 72 typically developing peers (mean age of 6 years and 10 months) matched on verbal mental age, Peppé and colleagues (2007) found significant group differences on 7 out of the 12 subtasks of the PEPS-C. In every case individuals with autism performed less well that their typically developing peers, although differences were especially marked in subtasks involving affective prosody. It is important to note that the PEPS-C does not assess every type of prosody. For example, it does not assess perception or production of lexical stress, an important aspect of linguistic prosody, a limitation acknowledged by Peppé (2012).

The McCann and Peppé review

In their comprehensive review article McCann and Peppé (2003) discussed the 15 previous empirical studies that were published on the topic of prosody and ASD between 1980 and 2002 (listed in chronological order in Table 2 of their paper as: Paccia & Curcio 1982; Baltaxe 1984; Baltaxe et al. 1984; McCaleb & Prizant 1985; Baltaxe & Guthrie 1987; Frankel et al. 1987; Fine et al. 1991; Erwin et al. 1991; Thurber & Tager-Flusberg 1993; Local & Wootton 1996; Fosnot & Jun 1999; Paul et al. 2000; Shriberg et al. 2001; Wang et al. 2001; Rutherford et al. 2002). The small number of previous studies indicates that prosody in ASD has been an under-researched area when compared with other aspects of speech and language. In their review, McCann and Peppé confirmed a link between prosodic difficulties and ASD but were not able to draw any firm conclusions regarding the nature or cause of this link. In fact, their main conclusion was that findings from these studies varied greatly. The authors suggested that this variability may relate to differences concerning definitions of prosody, diagnosis of ASD, sample sizes, participant profiles, and investigative methods.

McCann and Peppé (2003) emphasised that none of the studies they reviewed had incorporated comprehensive assessment of both expressive and receptive abilities making it "impossible to investigate issues concerning the relationship between receptive and expressive abilities." (p. 348). Knowing whether or not there is a relationship between receptive and expressive prosody in (at least some) individuals with ASD is important because it can assist in delineating amongst various possible causes of impairment. McCann and Peppé (2003), themselves, touched briefly on the possibility that a cognitive deficit relating to Theory of Mind might play a role in prosodic impairment in ASD, especially in relation to ineffective comprehension of others' prosody (they referenced Baron-Cohen 1995). However, they did not explain how this account could accommodate the wide range of prosodic impairments (both receptive and expressive), and contradictory findings, outlined in their review.

In investigating a comprehensive range of prosodic functions including both receptive and expressive prosody (referred to as perception and production of prosody) and both linguistic and pragmatic/affective prosody, Paul, Augustyn, Klin and Volkmar (2005) directly addressed a key concern raised by the McCann and Peppé (2003) review. Paul et al. (2005) examined 27 individuals with ASD and 13 typically developing peers using a battery of 12 subtests. Subtests covered perception and production of both grammatical and pragmatic/affective prosody. The subtests were outlined in an Appendix (which, incidentally, is a helpful resource for readers who may not be fully aware of the array of prosodic functions in English). Unfortunately, many of the subtests may have been too easy for participants. Five of the 12 subtests showed mean performance at almost 100% correct for both the ASD group and the typically developing group. Neither of the group means fell below 70% on any subtest. There were some group differences on tests of grammatical production of stress (i.e. lexical stress: 'CONduct' versus 'conDUCT') and pragmatic/affective processing of stress (i.e. emphatic or contrastive stress: 'I prefer BLUE ties on gentlemen'). These findings are not in line with Shriberg et al.'s earlier study that suggested that only pragmatic aspects of prosody are impaired in ASD. The only subtests that revealed group differences across both perception and production were those relating to pragmatic/affective processing of stress.

One of the key points highlighted in McCann and Peppé (2003) review is that the majority of the studies that examined expressive prosody relied predominantly on perceptual judgements of speech production rather than acoustic analyses. This is also true of the Paul et al. (2005) study. McCann and Peppé (2003) emphasised that perceptual judgements are valuable in that they reflect listeners' interpretations; however, determining the acoustic components of prosody (e.g. the relative contribution of pitch, loudness and duration) in natural speech exceeds the capabilities of human hearing. Certainly, perceptual judgements can be used to correctly identify atypical prosody; for example, when contrastivity has not been achieved in the pronunciation of a word like 'INcense'. However, listeners are not able to produce precise statistics relating to the relative prominence of pitch, loudness and duration. Any attempt to do so would result in variability from one listener to the next. Thus, perceptual analyses, alone, cannot provide adequate detail concerning the nature of atypical prosody in individuals with ASD. A precise and reliable understanding of atypical prosody is invaluable for understanding causal mechanisms and for the design of effective interventions. The next section of this chapter provides an overview of acoustic analyses of prosody.

Acoustic analyses of expressive prosody

As stated in the McCann and Peppé review, acoustic analyses of prosody provide a level of detail, objectivity and reliability that is beyond the capabilities of human hearing. In addition, acoustic analyses provide a way of testing listener perceptions. For example, in response to the wide array of descriptors that have been applied to atypical prosody in ASD, it has been stated that "Prosody to which the terms 'exaggerated' and 'monotonous' can both be applied suggests either a confusion of terminology or different manifestations." (Peppé, Cleland, Gibbon, O'Hare & Martinez Castilla 2011: p. 43) To illustrate, in the case of contrastivity across syllables in a word like 'INcense', exaggerated prosody suggests excessive use of pitch, loudness or duration to achieve prominence of the strong first syllable; whereas the term monotonous suggests a lack of prominence that leaves the first and second syllables with equal stress.

Contrary to their expectations, Hubbard and Traumer (2007) found that a small sample of children and young adults with autism (6–21 years) did not display decreased pitch range when imitating neutral-content phrases modelled with various emotional intonation (happy, sad, angry) compared with typically developing peers; in fact, they displayed greater pitch range. This finding was also reported by Diehl and colleagues (2009) who elicited narrative retellings from 21 children with high-functioning autism and 21 typically developing peers. They measured average fundamental frequency from 250 ms speech segments across each participant's entire narrative. The authors raised the important point that acoustic analyses of pitch, in particular, ought to consider the influence of gender and age on pitch when recruiting their participants and matching across ability groups because females and children tend to exhibit higher overall pitch and more variation in fundamental frequency (Henton 1989; Whiteside & Hodgson 2000). Certainly, the above-mentioned acoustic studies suggest that descriptions of atypical prosody in autism as being monotonic may not be accurate (at least not for the participants tested in the studies outlined above).

Using a syllable imitation task (from the Tennessee Test of Rhythm and Intonation Patterns: T-TRIP, Koike & Asp 1981) Paul and colleagues (2008) found small significant group differences in terms of syllable duration across 46 ASD speakers and 20 typical speakers (age range 7–28 years). While there were significant differences in acoustic length of stressed versus unstressed syllables for both groups, this difference was greater in the TD group compared to the group comprised of individuals with ASD. Another study to report differences in duration examined 11 participants with high-functioning autism and 9 typical peers (ranging in age from 7–18 years). In this study, Grossman, Bemis, Plesa Skwerer and Tager-Flusberg (2010) reported that the autism group had longer overall word productions. In observing the word productions of their autism group they stated: "...we noticed that participants often produced exaggerated pauses between the syllables... in stark contrast to the recordings of the TD control participants, who produced effortless enunciations that subjectively appeared briefer, less laboured, and more fluid in their transitions between syllables." (p. 787) Similar to the findings of Grossman and colleagues, Diehl and Paul's (2012) recent acoustic study reported that duration of utterance was the only acoustic feature to reveal group differences between children and adolescents with ASD and typically developing peers (all participants aged 8–17 years). Acoustic measures that did not reveal significant group differences were those pertaining to intensity and fundamental frequency.

A study by Van Santen and colleagues (2010) used imitation and picture-description to examine the production of prosody (lexical stress, emphatic stress and focus) in children with high-functioning autism and typical peers aged 4–8 years. Their results indicated that differences between the expressive prosody of those with autism and their typically developing peers do not result from the way individual prosodic features are realised; rather, they reflect differences in the relative contribution of prosodic features. Specifically, they stated that "...the key distinction between the TD and ASD groups does not reside in the overall strength with which prosodic contrasts are expressed but in a different balance of the degrees to which durational features and pitch features are used to express stress." (p. 231).

Acoustic analyses, while invaluable in providing detail, objectivity and reliability concerning the nature of component features of prosody such as pitch and duration, are more limited when it comes to understanding complex prosody such as that associated with irony.

Complex prosody

While acoustic features are likely play a role in the processing of any kind of prosody, complex prosody is also linked with interpretation of context and mood, as well as social aspects of communication. Few studies of prosody in ASD have tackled the phenomenon of complex prosody. One area of growing interest is irony (for a cognitive account of irony see Pexman 2008). Several studies have suggested that individuals with autism have difficulties with irony (MacKay & Shaw 2004; Martin & McDonald 2004). Wang, Lee, Sigman and Dapretto (2006) used fMRI to explore irony. Participants listened to brief scenarios (e.g. "When Jen sees his [bad/nice] haircut, she says, 'You look great'!") and were asked to determine whether the speaker was using irony. Children with ASD (18 males aged between 7 and 16 years of age) performed above chance but were not as accurate as their typically developing peers (18 peers aged 8–15 years of age) when it came to explicitly interpreting ironic remarks. The ASD group showed increased activation within the same neurological network observed for the TD group, namely, in the right inferior frontal gyrus and bilateral temporal areas. The researchers conceded that in a more naturalistic setting differences between individuals with ASD and their typically developing peers may be more striking.

In their study of irony in children with autism and typically developing peers, Pexman, Rostad, McMorris, Climie, Stowkowy and Glenwright (2011) reduced task demands by removing the need for participants to respond verbally and by allowing forced-choice responding. Similar to the findings of Wang et al. (2006) they observed some competence in detecting irony in children with autism. In particular, children with autism were competent on speaker belief and intent measures but exhibited more difficulty interpreting speaker humour. Of course, it is very difficult to disentangle the effects of prosody from those associated with context and mood, and social motivation when it comes to investigations of irony.

The relationship between prosody and other linguistic skills

It is interesting to ponder whether there is a relationship between prosody and other language skills in ASD. McCann, Peppé, Gibbon, O'Hare & Rutherford (2007) examined 31 children with high-functioning autism (mean age of 9.45 years). Correlational analyses using a composite measure of receptive prosody obtained from the PEPS-C, showed that receptive prosody was associated with performance on tests of receptive vocabulary (r = .779), receptive grammar (r = .585), expressive language (r = .717), nonverbal ability (r = .502), and chronological age (r = .598) in children with autism. Analyses of expressive prosody obtained from the PEPS-C revealed relationships with receptive grammar (r = .507) and expressive language (r = .498) in the same children. There was no relationship between either type of prosody and pragmatic ability, as measured by the Children's Communication Checklist (CCC: Bishop 1998). There was also no relationship between either type of prosody and production of segmental phonology, as measured by a test of consonant production in single word (GFTA-2: Goldman & Fristoe 2000). These results may reflect a causal or perhaps a bidirectional link between prosody and some forms of language but this cannot be determined without additional research.

Summary

The studies reviewed here were undertaken with different purposes and methodologies. While the somewhat divergent results necessitate a range of additional studies, one key point has emerged. It is now very clear that prosody is not affected in all individuals with ASD. None of the above-mentioned studies pre-screened their participants to ensure that they were investigating individuals with ASD who had (some kind of) prosodic impairment. This is reasonable if the aim is to gain an estimate of the number of individuals with ASD who have problems with prosody and some idea about the nature of those impairments. However, continued general recruitment of persons with ASD, combined with the modest sample sizes inherent in this area of research, is unlikely to advance our understanding of *why* some individuals with ASD experience problems with prosody. Nevertheless, researchers have begun to investigate the kinds of mechanisms which may underpin prosodic impairment in some individuals with ASD.

Possible mechanisms underpinning prosodic difficulties in ASD

Research addressing the underpinnings of prosodic impairment in ASD is in its infancy. Here, a brief overview of four possible mechanisms is provided: Theory of Mind deficits, motor speech impairments, atypical audio-vocal regulation, and deficient encoding of pitch. The overview is not intended as a comprehensive review of all the research that has been conducted into each of these mechanisms; rather, it is intended as a snapshot of some current research for each mechanism.

Theory of Mind deficits

It has been suggested that impaired Theory of Mind, which is considered by many to be a core feature of ASD, might be related to difficulties processing prosody, especially affective prosody and more complex types of prosody such as irony. Rutherford et al. (2002) used the term "Reading the mind in the voice" in the title of their study. They presented segments of speech (phrases and sentences) and asked participants to ascribe adjectives (correct versus foil) that pertained to basic emotions (e.g. 'joyous' versus 'scared'), social emotions (e.g. 'apologetic' versus 'hurried'), and speaker attitude (e.g. 'sarcastic' versus 'indifferent'). Their results showed that the Asperger/high-functioning-autism group had difficulty ascribing the correct adjectives when compared with controls.

Using a series of three experiments, each more cognitively demanding than the previous one, Chevallier, Noveck, Happe and Wilson (2011) challenged these findings. Their results indicated that both typically developing adolescents and those with ASD are capable of reading the mind in the voice even though the ASD group showed slower processing under more cognitively challenging conditions. Certainly, it seems unlikely that impaired Theory of Mind could account for the range of difficulties associated with linguistic (as opposed to affective) prosody that have been reported in the literature. Still, it might be interesting to pursue this line of research by recruiting participants with ASD who have Theory of Mind deficits and then undertaking a comprehensive investigation of their receptive and expressive prosody in both affective and linguistic domains. Similarly, it would be worthwhile to recruit participants with ASD who have clear prosodic deficits and then comprehensively examine their Theory of Mind abilities.

Motor speech impairments

Difficulties with a range of motor skills, including gross, fine and oral, have been observed in individuals with ASD. A recent study by Shriberg, Paul, Black and Van Santen (2011) investigated the possibility that it is impaired motor control that underlies prosodic deficits in ASD by using the Prosody-Voice Screening Profile (Shriberg et al. 1990) to elicit speech from 46 children with ASD, 13 children with speech delay, 15 participants with childhood apraxia of speech and 40 typically developing children (note the varying sample sizes). Results showed that children with ASD did not exhibit the slower speech, longer vowels and phonemic errors that are seen in motor speech disorders. Furthermore, acoustic analyses revealed pitch and intensity profiles in ASD that are not seen in motor speech disorders.

In providing discussion of alternative causal mechanisms of prosodic impairment in ASD, Shriberg and colleagues (2011) argued that individuals with ASD may lack the social imperative to 'tune-up' their speech so that it aligns closely with speakers in the community. Diehl and Paul (2012) described this as "a dearth of social motivation to 'talk just like' other speakers in the community" (p. 124). It is interesting to consider the processes that might be associated with 'tuning-up' one's speech so that it aligns with the ambient environment. Factors other than, or in addition to, social motivation may play a role. Arciuli and Paul (2012) discuss the possibility that an inability to detect statistical regularities in the environment (i.e. impaired statistical learning) may play a role when it comes to difficulties 'tuning-up' to input in the environment. Another possibility is that effective audio-vocal regulation may be required for 'tuning-up'.

Atypical audio-vocal regulation

Studies of post-lingual deafness and participants with cochlear implants indicate that control of loudness and pitch during speech production depends upon auditory feedback (e.g. Lane, Wozniak, Matthies, Svirsky, Perkell, O'Connell & Manzella 1997). Clearly, auditory feedback is used to modify one's vocalisations. It is thought that these modifications serve to increase intelligibility. For example, people speak more loudly when they are in a noisy environment (known as the Lombard effect). There is interest in the way auditory feedback alters speech in children with ASD. Russo, Larson and Kraus (2008) used the pitch-shift reflex paradigm to examine the way speakers modify their pitch when unexpected alterations to their speech occur during sustained vocalisation. Children wear headphones during vocalisation (e.g. sustained production of a vowel) so that pitch-shifted stimuli can be fed back. Typically developing individuals generally modify their speech in response to these perceived errors of vocalisation. In their assessment of 19 typically developing children and 18 children with ASD (aged range 7–12 years), Russo and colleagues (2008) found that 38% of children with ASD showed abnormally large responses to perturbed auditory feedback that was more than 1.65 standard deviations above the mean for typical peers. This was described as "a hyper-responsive audio-vocal system" (p. 119). The researchers hypothesised that this behaviour might result from overly sensitive perception or impaired vocal control. It is not known whether impaired audio-vocal regulation might be linked with deficient encoding of pitch.

Deficient encoding of pitch

The auditory brainstem processes frequency characteristics of speech such as pitch. Children with learning impairments that are language-based have been shown to exhibit atypical brainstem encoding of speech (e.g. Banai, Nicol, Zecker & Kraus 2005; Johnson, Nicol, Zecker & Kraus 2007). Russo, Skoe, Tromner, Nicol, Zecker, Bradlow and Kraus (2008) examined passively evoked brainstem responses when participants (21 children with ASD and 21 typically developing children) were listening to speech syllables that displayed different pitch contours. The stimuli consisted of a natural recording of a CV syllable that was manipulated to display a descending contour (220–130 Hz) and an ascending contour (130–220 Hz). Essentially, this manipulation captures the distinction between a statement and a question. The data revealed that although all children showed normal brainstem function in response to click stimuli, the ASD group showed impaired pitch tracking when listening to speech. Specifically, around 20% of the ASD group showed pitch tracking impairment that placed them 1.65 standard deviations from the mean of their group. The authors hypothesised that these brainstem deficiencies may be myelin-related and associated with disordered connectivity between brainstem and cortex (via reciprocal pathways to the limbic or auditory cortex). The authors suggested that this passively evoked brainstem response to pitch tracking could serve as an early screener of auditory brainstem function. They also reviewed previous findings indicating that pitch tracking in the brainstem appears to be experience dependent (more robust in musicians than non-musicians) but trainable (can be improved via short term training), which may have implications for early remediation of receptive prosody difficulties in those with autism.

Summary

The above-mentioned mechanisms have been put forward as explanations of why prosody might be impaired in some individuals with ASD. Much additional research is required before any of these mechanisms can be confirmed or disconfirmed. Moreover, just as we know that not every individual with ASD experiences problems with prosody, it seems clear that a range of prosodic difficulties emerge across the individuals that are affected. Accordingly, different mechanisms may underpin different prosodic impairments. For instance, it is difficult to justify investigation of whether Theory of Mind deficits directly underpin impaired production of contrastive lexical stress across syllables (e.g. in 'INcense' versus 'inCENSE') when the possibility of motor speech impairment and/or atypical audio-vocal regulation fits so much more comfortably with this type of production difficulty. Similarly, deficient encoding of pitch, alone, is unlikely to provide a satisfactory explanation as to why some individuals with ASD experience difficulties with irony. Pre-screening of participants with ASD in future studies, perhaps even in terms of the various types of prosodic impairment (linguistic versus affective; receptive versus expressive; word level versus phrase level), is needed to advance our understanding of the mechanisms underpinning prosodic difficulties.

Directions for future research

In addition to suggestions that have been made throughout the chapter, this section suggests two other avenues for future research. First, a better understanding of *typical* prosodic development would assist in identifying atypical prosody. Second, it would be valuable to explore the ways in which prosodic impairment might be addressed through remediation.

A better understanding of typical prosodic development

A leading researcher in prosody recently highlighted that "the lack of correctness yardsticks in prosody makes for particular problems in determining what is atypical" (Peppé 2009: p. 270–271). Clearly, we need a comprehensive understanding of prosodic processing in typically developing individuals. For example, at present, we know very little about the typical developmental time course of prosodic processing. A recent investigation of the developmental trajectory of lexical stress production in children aged 3–7 years and adults has revealed important findings (Ballard, Djaja, Arciuli, James & van Doorn 2012). A total of 73 typically developing children and 24 adults were asked to produce two strong-weak polysyllabic words (where the first syllable is more strongly stressed than the second) and two weak-strong polysyllabic words (where the second syllable is more strongly stressed than the first) in a picture-naming task. This resulted in 388 productions of which 325 met criteria for acoustic measurement. For the first and second syllables of each word, vowel duration, peak intensity and peak fundamental frequency were used to compute normalised Pairwise Variability Indices (PVIs: which provide a measure of stress contrastivity across syllables).

Results showed that duration and intensity were used consistently to mark lexical stress but fundamental frequency displayed more variability. Moreover, while the production of strong-weak words appears to be mastered in early childhood, mastery of weak-strong words appears to continue beyond the age of 7. This may reflect an interaction between higher-level linguistic processes (e.g. strong-weak is the dominant pattern of lexical stress in English) and the constraints of the maturing speech motor system (e.g. due to increases in subglottic pressure the physiological demand to produce rising contour is greater than falling contour). One of the reasons that this kind of research has not been undertaken previously is that acoustic analyses are much more time consuming than studies that rely on perceptual judgements. Yet, such data is directly relevant for studies of prosodic processing in ASD. For example, Ballard et al.'s findings demonstrate the clinical significance of this kind of research; it would seem inappropriate to attempt remediation designed to achieve adult-like stress contrastivity in weak-strong productions in young children (< 7 years).

An evidence-base for the treatment of prosodic impairment

A number of studies reviewed here suggest that at least some individuals with autism have problems with prosody and may benefit from intervention designed at improving their reception and/or production of prosody. Unfortunately, there is no solid evidence-base concerning treatment of impaired prosody, in otherwise typically developing individuals or in special populations. For instance, in a systematic review of research on children and adolescents with apraxia of speech (Childhood Apraxia of Speech: CAS), a population that exhibits prosodic impairment as a core feature (unlike ASD), Morgan and Vogel (2008: p. 7) stated "There are a wide range of treatment approaches reported in the literature, however the effectiveness of these interventions has not been stringently examined. Furthermore, only case study or case series investigations have been conducted, limiting the ability to generalise findings of existing studies to the broader population of children aged three to 16 years with CAS."

A recent study explored the effectiveness of explicit methods for inducing the production of particular patterns of lexical stress (Van Rees, Ballard, McCabe, Macdonald-D'Silva & Arciuli 2012). It incorporated the use of bisyllabic nonwords that are orthographically biased to either a strong-weak or a weak-strong pattern of lexical stress (based on the large-scale corpus analysis conducted by Arciuli, Monaghan & Seva 2010) along with principles of motor learning (as in Schmidt & Lee 2005). Fourteen typically developing children aged 5 to 13 years were randomly allocated using concealed allocation within blocks to a training or control group. The training group learned to produce particular patterns of lexical stress with strong maintenance and generalization to untrained stimuli. Patterns of stress production did not change in the control group. Additional research is required to investigate whether these kinds of explicit methods are useful in treating prosodic deficits in special populations such as children with CAS or ASD.

Another avenue for future research includes the remediation of deficits in receptive prosody.

Conclusion

Prosody serves a range of important functions during communication. Those who experience difficulties comprehending and/or producing prosody stand out from their peers. A number of methods have been used to investigate prosody in ASD, many of which have been outlined here. These include behavioural studies, acoustic analyses, electrophysiological measures, and brain imaging. The precise mechanisms underpinning prosodic impairment continue to be of great interest, with the bulk of recent studies focussing on the contribution of motor speech impairment, atypical audio-vocal regulation, or deficient pitch encoding. To date, findings are mixed. This may, in large part, reflect the fact that only some individuals with ASD experience problems with prosody and the fact that affected individuals display different types of prosodic impairment. Thus, general recruitment of persons with

ASD in studies that include small samples may not be the best way to advance our understanding of the specific mechanisms which underpin different prosodic deficits. Avenues for future research include increased effort to understand typical prosodic development for comparative purposes, and increased effort to explore the remediation of prosodic difficulties.

References

Arciuli, J., & Cupples, L. (2003). Effects of stress typicality during speeded grammatical classification. *Language and Speech, 46*(4), 353–374.

Arciuli, J. & Cupples, L. (2004). Effects of stress typicality during spoken word recognition by native and nonnative speakers of English: Evidence from onset gating. *Memory & Cognition, 32*, 21–30.

Arciuli, J., Monaghan, P., & Seva, N. (2010). Learning to assign lexical stress during reading aloud: Corpus, behavioural and computational investigations. *Journal of Memory and Language, 63*, 180–196.

Arciuli, J., & Paul, R. (2012). Sensitivity to probabilistic orthographic cues to lexical stress in adolescent speakers with ASD and typical peers. *Quarterly Journal of Experimental Psychology, 65*, 1288–1295.

Arciuli, J., & Slowiaczek, L. (2007). The where and when of linguistic word-level prosody. *Neuropsychologia, 45*, 2638–42.

Ballard, K., Djaja, D., Arciuli, J., James, D., & van Doorn, J. (2012). Developmental trajectory for production of prosody: Lexical stress contrastivity in children 3 to 7 years and adults. *Journal of Speech, Language, and Hearing Research, 55*, 1822–1835.

Baltaxe, C. (1984). Use of contrastive stress in normal, aphasic, and autistic children. *Journal of Speech and Hearing Research, 27*, 97–105.

Baltaxe, C., & Guthrie, D. (1987). The use of primary sentence stress by normal, aphasic and autistic children. *Journal of Autism and Developmental Disorders, 17*, 255–271.

Baltaxe, C., Simmons, J., & Zee, E. (1984). Intonation patterns in normal, autistic and aphasic children. In A. Cohen & M. van de Broecke (Eds.), *Proceedings of the 10th International Congress of Phonetic Sciences* (pp. 713–718). Dordrecht: Foris.

Banai, K., Nicol, T., Zecker, S., & Kraus, N. (2005). Brainstem timing: Implications for cortical processing and literacy. *Journal of Neuroscience, 25*, 9850–9857.

Baron-Cohen, S. (1995). *Mindblindness: An Essay on Autism and Theory of Mind.* Cambridge, MA: The MIT Press.

Bishop, D.V.M. (1988). Development of the Children's Communication Checklist (CCC): A method for assessing qualitative aspects of communicative impairment in children. *Journal of Child Psychology and Psychiatry, 39*, 879–891.

Chevallier, C., Noveck, I., Happe, F., & Wilson, D. (2011). What's in a voice? Prosody as a test case for the Theory of Mind account of autism. *Neuropsychologia, 49*, 507–517.

Cooper, N., Cutler, A., & Wales, R. (2002). Constraints of lexical stress on lexical access in English: Evidence from native and non-native listeners, *Language and Speech, 45*, 207–28.

Crystal, D. (2009). Persevering with prosody. *International Journal of Speech-Language Pathology, 11*, 257.

DeMeyer, M., Barton, S., DeMeyer, W., Norton, J., Allen, J., & Stelle, R. (1973). Prognosis in autism: A follow-up study. *Journal of Autism and Childhood Schizophrenia, 3,* 199–246.
Diehl, J., & Paul, R. (2009). The assessment and treatment of prosodic disorders and neurological theories of prosody. *International Journal of Speech-Language Pathology, 11,* 287–292.
Diehl, J., & Paul, R. (2012). Acoustic differences in the imitation of prosodic patterns in children with autism spectrum disorders. *Research in Autism Spectrum Disorders, 6,* 123–134.
Diehl, J., Watson, D., Bennetto, L., McDonough, J., & Gunlogson, C. (2009). An acoustic analysis of prosody in high-functioning autism. *Applied Psycholinguistics, 30,* 385–404.
Erwin, R., Van Lancker, D., Guthrie, D., Schwafel, J., Tanguay, P., & Buchwald, J.S. (1991). P3 responses to prosodic stimuli in adult autistic subjects. *Electroencephalography and Clinical Neurophysiology, 80,* 561–571.
Fear, B., Cutler, A., & Butterfield, S. (1995). The strong/weak syllable distinction in English. *Journal of the Acoustical Society of America, 97,* 1893–1904.
Fine, J., Bartolucci, G., Ginsberg, G., & Szatmari, P. (1991). The use of intonation to communicate in pervasive developmental disorders. *Journal of Child Psychology and Psychiatry, 32,* 771–782.
Fosnot, S., & Jun, S. (1999). Prosodic characteristics in children with stuttering or autism during reading and imitation. In *Proceedings of the 14th International Congress of Phonetic Sciences* (pp. 1925–1928).
Frankel, F., Simmons, J., & Richey, E. (1987). Reward value of prosodic features of language for autistic, mentally retarded, and normal children. *Journal of Autism and Developmental Disorders, 17,* 103–115.
Goldman, R., & Fristoe, M. (2000). *Goldman Fristoe-2 Test of Articulation.* Circle Pines, MN: American Guidance Service.
Grossman, R., Bemis, R., Plesa Skwerer, D., Tager-Flusberg, H. (2010). Lexical and affective prosody in children with high-functioning autism. *Journal of Speech Language and Hearing Research, 53*(3), 778–793.
Henton, C. (1989). Fact and fiction in the description of female and male pitch. *Language and Communication, 9,* 299–311.
Hubbard, K., & Traumer, D. (2007). Intonation and emotion in autistic spectrum disorders. *Journal of Psycholinguistic Research, 36,* 159–173.
Jarvinen-Pasley, A., Peppé, S., King-Smith, G., & Heaton, P. (2008). The relationship between form and function level receptive prosodic abilities in autism. *Journal of Autism and Developmental Disorders, 38,* 1328–1340.
Johnson, K., Nicol, T., Zecker, S., & Kraus, N. (2007). Auditory brainstem correlates of perceptual timing deficits. *Journal of Cognitive Neuroscience, 19,* 376–385.
Jusczyk, P., Cutler, A., & Redanz, N. (1993). Infants' preference for the predominant stress patterns of English words. *Child Development, 64,* 657–687.
Jusczyk, P., Houston, D., & Newsome, M. (1999). The beginnings of word segmentation in English-learning infants. *Cognitive Psychology, 39,* 159–207.
Kanner, L. (1943). Autistic disturbances of affective contact. *Nervous Child, 2,* 217–250.
Klopfenstein, M. (2009). Interaction between prosody and intelligibility. *International Journal of Speech-Language Pathology, 11,* 326–31.
Koike, K., & Asp, C. (1981). Tennesse Test of rhythm and intonation patterns. *Journal of Speech and Hearing Disorders, 46,* 81–87.

Lane, H., Wozniak, J., Matthies, M., Svirsky, M., Perkell, J., O'Connell, M., & Manzella, J. (1997). Changes in sound pressure and fundamental frequency contours following changes in hearing status. *Journal of the Acoustical Society of America, 101*, 2244–2252.

Laures, J., & Weismer, G. (1999). The effects of a flattened fundamental frequency on intelligibility at the sentence level. *Journal of Speech, Language, and Hearing Research, 42*, 1148–1156.

Lehiste, I. (1970). *Suprasegmentals*. Cambridge, MA: The MIT Press.

Local, J. & Wootton, T. (1996). On being echolalic: an analysis of the interactional and phonetic aspects of an autistic's language. *York Papers in Linguistics, 17*, 119–165.

MacKay, G., & Shaw, A. (2004). A comparative study of figurative language in children with autism spectrum disorders. *Child Language Teaching and Therapy, 20*, 13–32.

Martin, I., & McDonald, S. (2004). An exploration of causes of non-literal language problems in individuals with Asperger syndrome. *Journal of Autism and Developmental Disorders, 34*, 311–328.

McCaleb, P., & Prizant, B. (1985). Encoding of new versus old information by autistic children. *Journal of Speech and Hearing Disorders, 50*, 226–230.

McCann, J., & Peppé, S. (2003). Prosody in autism spectrum disorders: A critical review. *International Journal of Language and Communication Disorders, 38*(4), 325–350.

McCann, J., Peppé, S., Gibbon, F., O'Hare, A., & Rutherford, M. (2007). Prosody and its relationship to language in school-aged children with high-functioning autism. *International Journal of Language and Communication Disorders, 42*, 682–702.

Mehler, J., Jusczyk, P., Lambertz, G., Halsted, N., Bertoncinic, J., & Amiel-Tilson, C. (1988). A precursor of language acquisition in young infants. *Cognition, 29*, 143–178.

Morgan, J., & Demuth, K. (1996). *Signal to Syntax: Bootstrapping from Speech to Grammar in Early Acquisition*. Mahwah, NJ: Lawrence Erlbaum Associates.

Morgan, A., & Vogel, P. (2008). Intervention for childhood apraxia of speech. *Cochrane Database of Systematic Reviews, 3*(1): 48–66.

Paccia, J., & Curcio, F. (1982). Language processing and forms of immediate echolalia in autistic children. *Journal of Speech and Hearing Research, 25*, 42–47.

Paul, R., Augustyn, A., Klin, A., & Volkmar, F. (2005). Perception and production of prosody by speakers with autism spectrum disorders. *Journal of Autism and Developmental Disorders, 35*, 201–220.

Paul, R., Augustyn, A., Klin, A., Volkmar, F., & Cohen, D. (2000). Grammatical and pragmatic prosody perception in high-functioning autism. Paper presented at the Symposium for Research in Child Language Disorders. Madison, WI.

Paul, R., Bianchi, N., Augustyn, A., Klin, A., & Volkmar, F. (2008). Production of syllable stress in speakers with autism spectrum disorders. *Research in Autism Spectrum Disorders, 2*, 110–124.

Paul, R., Shriberg, L., McSweeney, J., Cicchetti, D., Klin, A., & Volkmar, F. Relations between prosodic performance and communication and socialization ratings in high functioning speakers with autism spectrum disorders. *Journal of Autism and Developmental Disorders, 35*(6), 861–869.

Paul, R., Fuerst, Y., Ramsay, G., Chawarska, K. & Klin, A., (2011). Out of the mouths of babes: Vocal production in infant siblings of children with ASD. *Journal of Child Psychology and Psychiatry, 52*, 588–598.

Pell, M., Monetta, L., Paulmann, S., & Kotz, S. (2009). Recognizing emotions in a foreign language. *Journal of Nonverbal Behaviour, 33*, 107–120.

Peppé, S. (2009). Why is prosody in speech-language pathology so difficult? *International Journal of Speech-Language Pathology, 11*, 258–271.

Peppé, S. (2012). Assessment of prosodic ability in atypical populations, with special reference to high-functioning autism. In V. Stojanovik, & J. Setter (Eds.), *Speech Prosody in Atypical Populations* (pp. 25–43). Guildford, UK: J&R Press.

Peppé, S., Cleland, J., Gibbon, F., O'Hare, A., & Martinez Castilla, P. (2011). Expressive prosody in children with autism spectrum conditions. *Journal of Neurolinguistics, 24*, 41–53.

Peppé, S., & McCann, J. (2003). Assessing intonation and prosody in children with atypical language development: The PEPS-C test and the revised version. *Clinical Linguistics and Phonetics, 17*, 345–354.

Peppé, S., McCann, J., Gibbon, F., O'Hare, A., & Rutherford, M. (2007). Receptive and expressive prosodic ability in children with high-functioning autism. *Journal of Speech, Language, and Hearing Research, 50*(4), 1015–1028.

Pexman, P. (2008). It's fascinating research: The cognition of verbal irony. *Current Directions in Psychological Science, 17*(4), 286–290.

Pexman, P., Rostad, K., McMorris, C., Climie, E., Stowkowy, J., & Glenwright, M. (2011). Processing of ironic language in children with high-functioning autism spectrum disorder. *Journal of Autism and Developmental Disorders, 41*, 1097–1112.

Rogers, S. (2006). Evidence-based intervention for language development in young children with autism. In T.C.W. Stone (Ed.), *Social and Communication Development in Autism Spectrum Disorders: Early Identification, Diagnosis, and Intervention*. New York, NY: The Guilford Press.

Russo, N., Larson, C., & Kraus, N. (2008). Audio-vocal system regulation in children with autism spectrum disorders. *Experimental Brain Research, 188*, 111–124.

Russo, N., Skoe, E., Trommer, B., Nicol, T., Zecker, S., Bradlow, A., & Kraus, N. (2008). Deficient brainstem encoding of pitch in children with Autism Spectrum Disorders. *Clinical Neurophysiology, 119*, 1720–1731.

Rutherford, M., Baron-Cohen, S., & Wheelwright, S. (2002). Reading the mind in the voice: A study with normal adults and adults with Asperger syndrome and high functioning autism. *Journal of Autism and Developmental Disorders, 32*, 189–194.

Samuelsson, C., Plejert, C., Nettelbladt, U., & Anward, J. (2011). The role of interactional prosody in language testing activities in Swedish. In V. Stojanovik & J. Setter (Eds.), *Speech Prosody in Atypical Populations* (pp. 45–69). Guildford, UK: J&R Press.

Shriberg, L., Kwiatkowski, J., & Rasmussen, C. (1990). *The Prosody-Voice Screening Profile*. Tucson AZ: Communication Skill Builders.

Shriberg, L., Paul, R., Black, L., & Van Santen, J. (2011). The hypothesis of apraxia of speech in children with autism spectrum disorder. *Journal of Autism and Developmental Disorders, 41*, 405–426.

Shriberg, L., Paul, R., McSweeney, J., Klin, A., Cohen, D., & Volkmar, F. (2001). Speech and prosody characteristics of adolescents and adults with high-functioning autism and Asperger syndrome. *Journal of Speech, Language, and Hearing Research, 44*, 1097–1115.

Shriberg, L., & Widder, C. (1990). Speech and prosody characteristics of adults with mental retardation. *Journal of Speech and Hearing Research, 33*, 627–53.

Simmons, J., & Baltaxe, C. (1975). Language patterns in adolescent autistics. *Journal of Autism and Childhood Schizophrenia, 5*, 333–351.

Slowiaczek, L. (1990). Effects of lexical stress in auditory word recognition. *Language and Speech, 33*, 47–68.

Schmidt, R.A., & Lee, T.D. (2005). *Motor Control and Learning: A Behavioural Emphasis* (4th ed.). Champaign, IL: Human Kinetics.
Thurber, C., & Tager-Flusberg, H. (1993). Pauses in the narratives produced by autistic, mentally-retarded, and normal children as an index of cognitive demand. *Journal of Autism and Developmental Disorders, 23,* 309–322.
Wang, A., Lee, S., Sigman, M., Dapretto, M. (2006). Neural basis of irony comprehension in children with autism: the role of prosody and context. *Brain, 129,* 932–943.
Van Kuijk, D. & Boves, L. (1999). Acoustic characteristics of lexical stress in continuous telephone speech. *Speech Communication, 27*, 95–111.
Van Rees, L., Ballard, K., McCabe, P., Macdonald-D'Silva, A., & Arciuli, J. (2012). Training production of lexical stress in typically developing children with orthographically biased stimuli and principles of motor learning. *American Journal of Speech-Language Pathology, 21*, 197–206.
Van Santen, J., Prud'Hommeaux, E., Black, L., & Mitchell, M. (2010). Computational prosodic markers for autism. *Autism, 14,* 215–236.
Wang, A., Dapretto, M., Hariri, A., Sigman, M., & Brookheimer, S. (2001). Processing affective and linguistic prosody in autism: An fMRI study. *Neuroimage, 13*, S621–S621.
Wetherby, A., Woods, J., Allen, L., Cleary, J., Dickinson, H., & Lord, C. (2004). Early indicators of autism spectrum disorders in the second year of life. *Journal of Autism and Developmental Disorders, 34,* 473–493.
Whiteside, S., & Hodgson, C. (2000). Some acoustic characteristics in the voices of 6- to 10-year-old children and adults: A comparative sex and developmental perspective. *Logopedics Phoniatrics Vocology, 25*, 122–132.
Wilson, D., & Wharton, T. (2006). Relevance and prosody. *Journal of Pragmatics, 38,* 1559–1579.
Wingfield, A., Lombardi, L., & Sokol, S. (1984). Prosodic features and the intelligibility of accelerated speech: Syntactic versus prosodic segmentation. *Journal of Speech and Hearing Research, 27,* 128–134.

SECTION 3

Literacy

CHAPTER 6

Reading for sound and reading for meaning in autism

Frith and Snowling (1983) revisited

Jon Brock & Nathan Caruana
Macquarie University

In their classic 1983 study, Frith and Snowling reported evidence for a dissociation in autism between intact semantic processing of single words, but relative difficulty on tests of sentence or paragraph comprehension. Here, we revisit the 7 experiments in Frith and Snowling's paper, in the light of the several dozen subsequent studies that have sought to replicate or extend their findings. We note that Frith and Snowling's results have stood the test of time remarkably well. There is, however, converging evidence that many of the semantic impairments previously considered to be "autism specific" may in fact be better accounted for by co-occurring language impairment.

> *"Reading skill is acquired quickly, but the children read monotonously and a story or moving picture is experienced in unrelated portions rather than its coherent totality."* (*Kanner 1943: p. 250*)

In his original description of 11 children with what he termed "autistic disorder", Leo Kanner (1943) noted a marked discrepancy between their fluent (if monotonous) reading and their apparent lack of comprehension of the material they had read. As with many of his observations, subsequent empirical research has been generally supportive of Kanner's views on reading skills in autism. In the 1960s, the term *hyperlexia* was coined to describe advanced decoding skills in the presence of intellectual disability (Huttenlocher & Huttenlocher 1973; Silberberg & Silberberg 1967) with researchers noting that many hyperlexics met criteria for autism (Healy, Aram, Horwitz & Kessle 1982). However, rather than being celebrated as a cognitive strength, or a signal of otherwise unrecognised intelligence, advanced reading skills were widely dismissed as mechanical "barking at print", in much the same way that echolalia, the rote repetition of other people's utterances, was considered to be meaningless and even problematic (see Roberts chapter, this volume).

A turning point came in 1983, with the publication in the Journal of Developmental Psychology of a paper by Uta Frith and Maggie Snowling, reporting a series of seven experiments testing autistic children's reading capabilities. Frith and Snowling concluded that the single word reading skills of autistic children were qualitatively similar to those of younger typically developing children at the same stage of reading acquisition. However, across several experiments, they found evidence for an inability to extract the broader meaning of connected text, precisely as Kanner had suggested.

Six years later, in *Autism: Explaining the Enigma*, Frith (1989) expanded on these findings, introducing the term 'central coherence' to describe the mechanism that "compels us human beings to give priority to understanding meaning" (p 101). Building on earlier theories put forward by Rimland (1964) and Hermelin and O'Connor (1970), she proposed that *weak* central coherence was the "red thread" running through many of the features of autism including social communication impairments as well as relative strengths on nonverbal tasks that required the meaning or Gestalt of the stimuli to be ignored. Current formulations of the weak central coherence account are somewhat less ambitious in scope (e.g. Happé & Frith 2006). Nonetheless, it remains one of three dominant cognitive accounts of autism (Rajendran & Mitchell 2007) and continues to influence theoretical and clinical approaches to the communication impairments associated with the disorder (e.g. Noens & van Berckelaer-Onnes 2005).

In this chapter, we revisit Frith and Snowling's 1983 study, describing each of the seven experiments and reviewing the studies of reading comprehension in individuals with autism that have been conducted in the intervening three decades that have attempted to replicate and extend their findings. We attempt to reconcile some apparently contradictory findings within this literature and conclude by discussing the relationship between reading comprehension and oral language comprehension more generally.

Participants

Frith and Snowling's autism group comprised of six boys and two girls, aged 9 to 17 years old, who demonstrated "the classic symptoms of autistic aloneness, cognitive/language deficits, and obsessional phenomena" (p. 331). At the time, there were no standardised autism diagnostic tools, with the authors relying on psychiatric diagnoses. The autistic children were selected to have a reading age of between 8 and 10 years according to the normative data of the British Abilities Scale (BAS) Word Reading Test (Elliott, Murray & Pearson 1979), which involved reading aloud single words. Full scale IQs, measured using the Wechsler Intelligence Scale for Children, ranged from 54 to 103.

In the majority of experiments, the performance of the autistic children was contrasted with that of two further groups of children, both matched to the autism group according to their performance on the BAS Word Reading Test. A typically developing control group included ten 9- to 10-year-old children (8 boys), described by their teachers as being of average ability. The dyslexia group were eight 10- to 12-year-old children (5 boys), who had all been referred to a dyslexia centre by their schools and were found to have poor reading skills for their age and IQ.

The Neale Analysis of Reading Ability

Frith and Snowling (1983) also reported the performance of autistic and dyslexic children on the Neale Analysis of Reading Ability (NARA), a popular standardized test in which children are required to read a short story aloud and then answer questions about the story (Neale 1958). The two groups performed at similar levels in terms of their reading accuracy, consistent with the fact that they were matched on word decoding skills. However, the autistic children achieved significantly lower scores for reading comprehension.

These findings are consistent with the results of other studies of autism using the NARA or NARA II. These have consistently shown reading comprehension to be significantly poorer than reading accuracy based on age-equivalent or age-standardized scores (Lockyer & Rutter 1969; Nation et al. 2006; Rutter & Bartak 1973. Similar results have also been reported on other tests of reading comprehension that likewise involve answering questions about sentences or passages that the participant has just read (Jones et al. 2009; Minshew, Goldstein, Muenz & Payton 1992; Minshew, Goldstein & Siegel 1995; Williams, Goldstein & Minshew 2006; see also but see Asberg, Kopp, Bergkelly & Gillberg 2010).

However, while the results are fairly consistent across studies, they may be less consistent across the individuals within those studies. Using the NARA II (Neale 1997), Nation, Clarke, Wright and Williams (2006) reported that 10 of 32 autistic children with measurable reading scores had impaired reading comprehension (standard scores <85) despite unimpaired reading accuracy. Only one child showed the opposite pattern, meaning that the overall trend was again for poorer comprehension than decoding. Nonetheless, the majority of children had similar scores for decoding and comprehension. Further correlational analyses showed that reading comprehension was strongly predicted by oral language comprehension skills.

In a more recent study, Norbury and Nation (2011) divided their sample of 27 adolescents with autism (26 male) according to whether or not they had oral language impairment, defined in terms of clinical records and performance below -1.25 SD on the recalling sentences subtest of the Clinical Evaluation of Language Fundamentals (Semel, Wiig & Secord 2006). The subgroup with language impairment had significantly lower reading comprehension scores than age-matched typically developing controls. In contrast, those *without* language impairment had age-appropriate reading comprehension.

The link between oral language skills and reading comprehension in autism was further emphasized in another recent study by Huemer and Mann (2010), using the Gray Oral Reading Test-Revised, 4th edition, which follows a similar format to the NARA. Factor analysis of pooled data from children with autism or dyslexia revealed two distinct factors: reading accuracy and rate loaded onto one factor, along with other measures of decoding; while reading comprehension loaded onto a second factor, alongside measures of spoken language comprehension.

This relationship between reading comprehension and oral language skills is an issue we return to at the end of the chapter. For now, suffice it to say that there is clear and fairly consistent evidence from studies using a wide range of standardized tests to support Frith and Snowling's (1983) view that reading comprehension can dissociate from decoding skills in that individuals with autism tend to have reading comprehension difficulties that are more severe than can be explained in terms of impaired decoding skills alone. What standardized tests fail to address, however, is the underlying mechanism of this comprehension impairment. Thus, in the seven experiments reviewed below, Frith and Snowling attempted to tease apart different explanations for comprehension difficulty, looking at processing of progressively larger sections of text, from single words through to extended passages of prose.

Experiment 1: Words/Nonwords

The first three experiments in Frith and Snowling's paper involved reading of single words. Frith and Snowling reasoned that, if children with autism were merely "barking at print", then their pattern of reading performance across different classes of lexical material would be different to typically developing children at the same level of reading skill.

Experiment 1 was motivated by Coltheart's *dual route* model of reading (Coltheart 1978). According to this model, regular words such as "cat" or "house" can be read successfully either by being recognized whole (the lexical route) or being sounded out letter by letter (grapheme phoneme conversion). For irregular words, such as "yacht", the usual letter-to-sound rules do not work, and so reading relies heavily on the lexical route. In contrast, unfamiliar words or nonwords such as "blench" must be sounded out because it is impossible to recognize whole a word that has not been seen before. Contrasting a child's ability to read nonwords with their reading of irregular real words thus provides a metric of the relative strengths of the two different routes.

Figure 1 shows the pattern of performance of the three groups across regular words, irregular words, and nonwords. Compared to typically developing children, those with dyslexia were significantly poorer at reading nonwords. They also showed little difference between regular and irregular words. Within the dual route framework, this pattern of results suggests an inability to sound out words that cannot be recognized whole. In contrast, the children with autism showed almost identical patterns of performance to the typically developing children across the different types of word.

A number of subsequent studies have contrasted word and nonword reading in autistic individuals. Minshew et al. (1994) tested high-functioning adolescents and young adults on subtests of the Woodcock Reading Mastery Test – Revised (Woodcock 1987). Consistent with Frith and Snowling's results, performance was similar for word reading (Word Identification) and nonword reading (Word Attack), with standardized scores slightly above age-appropriate levels.

Other researchers have reported cases of children with very poor nonword reading, in spite of skilled word reading (Aaron, Fantz & Manges 1990). For example, Nation et al. (2006) identified 5 out of 32 autistic children in their sample who were at floor on nonword reading, despite having a standardized score of at least 95 for word reading. Similarly, Newman et al. (2007) reported considerable variation in nonword reading within autism. In particular, the ability to read nonwords differentiated autistic children with hyperlexia from those who did not meet criteria for hyperlexia.

Surprisingly few studies have investigated the regular / irregular distinction in autistic children. Welsh, Pennington and Rogers (1987) reported that five children with autism and hyperlexia performed better on regular than irregular words. Although the authors claimed that this was evidence for a dysfunctional lexical route, the absence of a control group makes the data difficult to interpret (note that the typically developing children tested by Frith and Snowling also showed this pattern of results). Moreover, the children showed significant effects of word frequency, which according to Coltheart's (1978) model can only be explained in terms of a functioning lexical route.

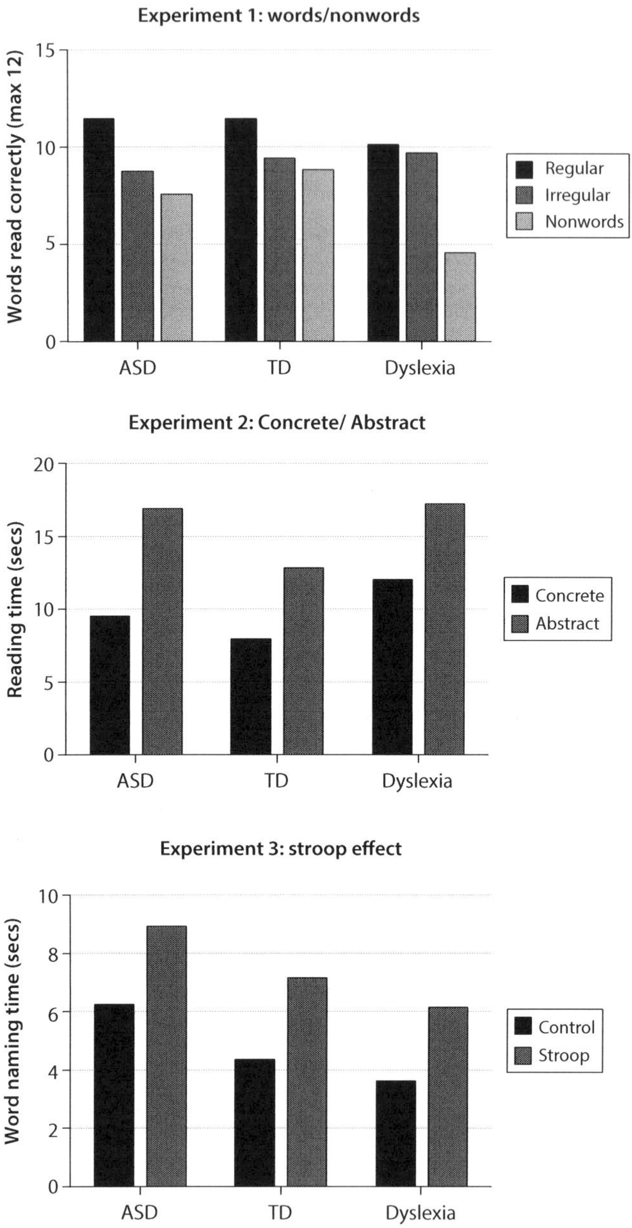

Figure 1. Group means in Experiments 1, 2, and 3

Experiment 2: Abstract/Concrete words

In their second experiment, Frith and Snowling examined the concreteness effect, whereby concrete or highly imagable words are easier to read than abstract words (Richardson 1975). Again, the reasoning was that, if children with autism are merely "barking at print" without processing the meaning of the words, then they should not show a concreteness effect.

To test this prediction, children were given lists of 12 concrete and 12 abstract words to read aloud. The word lists were matched for word frequency and length – factors that are known to affect reading accuracy and speed. Any differences in performance could then be attributed to semantic processing. In fact, very few errors were made by any of the children, but concrete words were read significantly faster than abstract words (see Figure 1). Importantly, this concreteness effect on reading speed did not interact with group membership. If anything, autistic children showed an increased concreteness effect on response times – contrary to the prediction.

There have, to our knowledge, been no attempts to directly replicate Frith and Snowling's Experiment 2. Reduced concreteness effects in autism have been reported in studies of memory for word lists, perhaps reflecting differences in encoding strategy (Toichi & Kamino 2003). In contrast, other studies have reported typical concreteness effects in tests of vocabulary knowledge (Hobson & Lee 1989). Perhaps the closest to a replication comes from a study by Eskes, Bryson & McCormick (1990) investigating the concreteness effect on reading using a Stroop interference paradigm. This study was a response to Frith and Snowling's Experiment 3, which is described next.

Experiment 3: Stroop interference

In the Stroop paradigm (Stroop 1935), participants are presented with a list of words or character strings typed in different ink colours. Response times for naming the ink colours are considerably slower if the words themselves are incongruous colour words (e.g. the word "GREEN" written in red ink). Given that participants are instructed to ignore the words themselves, this suggests that access to the meanings of the words is automatic and obligatory (Posner & Snyder 1975) and the Stroop task therefore provides a test of "capture by meaning" (cf. Shah & Frith 1983). In fact, Frith and Snowling (1983) found that the size of the interference effect was similar across the three groups (see Figure 1).

Similar results have been reported in six replication studies (Bryson 1983; Christ, Holt, White & Green 2007; Eskes, Bryson, McCormick 1990; Goldberg et al. 2005; Lopez, Lincoln, Ozonoff & Lai 2005; Ozonoff & Jensen 1999). A seventh study *did* report a reduced interference effect in children with autism (Adams & Jarrold 2009), although it is unclear why these results differed from those of other studies.

The most comprehensive investigation was conducted by Eskes et al. (1990). Like Frith and Snowling, these authors reported that children with autism showed a similar interference effect to typically developing controls when naming the colours of incongruent colour words. They also showed similar interference effects from colour associates (e.g. the word GRASS written in brown). Moreover, as noted above, the autistic children showed increased interference from concrete compared with abstract words (e.g. TABLE vs. LIFE). Again, the magnitude of this concreteness effect was comparable to that shown by control children. These findings indicate that the presence of the Stroop effect extends beyond the effects of colour words and that individuals with autism do process the meanings of the individual words they hear.

Experiment 4: Final 's'

Frith and Snowling's first three studies failed to find any evidence of atypical single word processing. In their fourth and fifth experiments, they moved on to investigate the effect of sentence context on the interpretation of single words. In both experiments, participants were required to read aloud sentences containing ambiguous words that could be pronounced in more than one way. The pronunciation they gave then indicated how they had interpreted the sentence.

In Experiment 4, the critical words were nonwords such as "bippis" that ended in a letter "s" preceded by a vowel. In some sentences (e.g. "All these bippis…"), the participants were expected to infer that the final "s" was a plural marker and so should be pronounced with a voiced /z/ sound (as in "hippos"). In other sentences (e.g. "One yellow bippis…"), the novel word was a singular noun and the "s" was to be pronounced with an unvoiced /s/ (as in "proboscis"). Because the word was a nonword, children had to use the syntactic context of the sentence to determine whether to leave the "s" voiced or unvoiced.

Children with autism were sensitive to this syntactic manipulation, being much more likely to give the voiced /z/ in plural contexts (see Figure 2). Frith and Snowling did not test the typically developing or dyslexic children on this task. However, they noted that, numerically, the performance of the autistic children was very similar to that of typically developing children aged 8- to 10 years

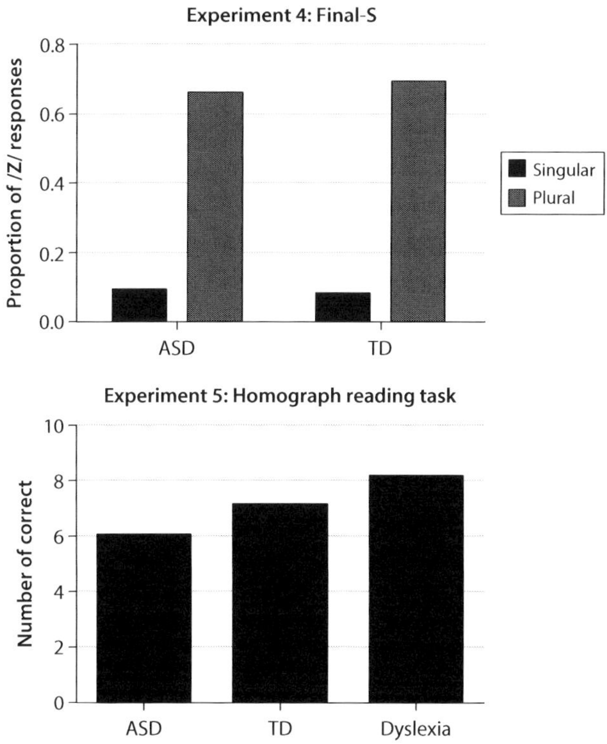

Figure 2. Group means in Experiments 4 and 5

(the reading age of the autistic children) in a previous study (Campbell & Besner, 1981). Frith and Snowling concluded, therefore, that "children with autism can be sensitive to syntactic constraints" (p. 336). To our knowledge, no attempts have been made to replicate this experiment.

Experiment 5: Homographs

Undoubtedly the most influential experiment in the series was Experiment 5, in which participants were required to read aloud sentences containing homographs – written words that have multiple meanings associated with the same orthographic form. Crucially, the homographs chosen by Frith and Snowling all had different pronunciations associated with their different meanings. For example, the word "*bow*" is pronounced differently in the sentences.

> *"Tom was an Indian and pretended to have arrows and a bow."*
> *"Before he began his speech he made a bow."*

For four of the five homographs used in the test (bow, row, tear, lead), children with autism consistently gave the most common pronunciation, regardless of contextual cues. Children with dyslexia and typically developing children performed significantly better, although as Figure 2 shows, the difference in terms of actual number of errors was relatively small.

The fifth homograph, "read", was pronounced accurately across both contexts by all of the autistic children. Notably, "read" is a verb, whereas the other homographs were all nouns in both contexts (although they could all be verbs in other syntactic contexts). Perhaps more importantly, the two pronunciations of "read" correspond to different tenses of the same verb stem as opposed to completely unrelated meanings, as was the case for the other homographs. Thus the contextual cues are syntactic rather than semantic and the unimpaired performance on this homograph is entirely consistent with the apparently normal performance on the "bippis" task described above (Experiment 4). Frith and Snowling argued, therefore, that they had identified "a failure to utilize semantic context in the absence of syntactic cues" (p. 339).

In 1986, Snowling and Frith reported a follow-up study, using similar stimuli but adding a second condition in which the homographs came before the disambiguating context (e.g. "He took a bow when everybody clapped"). A further adaptation was that the whole experiment was administered twice, with a training session between the first and second runs, in which participants were alerted to the ambiguous nature of the words and coached in their alternative meanings. Overall, children with autism performed at a similar level to intellectually disabled control children, with variation in performance linked to verbal mental age rather than diagnosis. As pointed out by Happé (1997), the training session changed the nature of the task, meaning that it was no longer a test of natural reading comprehension. Nonetheless, the 1986 study further highlights the importance of language level in reading comprehension.

A further four studies have been conducted using Snowling and Frith's stimuli, but without the training session. Although none of these studies directly assessed knowledge of the alternative meanings of the homographs, participant groups were matched on verbal IQ (Burnette et al. 2005; Jolliffe & Baron-Cohen 1999; López & Leekam 2003) or were selected such that those in the autism group had larger receptive vocabularies than control participants (Happé 1997). Results were broadly in line with Frith and Snowling's original report, with autistic individuals making more pronunciation errors than controls. This was true whether researchers considered only the participants' first responses or allowed them to correct any pronunciation errors. One slight anomaly is that Happé (1997) found evidence for impairment when the context preceded the homograph but not when it came after. The most likely explanation for this finding is that the control children in this study were considerably younger than those with autism and may have been less adept at reading ahead to work out what the correct meaning was.

Another important issue is the extent to which performance varies across individuals. In Frith and Snowling's original study, all eight children with autism consistently gave the wrong pronunciation for the subordinate meaning. However, given the low levels of performance across all three groups, this impressive consistency may have been a function of floor effects. In other studies, with overall higher levels of performance, the reported standard deviations indicate considerable variability. Indeed, because only four or five trials were administered per condition, it is possible to work out the exact distribution of scores for each condition. Figure 3 shows that, across the three studies conducted by Happé (1997), Jolliffe and Baron-Cohen (1999) and López and Leekam (2003), 40% of participants with ASD pronounced the subordinate meaning correctly on every single trial. In other words, group differences were driven by a subgroup of individuals with autism who perform poorly, rather than reflecting a 'universal' characteristic of autism (cf. Happé 1997).

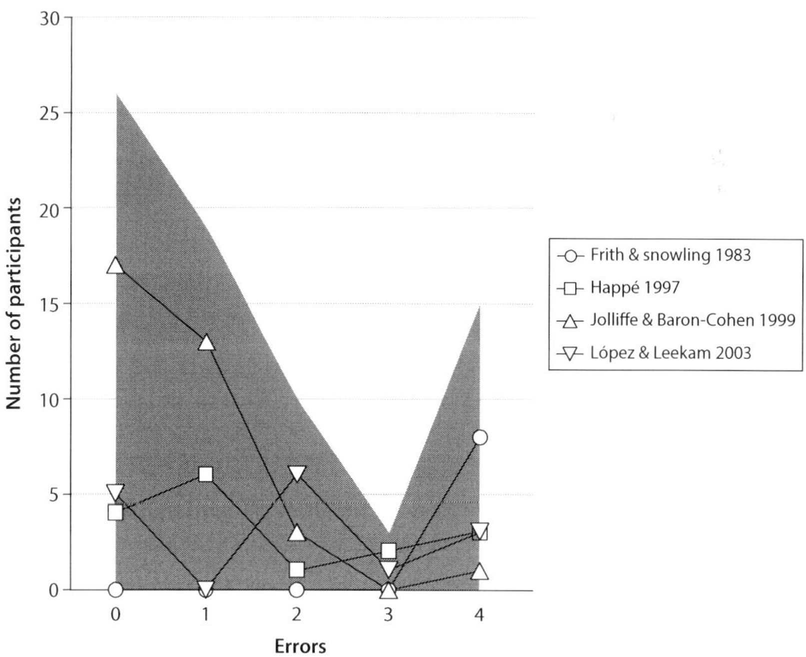

Figure 3. Number of errors made by participants with autism in four studies of homograph reading (context first, rare pronunciation condition). Shaded area shows the combined sample across all four studies

The reason for the small number of trials in the homographs task is that appropriate homographs are relatively rare in English. The majority of homographs are like "bank", having the same pronunciation for both meanings, making it impossible to know which meaning was intended, or they rely on subtle prosodic differences (e.g. "INcense" versus "inCENSE") that may in themselves be challenging for some individuals with autism (see chapter on prosody by Arciuli, this issue). Thus, in a recent and currently unpublished study, we investigated homograph reading in Israeli children with autism whose primary written language was Hebrew – a much richer source of homographs (Brock, Sukenik & Friedmann 2012). As in the studies of English-speaking individuals, we found considerable variation in performance, with some children making multiple errors and others performing almost perfectly. Homograph reading accuracy was predicted by children's age and autism severity (according to the Childhood Autism Ratings Scale; Schopler, Reichler, DeVellis & Daly 1980), their reading speed, their knowledge of the meanings of written words, and their ability to name pictures. These results provide further evidence for a link between reading comprehension and both decoding skills and oral language abilities.

Experiment 6: Gap test

In Experiment 6, participants completed the Gap test (McLeod 1970) in which they were required to read a section of text and write in the missing word, as in the example below:

There was a chest of ______ *and a cupboard to put things* _______.

There was no time limit, children were encouraged to guess, and they were not penalized for spelling errors. Even so, children with autism made many more errors than those in the other two groups. These were predominantly in the same syntactic class (noun, verb, adjective) as the correct word, suggesting that the difficulties were semantic rather than syntactic in nature (see Figure 4).

Similar results are found in other studies using gap tests that are part of standardized assessments of reading achievement. Using the Passage Completion subtest of the Woodcock Reading Mastery Test, Minshew and colleagues found that individuals with autism perform worse than age- and IQ-matched controls, despite performing at similar levels on measures of reading decoding (Minshew et al. 1995; Minshew, Goldstein & Siegel 1997; Williams et al. 2006). More recently, Newman et al. (2007) administered the Passage Comprehension subtest of the Woodcock-Johnson Tests of Achievement III, which is also similar in format. Once differences in single word reading had been controlled for statistically, children with autism performed significantly worse than typically developing children, regardless of whether or not they met criteria for hyperlexia.

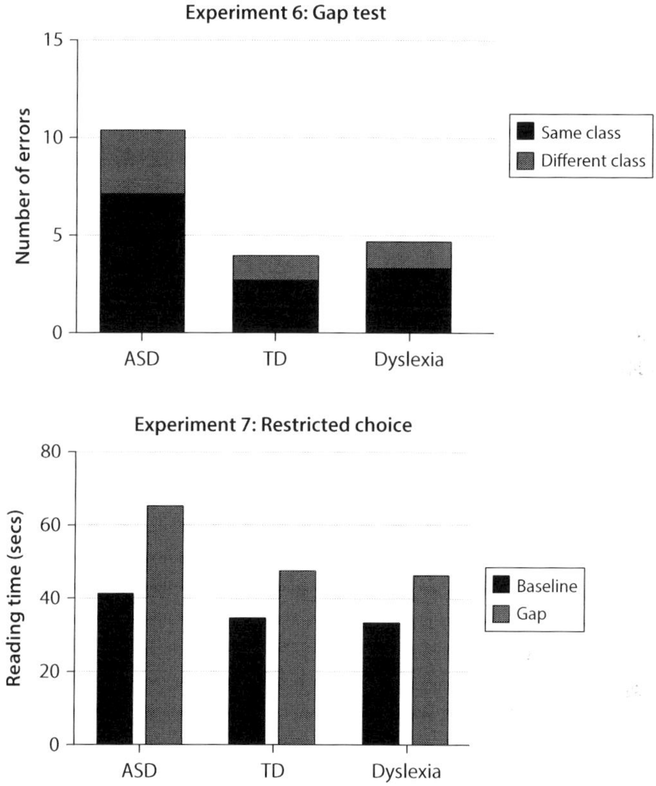

Figure 4. Group means in Experiments 6 and 7

Experiment 7: Restricted choice

Experiment 7 was a development of Experiment 6. Participants were again required to read passages. This time, however, they read aloud and, at various points in the passage, had to choose one from three words. In each case, the three words were all from the same word class (all prepositions, all verbs, or all nouns) so there were no syntactic cues.

> *Tom could swim/hear/heat something else, nearby. Was it a water rat? He looked in the holes/drawers/books in the riverbank.*

As in Experiment 6, children with autism made more errors than dyslexic or typically developing children. They were also slower to read those sentences containing choices, despite not differing significantly on time overall (see Figure 4).

In a follow-up study, Snowling and Frith (1986) developed a slightly more nuanced version of Experiment 7, in which the word choices included the correct word, an entirely implausible word, and a word that was plausible given the sentence context but inconsistent with the broader story context.

> *In early summer, five tiny babies were born. After only four days, their mother/friends/records led them to the pond for their first swimming lesson.*

Children with autism performed at a similar level to intellectually disabled control children of comparable verbal mental age (receptive vocabulary knowledge). However, as was found for the other tasks conducted by Snowling and Frith (1986), performance varied as a function of verbal mental age.

Somewhat similar results were reported in the recent study by Norbury and Nation (2011) using essentially the same task (although children were also asked comprehension questions throughout the task). Mirroring the results on the NARA, mentioned earlier, autistic children with language impairment performed significantly worse than age-matched typically developing children, whereas those with age-appropriate language were unimpaired. Thus, again, there is clear evidence for variation in reading comprehension linked to oral language skills, this time at the level of paragraph comprehension.

Discussion

The results of Frith and Snowling's 1983 study can be summarized as follows: First, on tests that involved single word reading, autistic children resembled younger typically developing children who were matched on their ability to read single words. Although this sounds somewhat circular, the notion that autistic children merely "barked at print" would have led one to predict *qualitative* differences in single word reading. Instead, the autistic children showed typical patterns of reading performance across regular, irregular, and novel words (Experiment 1); and across concrete and abstract words (Experiment 2). They also evidenced typical interference from colour words (Experiment 3).

Second, and in contrast to their single-word reading, the autistic children demonstrated clear difficulties when required to process multi-word text. They showed a reduced influence of sentence context on reading homographs (Experiment 5), and had difficulty producing or choosing suitable words that would complete the text (Experiments 6, 7). There was, however, no evidence for difficulties in using sentence context to determine the syntactic class of a word (Experiments 4, 5 and 6). Together, these observations led Frith and Snowling to conclude thus:

> *So far, we can state only that we traced the deficit to a failure to utilize semantic context in the absence of syntactic cues. Also, we hypothesize that this failure cannot be reduced to a failure of semantic access to individual words.*

As we have seen, Frith and Snowling's results have stood the test of time remarkably well, with similar findings being reported in numerous studies using the same or equivalent tests of reading ability. Basic decoding skills are of course a prerequisite for reading comprehension, but it is clear that many children and adults with autism struggle on tests of reading comprehension despite having relatively strong decoding skills.

In addition to the replication studies reviewed above, Frith and Snowling's conclusions have also been supported by results from other paradigms. For example, evidence for typical processing of word meaning comes from studies using semantic priming paradigms in which the response to a word is facilitated if it is preceded by a semantically related word (Kamio & Toichi 2000; López & Leekam 2003; Toichi & Kamio 2001; but see Kamio et al. 2007). Evidence for reduced context effects at the sentence level comes from studies indicating that the N400 brain response of individuals with autism is insensitive to whether a written word is congruent or incongruent with the preceding sentence context (Braeutigam et al. 2008; Pijnacker et al. 2011; Ring, Sharma, Wheelwright & Barrett 2007).

Despite the converging evidence at the group level, it has also become evident that not all individuals are affected in this way. As we have seen, some studies with high functioning autistic participants have failed to find evidence of reduced context effects in reading comprehension. Others have found significant impairment only in a subgroup of individuals with autism. Across these studies the most consistent predictor of within-group variability in test performance is the individual's oral language level or, alternatively, their degree of language impairment. This is the case for performance on the NARA (Nation et al. 2006; Norbury & Nation 2011) and similar tests (Huemer & Mann 2010); the Restricted Choice test (Snowling & Frith 1986; Norbury & Nation 2011); and, indeed, the homograph test (Snowling & Frith 1986; Brock et al. 2012).

Notably, the same pattern has also been observed in studies of spoken sentence comprehension. Norbury (2005), for example, asked participants to listen to sentences containing homophones – ambiguous *spoken* words – and then decide whether the sentence matched a picture corresponding to one of the meanings of the homophone (e.g. *"John fished from the bank"* followed by a picture of money). Children with autism who had age-appropriate language skills performed at the same level as their typically developing peers (see also Henderson, Clarke & Snowling 2011). Autistic children who had language difficulties performed poorly on the test, but so too did non-autistic children with specific language impairment.

An identical pattern of results was reported by Brock, Norbury and Einav (2008) using a language-mediated eye-movement paradigm, whereby context effects were indexed by participants' tendency to look at objects on a computer display that were consistent or inconsistent with the context of sentences they were listening to. Again, the magnitude of context effects varied as a function of oral language ability, independent of autism diagnosis.

Thus, we have two apparently conflicting sets of results. On the one hand, there are the many studies reporting evidence for reading comprehension difficulties and reduced sensitivity to context in autism, even when carefully controlling for verbal IQ or verbal mental age. On the other hand, there are a growing number of studies showing that variation in context effects and comprehension performance is primarily a function of oral language skill, rather than autism diagnosis.

Reconciling these findings is far from straightforward. One possibility is that individuals with autism experience additional comprehension difficulties that cannot be explained in terms of language impairments or poor decoding skills. Exactly what that additional deficit might be, however, remains somewhat mysterious. While the results seem to be fairly consistent across studies using the same task, there is no obvious "fine cut" between the comprehension tasks that reveal group differences and those that do not. Frith and Snowling's original suggestion of a basic deficit in "context processing", as envisaged in the weak central coherence account, runs up against the findings from the eyetracking (Brock et al. 2008) and homophone tasks (Norbury 2005). Happé's (1997) suggestion that individuals with autism have difficulty "extracting higher level meaning" might allow for intact *local* context effects within sentences in these studies, and is certainly consistent with the evidence reviewed earlier that autistic individuals are unable to make the inferences required to join two sentences into a coherent narrative (e.g. Jolliffe & Baron-Cohen 1999; Minshew et al. 1995). However, it is inconsistent with findings from studies using the Restricted Choice task – choosing a word that is coherent with the story context rather than just the sentence context is related to language ability rather than autism diagnosis (Norbury & Nation 2011; Snowling & Frith 1986).

There are other factors to consider. Certain reading comprehension tasks might prove difficult for individuals with autism for reasons unrelated to their reading comprehension. For example, a number of studies have reported that individuals with autism have difficulty answering questions that involve inferences about events that are implied but not explicitly stated in the text (Dennis et al. 2001; Jolliffe & Baron-Cohen 1999; Minshew et al. 1992, 1995; Norbury & Nation 2011; Williams et al. 2006; see also Ozonoff & Miller 1996). However, Saldana and Frith (2007) found that, despite performing poorly on a conventional test of reading comprehension, children with autism did appear able to make text-based inferences because they were quicker to read sentences that had been primed by an inference generated earlier in the text. Again, it is not entirely clear what specific task demands are relevant. Nonetheless, it is important to recognize that scores on many reading comprehension tests may underestimate the true levels of comprehension of autistic children.

A further important consideration may be the nature of the task used for matching. Given the uneven profile of language skills, matching participants on one measure is likely to leave groups unmatched on other linguistic skills that are more directly relevant to reading comprehension (Jarrold & Brock 2004). Many of the studies reporting significant group differences have matched groups on either receptive vocabulary knowledge or an omnibus measure of verbal IQ. In contrast, studies emphasizing the link between reading comprehension and oral language skills have tended to include measures of sentence-level comprehension or production.

Ultimately, this discussion leads us to question the value of attempts to identify "autism-specific" impairments of reading – or anything else for that matter. A more fruitful approach might be to focus on individual variation, within autism and across diagnostic groups (Brock 2011). In the case of reading, the aim should be to investigate and identify the factors that contribute towards good reading and reading comprehension, regardless of a child's diagnostic status. As Norbury and Nation (2011) point out, there is also much to be gained by considering reading comprehension in autism in the light of the extensive body of research on individual differences in non-autistic readers, where the link between reading comprehension and general language processes has long been recognised (e.g. Catts, Adlof, & Ellis-Weismer 2006; Hoover & Gough 1990). An important goal for future autism research is to determine the precise aspects of oral language that contribute to variation in reading comprehension – and the cognitive mechanisms that mediate this relationship.

References

Aaron, P.G., Frantz, S.S., & Manges, A.R. (1990). Dissociation between comprehension and pronunciation in dyslexic and hyperlexic children. *Reading and Writing, 2*, 243–264.

Adams, N.C. & Jarrold, C. (2009). Inhibition and the validity of the Stroop task for children with autism. *Journal of Autism and Developmental Disorders, 39*, 1112–21.

Asberg, J., Kopp, S., Berg-Kelly, K., & Gillberg, C. (2010). Reading comprehension, word decoding and spelling in girls with autism spectrum disorders (ASD) or attention-deficit/ hyperactivity disorder (AD/ HD): Performance and predictors. *International Journal of Language & Communication Disorders, 45*, 61–71.

Braeutigam, S., Swithenby S.J., Bailey A.J. (2008). Contextual integration the unusual way: A magnetoencephalographic study of responses to semantic violation in individuals with autism spectrum disorders. *European Journal of Neuroscience, 27*, 1026–36.

Brock, J. (2011). Complementary approaches to the developmental cognitive neuroscience of autism – Reflections on Pelphrey et al. (2011). *Journal of Child Psychology and Psychiatry, 52,* 645–646.

Brock, J., Norbury, C.F., Einav, S., & Nation, K. (2008). Do individuals with autism process words in context? Evidence from language-mediated eye-movements. *Cognition, 108,* 896–904.

Brock, J., Sukenik, N., & Friedmann, N. (2012). *Autistic Children's Reading of Homographs: Insights from Hebrew.* Manuscript submitted for publication.

Bryson, S.E. (1983). Interference effects in autistic children: Evidence for the comprehension of single stimuli. *Journal of Abnormal Psychology, 92,* 250–254.

Burnette, C.P., Mundy, P.C., Meyer, J.A., Sutton, S.K., Vaughan, A.E., & Charak, D. (2005). Weak central coherence and its relations to theory of mind and anxiety in autism. *Journal of Autism and Developmental Disorders, 35,* 63–73.

Campbell, R. & Besner, D. (1981). This and thap – Constraints on the pronunciation of new, written words. *Quarterly Journal of Experimental Psychology, 33,* 375 – 396.

Catts, H., Adlof, S.M., & Ellis-Weismer, S. (2006). Language deficits in poor comprehenders: A case for the Simple View of reading. *Journal of Speech, Language, and Hearing Research, 49,* 278–293.

Christ, S.E., Holt, D.D., White, D.A., & Green, L. (2007). Inhibitory control in children with autism spectrum disorder. *Journal of Autism and Developmental Disorders, 37,* 1155–1165.

Coltheart, M. (1978). Lexical access in simple reading tasks. In G. Underwood (Ed.), *Strategies of Information Processing.* London: Academic Press.

Dennis, M., Lazenby, A.L., & Lockyer, L. (2001). Inferential language in high-functioning children with autism. *Journal of Autism and Developmental Disorders, 31,* 47–54.

Elliott, C.D., Murray, D.J. & Pearson, L.S. (1979). *The British Ability Scales.* Slough, Bucks: NFER.

Eskes, G., Bryson, S., & McCormick, T. (1990). Comprehension of concrete and abstract words in autistic children. *Journal of Autism and Developmental Disorders, 20,* 61–73.

Frith, U., & Snowling, M. (1983). Reading for meaning and reading for sound in autistic and dyslexic children. *Journal of Developmental Psychology, 1,* 329–342.

Frith, U. (1989). *Autism: Explaining the Enigma.* Oxford: Blackwell.

Goldberg, M.C., Mostofsky, S.H., Cutting, L.E., Mahone, E.M., Astor, B.C., Denckla, M.B., et al. (2005). Subtle executive impairment in children with autism and ADHD. *Journal of Autism and Developmental Disorders, 35,* 279–293.

Happé, F.G.E. (1997). Central coherence and theory of mind in autism: Reading homographs in context. *British Journal of Developmental Psychology, 15,* 1–12.

Happé, F.G.E., & Frith, U. (2006). The weak coherence account: Detail-focused cognitive style in autism spectrum disorders. *Journal of Autism and Developmental Disorders, 36,* 5–25.

Healy, J.M., Aram, D.M., Horwitz, S.J., & Kessler, J.W. (1982). A study of hyperlexia. *Brain and Language, 9,* 1–23.

Henderson, L.M., Clarke, P.J., & Snowling, M.J. (2011). Accessing and selecting word meaning in autism spectrum disorder. *Journal of Child Psychology and Psychiatry, 52,* 964–973.

Hermelin, N., & O'Connor, N. (1970). *Psychological Experiments with Autistic Children.* Oxford: Pergamon Press.

Hobson, R.P., & Lee, A. (1989). Emotion-related and abstract concepts in autistic people: Evidence from the British Picture Vocabulary Scale. *Journal of Autism and Developmental Disorders, 19,* 601 – 623.

Hoover, W.A. & Gough, P.B. (1990). The simple view of reading. *Reading and Writing, 2,* 127–160.

Huemer, S. & Mann, V. (2010). A comprehensive profile of decoding and comprehension in Autism Spectrum Disorders. *Journal of Autism and Developmental Disorders, 40,* 485–493.

Huttenlocher, P., & Huttenlocher, J. (1973). A study of children with hyperlexia. *Neurology, 23,* 1107–1116.

Jarrold, C., & Brock, J. (2004). To match or not to match? Methodological issues in autism-related research. *Journal of Autism and Developmental Disorders, 34,* 81–86.

Jolliffe, T., & Baron-Cohen, S. (1999). A test of central coherence theory; linguistic processing in high-functioning adults with autism or Asperger's syndrome: Is local coherence impaired? *Cognition, 71,* 149–185.

Jones, C.R.G., Happé, F.G.E., Golden, H., Marsden, A.J.S., Tregay, J., Simonoff, E., Pickles, A., Baird, G., & Charman, T. (2009). Reading and arithmetic in adolescents with autism spectrum disorders: Peaks and dips in attainment. *Neuropsychology, 23,* 718–728.

Kamio, Y., Robins, D., Kelley, E., Swainson, B., & Fein, D. (2007). Atypical lexical/semantic processing in high-functioning Autism Spectrum Disorders without early language delay. *Journal of Autism and Developmental Disorders, 37,* 1116–22.

Kamio, Y., & Toichi, M. (2000). Dual access to semantics in autism: Is pictorial access superior to verbal access? *Journal of Child Psychology and Psychiatry, 41,* 859–867.

Kanner, L. (1943). Autistic disturbances of affective contact. *Nervous Child, 2,* 217–250.

Kaufman, A.S., & Kaufman, N.L. (1985). *Kaufman Test of Educational Achievement.* Circle Pines, MN: American Guidance Service.

Lockyer, L., & Rutter, M. (1969). A five to fifteen year follow-up study of infantile psychosis III. Psychological aspects. *British Journal of Psychiatry, 115,* 865–882.

Lopez, B.R., Lincoln, A.J., Ozonoff, S. & Lai, Z. (2005). Examining the relationship between executive functions and restricted, repetitive symptoms of Autistic Disorder. *Journal of Autism and Developmental Disorders, 35,* 445 – 460.

López, B., & Leekam, S.R. (2003). Do children with autism fail to process information in context? *Journal of Child Psychology and Psychiatry, 44,* 285–300.

McLeod, J. (1970). *GAP Reading Comprehension Test.* London: Heinemann Educational.

Minshew, N.J., Goldstein, G., & Siegel, D.J. (1995). Speech and language in high functioning autistic individuals. *Neuropsychology, 9,* 255–261.

Minshew, N.J., Goldstein, G., Taylor, H.G., & Siegal, D.J. (1994). Academic achievement in high functioning autistic individuals. *Journal of Clinical and Experimental Neuropsychology, 16*(2), 261–270.

Minshew, N.J., Goldstein G., Muenz L.R., Payton, J.B. (1992). Neuropsychological functioning in non-mentally retarded autistic individuals. *Journal of Clinical and Experimental Neuropsychology, 14,* 749–761.

Minshew, N.J., Goldstein, G., & Siegel, D. (1997). Neuropsychologic functioning in autism: Profile of a complex information processing disorder. *Journal of the International Neuropsychological Society, 3,* 303–316.

Nation, K., Clarke, P., Wright, B., & Williams, C. (2006). Patterns of reading ability in children with autism spectrum disorder. *Journal of Autism and Developmental Disorders, 36,* 911–919.

Neale, M.D. (1958). *Neale Analysis of Reading Ability.* London: Macmillan.

Neale, M.D. (1987). *Neale Analysis of Reading Ability – Revised.* Windsor: NFER-Nelson.

Newman, T.M., Macomber, D., Naples, A.J., Babitz, T., Volkmar, F., Grigorenko, E.L. (2007). Hyperlexia in children with autism spectrum disorders. *Journal of Autism and Developmental Disorders, 37,* 760–774.

Noens, I.L., & van Berckelaer-Onnes, I.A. (2005). Captured by details: Sense-making, language and communication in autism. *Journal of Communication Disorders, 38,* 123–141.

Norbury, C.F., & Nation, K. (2011). Understanding variability in reading comprehension in adolescents with autism spectrum disorders: Interactions with language status and decoding skill. *Scientific Studies of Reading, 15,* 191–210.

Norbury, C.F. (2005). Barking up the wrong tree? Lexical ambiguity resolution in children with language impairments and autistic spectrum disorders. *Journal of Experimental Child Psychology, 90,* 142–171.

Ozonoff, S., & Jensen, J. (1999). Brief report: Specific executive function profiles in three neurodevelopmental disorders. *Journal of Autism and Developmental Disorders, 29,* 171–177.

Ozonoff, S., & Miller, J.N. (1996). An exploration of right-hemisphere contributions to the pragmatic impairments of autism. *Brain and Language, 52,* 411–434.

Pijnacker, J., Geurts, B., Van Lambalgen, M., Buitelaar, J.K., & Hagoort, P. (2011). Reasoning with exceptions: An event-related brain potentials study. *Journal of Cognitive Neuroscience, 23,* 471–480.

Posner, M.I., & Snyder, C.R.R. (1975). Facilitation and inhibition in the processing of signals. In P.M.A. Rabbit & S. Dornic (Eds.) *Attention and performance.* New York, NY: Academic Press.

Rajendran, G., & Mitchell, P. (2007). Cognitive theories of autism. *Developmental Review, 27,* 224–260.

Richardson, J.T.E. (1975). Concreteness and imageability. *Quarterly Journal of Experimental Psychology, 27,* 235–249.

Rimland, B. (1964). Infantile Autism: the Syndrome and its Implications for a Neural Theory of Behavior. Chicago, IL: Appleton-Century-Crofts.

Ring, H., Sharma, S., Wheelwright, S. & Barrett, G. (2007). An electrophysiological investigation of semantic incongruity processing by people with Asperger's syndrome. *Journal of Autism and Developmental Disorders, 37,* 281–290.

Rutter, M., & Bartak, L. (1973). Special education treatment of autistic children: A comparative study. II Follow-up findings and implication for service. *Journal of Child Psychology and Psychiatry, 14,* 241–270.

Saldana, D., & Frith, U. (2007). Do readers with autism make bridging inferences from world knowledge? *Journal of Experimental Child Psychology, 96,* 310–319.

Schopler, E., Reichler, R.J., DeVellis, R.F., & Daly, K. (1980). Toward objective classification of childhood autism: Childhood Autism Rating Scale (CARS). *Journal of Autism and Developmental Disorders, 10,* 91–103.

Semel, E., Wiig, E., & Secord, W. (2006). *Clinical Evaluation of Language Fundamentals* (4th ed.). London: Harcourt.

Shah, A. & Frith, U. (1983). An islet of ability in autistic children- a research note. *Journal of Child Psychology and Psychiatry, 24,* 613–620.

Silberberg, N., & Silberberg, M. (1967). Hyperlexia – Specific word recognition skills in young children. *Exceptional Children, 34,* 41–42.

Snowling, M., & Frith, U. (1986). Comprehension in "hyperlexic" readers. *Journal of Experimental Child Psychology, 42,* 392–415.

Stroop, J. (1935). Studies of interference in serial verbal reactions. *Journal of Experimental Psychology, 18,* 643–662.

Toichi, M., & Kamio, Y. (2001). Verbal association for simple common words in high-functioning autism. *Journal of Autism and Developmental Disorders, 31,* 383–490.

Toichi, M. & Kamio, Y. (2003). Long-term memory in high-functioning autism: Controversy on episodic memory in autism reconsidered. *Journal of Autism and Developmental Disorders, 33,* 151–161.

Welsh, C.M., Pennington, B.F., & Rogers, S. (1987). Word recognition and comprehension skills in hyperlexic children. *Brain and Language, 32,* 76–96.

Williams, D.L., Goldstein, G., Minshew, N.J. (2006). Neuropsychologic functioning in children with autism: Further evidence of disordered complex information processing. *Child Neuropsychology, 12,* 279–298.

Woodcock, RN. (1987). *Woodcock Reading Mastery Tests-revised Examiner's Manual.* Circle Pines, MN: American Guidance Service.

CHAPTER 7

Language and literacy subtypes in young children with a high-functioning autism spectrum disorder

Diane Jacobs & Amanda Richdale
LaTrobe University

Individuals diagnosed with an Autism Spectrum Disorder (ASD) present with language and reading abilities that range from far below average to far above average. There is a lack of research investigating the classification of children diagnosed with a high-functioning ASD (HFASD) according to language and reading ability. The present study aimed to explore the language and reading profiles within a group of young children diagnosed with a HFASD and to establish whether or not the language and reading profiles identified within this group were similar to those seen in age-matched children without a diagnosis of ASD. The results showed that children diagnosed with a HFASD present with language and reading ability profiles similar to those of non-ASD peers. Furthermore, regression analyses revealed that the predictors of decoding and also reading comprehension were similar for children with HFASD and their non-ASD peers.

Introduction

High-functioning autism spectrum disorder (HFASD) is an umbrella term describing individuals with Autistic Disorder, Pervasive Developmental Disorder Not Otherwise Specified, or Asperger's Disorder who have a full scale IQ in the normal range (i.e. >70). Individuals diagnosed with Autistic Disorder exhibit early language delay, while for those with Asperger's Disorder there is no clinically significant language or cognitive delay; high-functioning individuals with PDDNOS may or may not have early language delay (American Psychological Association 2000). Individuals with HFASD are believed to have a better prognosis than those with an Autism Spectrum Disorder (ASD) and co-morbid intellectual disability. Despite this better prognosis, life-long problems are evident in the core areas required for a DSM-IV-TR (APA 2000) diagnosis, namely social relationships, social understanding and imagination, language and social communication, and adaptive functioning (Howlin 2003; Tager-Flusberg, Paul & Lord 2005).

Structural language skills in individuals with HFASD

Six speech-language subtypes have been identified within preschool and school-aged speech-language impaired populations with four of these (verbal auditory agnosia, phonologic-syntactic disorder, lexical-syntactic disorder, and semantic-pragmatic disorder) found in same-aged ASD populations (Rapin, Dunn, Allen, Stevens & Fein 2009). The phonologic-syntactic subtype parallels the deficits currently associated with specific language impairment (SLI), which refers to children aged 3 years and older who have a congenital language delay or disorder with no obvious accompanying condition. Whether or not some children with HFASD are phenotypically similar to children with SLI is a matter of debate (Leyfer, Tager-Flusberg, Dowd, Tomblin & Folstein 2008; Tager-Flusberg 2006; Whitehouse, Barry & Bishop 2007, 2008). Additionally, the language profiles of individuals diagnosed with a HFASD include those with adequate or advanced structural language skills that parallel those of typically developing peers (Rapin et al. 2009). Therefore, language profiles may not assist with the diagnosis of HFASD nor differentiate between Autistic Disorder, Pervasive Developmental Disorder Not Otherwise Specified, or Asperger's Disorder when full scale IQ is within the normal range. Instead, language deficits when present may be viewed as co-morbidity rather than core diagnostic symptomatology. That said, to date, no previous study has attempted to identify the full range of language profiles nor their accompanying literacy abilities in individuals with HFASD. The current study was designed to address this gap in the literature. Specifically, we sought to identify whether or not the range of language and literacy subtypes found within the typically developing population could be found within a group of young individuals with HFASD. We also sought to establish whether the same variables can be used to predict literacy ability in typically developing and HFASD groups.

Reading skills of individuals with a HFASD

Like spoken language skills, reading skills vary within the general population. Children with SLI may have a comorbid reading disability (Catts, Adolf, Hogan & Weismer 2005). Similarly, otherwise typically developing children may present with a specific reading disability (SRD) despite having at least average intelligence, intact perceptual skills, no frank neurological deficits, no socioemotional dysfunction, and no environmental differences or deprivation (Vellutino 1979). Most individuals with a diagnosis of SRD exhibit deficits in decoding or word recognition but comprehension problems can also co-occur (Adlof, Catts & Little 2006).

Approximately 10% of children aged 7 to 10 years who are otherwise typically developing exhibit poor reading comprehension with adequate decoding and are referred to as 'poor comprehenders' (Stothard & Hulme 1992).

The typical reading profile reported in HFASD is one of adequate decoding combined with impaired reading comprehension, that is, a 'poor comprehender' profile. For example, Minshew, Goldstein and Siegel (1995) reported age appropriate decoding scores (word and nonword reading) but low average passage comprehension for 62 HFASD individuals with a mean age of 17 years. Church, Alisanski, and Amanullah (2000) found that teachers reported good decoding but poor reading comprehension for children with Asperger's Disorder within the later primary school years. However, children with HFASD may also present with poor decoding (Manjiviona 2003; Mayes & Calhoun 2008), resembling children with SRD. Hence, two different reading impaired profiles comprising either poor reading comprehension or poor decoding can be identified in this population (which may exist in combination with poor comprehension although the studies cited did not report on comorbidity of decoding and comprehension difficulties aside from a single case study report in Manjiviona 2003).

Additionally, some individuals with HFASD have average or above decoding and reading comprehension. For example, Griswold, Barnhill, Myles, Hagiwara and Simpson (2002) reported average to significantly above average word reading and passage reading comprehension scores for some of 21 children and adolescents diagnosed with Asperger's Disorder. Similarly, Goldstein, Minshew and Siegel (1994) noted average or above decoding and reading comprehension scores for some children and adolescents with HFASD.

Predictors of reading

In typically developing children, cognition, visual perception, phonology, and spoken language have been identified as predictive of concurrent and future reading proficiency (Scarborough 1998; Swanson, Trainin, Necoechea & Hammill 2003). Visual perception and phonology have the strongest relationship with decoding whilst spoken language has the strongest association with reading comprehension. Moderate to large correlations have also been reported between full scale IQ and each of word reading, nonword reading, and reading comprehension (Scarborough 1998).

Decoding requires intact visual perceptual and phonological processing abilities. Visual perception is needed for print and word pattern recognition in order to identify and recall sight words using graphophonemic knowledge, whilst phonological processing skills are required for the detection and discrimination of phonemes which are then linked to graphemes (Ehri 2002). Phonological processing encompasses phonological awareness (PA), rapid automatised naming (RAN), and phonological memory (PM). PA is the discernment or overt appreciation of the phonological composition or sound structure of words within one's language (Torgeson, Wagner & Rashotte 1994). This enables individuals to link the spoken word form to its written representation (Gillon 2004) and is central to the development of decoding and spelling, thus allowing the comprehension and composition of written text. RAN involves the ability to rapidly and easily access and retrieve phonological information stored in long-term memory (Wolf & Bowers 1999). It requires the perception and identification of a visual stimulus and retrieval of its phonological representation from the lexicon. PM refers to the temporary encoding and storage of phonological information in short-term memory. It scaffolds the long-term acquisition of the phonological structure of language. Those with PM deficits may experience difficulty either learning the sound composition of new words or storing sounds when decoding longer words (Baddeley, Gathercole & Papagno 1998).

The majority of children with SRD, and children with SLI who have comorbid decoding problems, exhibit phonological processing deficits resulting in poor decoding (Catts et al. 2005). Conversely, a very small percentage of individuals experience decoding difficulties due to visual-perceptual deficits.

To understand written discourse, spoken language skills including syntactic, semantic, and narrative abilities are required (Catts, Fey, Zhang & Tomblin 1999). Semantic knowledge helps readers to predict upcoming words based on the comprehension of previously read material, whilst sensitivity to syntax supports decoding and comprehension via the use of linguistic context to predict upcoming sentence elements (Catts & Kamhi 2005). Narrative ability allows the reader to organise, predict, and interpret information at text level (Catts et al. 1999). Finally, pragmatic knowledge ensures that the higher-order language skills of analysis, evaluation, and problem solving combine with inferential rule knowledge to allow the 'old' information of general knowledge and understanding of the preceding text and its situational context to be combined with new text information (Tunmer & Hoover 1992).

Children diagnosed with SRD typically exhibit reduced comprehension of written material as a result of poor decoding ability rather than oral language comprehension difficulties (Adlof et al. 2006). Conversely, children diagnosed with SLI are at increased risk of reduced reading comprehension as a result of poor oral language comprehension skills with 50% or more identified as having poor reading comprehension (Catts & Kamhi 2005). Thus, children diagnosed with SRD present with a different language and reading ability profile than children diagnosed with SLI, while children with comorbid SLI-SRD will present with the combined profiles.

Literacy predictors in HFASD

The basis of adequate decoding ability in children with ASD remains unclear; both phonological and visual-based explanations have been examined. Frith and Snowling (1983) reported adequate nonword reading and correct morpho-phonological production (plural 's') for children with Autistic Disorder and concluded that those who could read did not have impaired phonological abilities. Similarly, Minshew et al. (1995) found that adolescents with HFASD had significantly better word attack skills, the ability to sound out nonsense and low frequency words, than typically developing controls matched for age and full scale IQ. Nonword and low frequency word reading is a skill often assessed in PA testing, hence this strength may reflect good PA skills in children with ASD.

More recent research has found poor PA skills in HFASD children compared with typically developing peers. Twenty-three HFASD children aged 5–12 years (Hooper, Poon, Marcus & Fine 2006), and 20 individuals aged 8–19 years (Newman, Macomber, Naples, Babitz, Volkmar & Grigorenko 2006) performed more poorly on PA composite tasks than did their typically developing peers. Likewise, Gabig (2010) reported that 14 children with autism aged 5 to 7 years performed significantly poorer than 10 same-aged, typically developing peers on two PA tasks, elision and sound blending tasks. PA was not related to word and nonword reading for the autism group. Thus, the relationship between PA and literacy is unclear for children with a HFASD.

In HFASD, verbal ability (verbal IQ and spoken language) is associated with PM. Average PM is reported for individuals with average language skill and below average PM for those with below average language ability (Bishop, Mayberry, Maley, Wong, Hill & Hallmayer 2004; Kjelgaard & Tager-Flusberg 2001). However no studies have investigated the predictive relationship of PM to literacy in individuals with ASD.

Studies examining RAN in individuals with HFASD have reported inconsistent results. Newman et al. (2006) reported that RAN in 20 young people with HFASD aged 8 to 19 years did not differ from those of younger typically developing students matched for word reading ability, whilst Hooper, Poon, Marcus and Fine (2006) found that 23 HFASD children aged 5–12 years performed poorer than same-aged peers. Hence, the RAN abilities in children with HFASD remain unclear.

Overall, the investigation of phonological processing in children with HFASD has produced varied results but PA abilities appear to be impaired in at least some individuals. It may be that HFASD individuals with poor phonological processing skills are also those who exhibit poor decoding abilities and thus have a SRD profile. Alternatively, it could be that for some individuals with HFASD skills other than phonological processing underpin good decoding. The most likely candidate is visual spatial skills.

Both visual memory and knowledge of visual-spatial relationships are visual perceptual skills and low-level visual perceptual abilities are reported to be a relative strength in HFASD. Some researchers have attributed the superior word and nonword decoding found in ASD to well-developed visual memory (Williams, Goldstein & Siegel 2006). Adequate ability has been found for immediate and delayed visual recognition and visuo-spatial short-term memory (Ozonoff & Strayer 2001; Williams et al.). Similarly, visual-spatial abilities as indicated by Wechsler IQ profiles have been reported as a strength in some children with HFASD (Siegel, Minshew & Goldstein 1996). Thus, superior word recognition skills in HFASD children may result from advanced visual memory ability rather than phonological processing skill. That said, both phonological processing and visual-perceptual skills may be important for decoding, just as they are for typically developing children. Whether or not both phonological processing and visual perception are associated with reading in HFASD is unknown.

Reading comprehension

Studies investigating the association between spoken language and reading comprehension indicate that reduced reading comprehension in ASD stems from semantic rather than syntactic deficits (Saldana, Carreiras & Frith 2009; Wahlberg & Magliano 2004). Individuals with ASD reportedly use syntactic but not semantic information to aid reading comprehension (Frith & Snowling 1983) and exhibit greater difficulty inferring information from text than typically developing peers, resulting in the breakdown of the comprehension of written information (Minshew et al. 1992; Rumsey & Hamburger 1988). Syntactic comprehension and expression are typically regarded as relative strengths in verbal children with ASD with development following a normal pattern, albeit at a reduced rate (Tager-Flusberg 1981a). Conversely, semantics is almost universally identified as an area of difficulty for individuals with ASD especially at sentence level. Particular deficits are noted for the comprehension of semantic relationships, figurative or non-literal language, inference, and ambiguous language (Lewis, Murdoch & Woodyatt 2007; Minshew et al. 1992).

Last, the impact of pragmatic language ability on reading comprehension is unknown. Pragmatic deficits are a hallmark of ASD with difficulties present across a range of contextual variations and settings and deficits greater than predicted by structural language abilities (Bishop & Norbury 2002; Volden, Coolican, Garon, White & Bryson 2009). That said, whether or not social language (pragmatics) or even structural language abilities (syntax, semantics) have the same relationship with reading comprehension for HFASD as in typically developing children is unknown.

The current study

For children with ASD, language and reading skill show similar patterns to those found in the general population; that is, typical, SRD, and SLI profiles are reported. However, whilst mixed language and reading profiles appear to exist in ASD, it is unknown whether children with HFASD show similar heterogeneity in their language and literacy profiles. Furthermore, no previous research has examined the predictors of both decoding and reading comprehension in a single sample of HFASD children. Hence, it is unknown whether the predictors of reading development are the same for HFASD children as they are in the broader population. These questions are pertinent to our understanding of the development of literacy in the HFASD population and the application of appropriate reading interventions when required.

The aims of this study were to: (1) Investigate the presence of language and reading subtypes within a young HFASD population; (2) Examine the predictors of reading in HFASD versus non-ASD samples.

Method

Participants

Children ($N = 168$) aged 6 to 8 years in their second (Year 1) or third (Year 2) of schooling participated in this study. There were four groups of children (HFASD, SRD, SLI, TD), each with 42 children (see Table 1). The groups did not differ significantly on age, $F(3, 164) = 1.10, p = .13$ or number of children in Year 1 or Year 2, $\chi^2(3) = .48, p = .92$. The groups did differ in the number of males and females in each group, $\chi^2(3) = 35.82, p < .001$, and number of children with English as a second language, $\chi^2(3) = 32.47, p < .001$. Examination of standardised residuals (> 2.0) showed that these differences were due to more boys in the HFASD group and more girls in the typically developing (TD) group, and more children with English as a second language background in the SLI group than in other groups. For those children exposed to two languages, SLI was diagnosed once it had been established that the child's skills in the non-English language were poorer than or equal to skills within the English language.

Table 1. Descriptive variables for the four diagnostic groups

	HFASD	SRD	SLI	TD
Age (months)	93.31 ± 8.46	95.07 ± 7.92	91.38 ± 7.22	91.76 ± 7.64
Males	38	26	32	13
Females	4	16	10	29
Year 1 (*n*)[1]	19	18	21	20
Year 2 (*n*)[2]	23	24	21	22
English Second Language	2	2	19	6

[1]Second year of school
[2]Third year of school

Diagnosis of HFASD was confirmed by examining the children's diagnostic reports. According to their reports, the children all had a score > 30 on the Childhood Autism Rating Scale (Schopler, Reichler & Renner 1998). All children were attending a mainstream primary school and the majority (34) received government funded integration support within the school system.

Three criteria were required for inclusion in the SRD group. First, children must have participated in The Reading Recovery Program, a federally funded reading intervention program, for Year 1 students with reading difficulties. Second, children had to have a current decoding difficulty defined as a reading accuracy score of at least 1.0 *SD* below the mean on the Neale Analysis of Reading Ability – Third Edition (Neale-III; Neale 1999), which is consistent with previous research (McArthur, Hogben, Edwards, Heath & Mengler 2000; Meyer, Wood, Hart & Felton 1998). Third, decoding difficulties had to occur in combination with at least average full scale IQ, which is also consistent with previous research (Rutter & Yule 1975; Vellutino, Scanlon & Lyon 2000).

At the time of their acceptance into the study all children in the SLI group had a diagnosis of severe language disorder by a Speech-Language Pathologist. The children met criteria for additional funded school support for severe language disorder:[1] (1) a score ≥ 2*SD* below the mean for the student's age on two standardised language tests; (b) the severity of the disorder could not be accounted for by hearing impairment, social emotional factors, English as a Second Language, or cultural factors; (c) a history of early language delay and difficulties; and (d) a nonverbal IQ ≤ 1.0 *SD* below the mean on two intellectual tests one of which had to be from one of the Wechsler scales.

1. Since this study was completed the criteria for funded school support for language disorder have changed and students must now have a score of ≥ 3*SD* below the mean on two standardised language tests

TD children had no identified concerns prior to, or at the point of entry into the study. All children had an average verbal IQ, nonverbal IQ, and full scale IQ as confirmed either prior to the study or during their participation in the study.

Materials

Full scale IQ was assessed using the Wechsler Abbreviated Scale of Intelligence (Wechsler 1999), or the Wechsler Pre-School and Primary Scale of Intelligence – Revised (Wechsler 1992), or the Wechsler Intelligence Scale for Children – Third edition (WISC-III; Wechsler 1991).

Visual perception was assessed using the Test of Visual-Perceptual Skills (non-motor) – Revised (Gardner 1996) (TVPS-R). The TVPS-R comprises seven subtests: Visual Discrimination, Visual Memory, Visual-Spatial Relationships, Visual Form-Constancy, Visual Sequential-Memory, Visual Figure-Ground, and Visual Closure, where test items involve abstract forms. Subtest items are scored as correct or incorrect and then summed and the scores are converted to standards score based on the individual's age. The seven, scaled scores are summed to calculate an overall visual perceptual quotient.

Three areas of spoken language were assessed: semantics, syntax, and pragmatics. Semantics and syntax examine structural language whilst pragmatics assesses social language. Semantics was assessed via the Peabody Picture Vocabulary Test-III (PPVT-III); Dunn & Dunn 1997), the Expressive Vocabulary Test (EVT; Williams 1997), the Clinical Evaluation of Language Fundamentals – Third Edition (CELF-3; Semel, Wiig & Secord 1995), and the Bus Story (Renfrew 1995).

The CELF-3 does not provide standard scores for semantics and syntax. Thus two subtests that specifically examined semantics, the Concepts and Directions subtest and the Word Classes subtest, were averaged to develop a semantics score. A Semantics Composite was then developed using the scores from CELF-3 semantics, PPVT, EVT, and the Bus Story information recall. CELF-3 semantics standard scores ($M = 10$, $SD = 3$) were converted as outlined in Sattler (2001) to be equivalent to those of the other semantics variables ($M = 100$, $SD = 15$). The four scores were then summed and averaged to form the new Semantics Composite. A Syntax Composite was developed by averaging the Sentence Structure, Word Structure, Recalling Sentences, and Formulated Sentences subtest scores from the CELF-3. This score ($M = 10$, $SD = 3$) was then converted as outlined in Sattler (2001) to have a mean of 100 and a *SD* of 15.

Pragmatics was examined using the Pragmatics Profile of Everyday Communication Skills in School-Aged Children (Dewart & Summers 1995). The profile provides qualitative, not normative data. To obtain comparison scores, the number of items on which parents identified adequate skill was summed for each participant giving a maximum score of 29 and a minimum score of 0. These scores were converted into percentages that were compared across groups. Higher percentage scores indicated better pragmatic ability.

The Comprehensive Test of Phonological Processing (CTOPP; Wagner, Torgesen & Rashotte 1999) and the Sutherland Phonological Awareness Test (SPAT; Neilson 1995) were completed as measures of PA. As both have the same *M* (100) and *SD* (15) results were summed and then averaged to form a single PA composite score. Additionally, the CTOPP was used to examine PM and RAN.

The Woodcock Reading Mastery Tests – Revised, Form G, (WRMT-R; Woodcock 1997) and the Neale-III (Neale 1999) measured reading ability at word and paragraph level respectively. A Decoding Composite was calculated by averaging the standard score results ($M = 100$, $SD = 15$) obtained from the Word Identification and Word Attack subtests from the WRMT-R and the Accuracy Scale of the Neale-III. A Comprehension Composite was formulated using the Word Comprehension subtest of the WRMT-R and the Comprehension Scale of the Neale -III. Neale-III standard scores were calculated using *M* and *SD* data provided within the test manual.

Procedure

Ethical approval was obtained from RMIT University Faculty of Applied Science Human Research Ethics Sub-Committee and the Department of Education and Training. Participants were volunteers obtained via schools, private practitioners, or advertisement.

Participants were assessed at the RMIT University Psychology Clinic, at their school, or in their home, depending on family preference. Children were tested in either a one-to-one situation or with a parent present. The children completed tests of cognition, visual-perception, phonological processing, formal language, and reading over two or three sessions ranging from 60 to 90 minutes in length, excluding breaks.

Analysis

To investigate group differences on a single dependent variable a single-factor between-subjects analysis of variance (ANOVA) was used. If a covariate was introduced analysis of covariance was conducted (ANCOVA). Group comparisons for conceptually related tasks were completed using a single-factor, between subjects, multivariate analysis of variance (MANOVA), or when a covariate was used, a multivariate analysis of covariance (MANCOVA). Multivariate analysis was used to protect against inflated Type 1 error from completing multiple ANOVA or ANCOVA tests for correlated dependent variables. Post-hoc testing of any relationships among the groups was completed using the Tukey HSD procedure for ANOVA and MANOVA, and pair-wise comparisons with Bonferroni adjusted α levels for ANCOVA and MANCOVA. Finally, hierarchical multiple regression analyses were conducted to assess the contribution of the following factors to decoding and reading comprehension for the HFASD and non-HFASD groups: cognition, visual perception, PA, PM, RAN, semantics, syntax, and pragmatic measures identified in the literature as possible predictors of literacy.

Results

To address the aims of the study and examine the presence of language and/or reading difficulties across the four original diagnostic groups (HFASD, SRD, SLI, and TD), language/reading ability groups were created. Regardless of their original diagnosis, children were assigned to language and reading ability groups on the basis of their current language (CELF-3 total score; CELF-T), Reading (Neale-III passage reading score) and nonverbal IQ (NVIQ) scores. Passage reading rather than word reading was chosen as this equates best to functional reading skill. Consistent with definitions used in previous research in the UK (Bishop & Edmundson 1987), USA (Catts 1993), Canada (Beitchman, Nair, Clegg, Ferguson & Patel 1986), and Australia (McArthur et al. 2000), CELF-T and Neale-III standard scores > 1 SD below the mean (< 85) were used to represent language and literacy impairment respectively.

Four ability groups were identified ('A' refers to ability group; ASLI, ASRD, ALIRD and ATD). Children with a: (1) CELF-T score of < 85, Neale-III accuracy score > 85, and a nonverbal IQ ≥ 85 were classified as ASLI, those with specific language impairment but no reading disorder ($n = 23$); (2) CELF-T > 85, Neale-III reading accuracy score < 85, and a nonverbal IQ ≥ 85 were classified as ASRD, those without specific language impairment but with a reading disorder ($n = 32$); (3) CELF-T and Neale-III reading accuracy score < 85 and a nonverbal IQ ≥ 85 were classified as combined language impairment-reading disability (ALIRD), those with both a specific language impairment and a reading disorder ($n = 47$); and (4) CELF-T and Neale-III reading scores above 85 and nonverbal IQ ≥ 85 were classified as ATD, those who were typically developing ($n = 63$). The original HFASD diagnostic group showed the greatest reading and language heterogeneity and was spread across the four language-reading ability groups. About a third of the original SRD group and two thirds of the original SLI group had both language and literacy deficits. One SRD child met criteria for SLI. It is important to note that three HFASD students with a nonverbal IQ < 85 were omitted from further analysis. It can be seen from Table 2 that 10 subgroups were formed. As there was only one SRD child in the ASLI group, this child was omitted from further analyses resulting in 9 subgroups.

Table 2. Cross-tabulation of the number of participants in each of the diagnostic and ability groups

Original diagnostic group	Ability group				Total (*n*)
	ASLI	ASRD	ALIRD	ATD	
HFASD	9	5	4	21	39
SRD	1	27	14	–	42
SLI	13	–	29	–	42
TD	–	–	–	42	42
Total (*n*)	23	32	47	63	165

Table 3 outlines the mean and *SD* on all measures for the 9 subgroups.

We examined the predictors of decoding and reading comprehension for HFASD versus non-ASD children. Given the small sample size for some diagnostic-ability groups and that a primary aim was to determine if the predictors of literacy ability in HFASD children was similar to that found in children in general, participants were grouped according to ASD status; (i.e. HFASD versus non-ASD) with both the HFASD and non-ASD groups comprising children from the varied ability groups (i.e. SLI, SRD, LIRD, and TD). Simple regression analyses were then run to identify the predictors of decoding and reading comprehension first for the non-ASD group ($n = 138$) and then for the HFASD group ($n = 39$).

As previous research has identified cognition as having a moderate correlation with literacy, full scale IQ was entered at step 1 of the analysis for decoding. Full scale IQ accounted for 32.3% of the variance in decoding for the HFASD sample and 38.2% of the variance for the non-ASD sample. PA was entered at step 2 as it has been identified as a significant predictor of decoding for non-ASD children; PA accounted for an additional 17.4% of the variance in decoding for the HFASD group and 21.3% for the non-ASD group. Once full scale IQ and PA were entered into the regression the remaining predictor variables were entered into the regression individually to establish whether or not they contributed any additional unique variance to the model. For the non-ASD group PM, RAN, and semantics each added a small amount of unique variance. Conversely, for the HFASD group no other predictor variables were significant. However, the amount of variance accounted for by PM and RAN for the HFASD group was similar to that of the non-ASD group. Hence, it could be that given a larger HFASD sample both PM and RAN would be identified as significant predictors of decoding for HFASD children too (see Table 4).

Table 3. Mean and SD of scores on cognition, visual-perception, language, and literacy tests for the 9 ability subgroups

Measures[1]	ASLI		ASRD		ALIRD			ATD	
	HFASD ($n = 9$)	SLI ($n = 13$)	HFASD ($n = 5$)	SRD ($n = 27$)	HFASD ($n = 4$)	SLI ($n = 29$)	SRD ($n = 14$)	HFASD ($n = 21$)	TD ($n = 42$)
Full scale IQ	86.67 (4.58)	86.69 (6.74)	98.80 (7.79)	94.04 (5.52)	84.75 (5.25)	84.21 (6.75)	90.79 (3.93)	103.41 (12.69)	104.48 (12.89)
TVPS-R	79.00 (8.79)	106.54 (13.44)	101.80 (28.84)	99.44 (16.23)	80.00 (18.85)	95.52 (18.38)	98.86 (14.58)	113.75 (17.53)	117.12 (11.63)
PA	98.83 (16.29)	88.31 (10.61)	98.70 (22.30)	91.93 (11.47)	88.63 (12.59)	78.97 (11.89)	88.57 (15.96)	111.28 (15.29)	110.06 (15.31)
PM	90.67 (8.28)	80.54 (6.84)	85.60 (11.70)	94.89 (11.68)	82.00 (10.10)	80.97 (6.63)	87.14 (10.49)	100.33 (12.60)	100.57 (11.69)
RAN	97.00 (28.67)	106.00 (8.03)	89.80 (13.18)	97.11 (11.39)	83.50 (6.25)	94.83 (12.95)	88.36 (17.46)	106.94 (10.62)	107.83 (9.71)
Semantics	81.85 (9.17)	74.62 (5.38)	94.80 (6.12)	86.49 (7.87)	74.34 (2.51)	76.24 (8.84)	82.59 (4.87)	98.88 (9.93)	99.34 (9.97)
Syntax	6.36 (1.23)	4.71 (.87)	9.60 (2.21)	9.30 (1.11)	4.50 (1.36)	5.14 (1.34)	7.13 (.82)	10.89 (2.07)	10.92 (2.20)
Pragmatics[2]	38.62[3] (23.31)	52.59[4] (8.20)	38.62[5] (9.25)	70.42[6] (14.14)	38.79[7] (15.77)	55.32[8] (17.18)	75.43[9] (18.47)	76.63[10] (25.96)	92.81[11] (9.69)
Decoding	96.89 (6.54)	93.95 (5.68)	89.00 (9.74)	87.14 (6.05)	86.42 (4.27)	83.03 (5.76)	84.86 (6.57)	110.70 (14.85)	109.23 (13.31)
Reading Comprehension	89.78 (9.20)	86.92 (4.76)	86.20 (8.02)	84.83 (4.05)	80.75 (2.90)	79.86 (4.85)	83.04 (5.19)	103.87 (14.23)	104.04 (13.41)

[1] higher score equals better performance for all measures,
[2] percentage scores,
[3] $n = 5$
[4] $n = 12$
[5] $n = 5$
[6] $n = 27$
[7] $n = 4$
[8] $n = 24$
[9] $n = 8$
[10] $n = 19$
[11] $n = 35$

Table 4. Regression models for decoding for the HFASD and non-ASD groups

	HFASD ($n = 39$)	Non-ASD ($n = 138$)
Variable entered	**Variance**	**Variance**
Full scale IQ	32.3%	38.2%
PA	17.4% (48.5%)	21.3% (59.5%)
PM	2.3% (ns)	2.5% (61.7%)
RAN	5.2% (ns)	5.3% (64.6%)
Semantics	<1% (ns)	3.4% (62.7)
Syntax	<1% (ns)	<1% (ns)
Visual-perception	4.7% (ns)	1.2% (ns)

For reading comprehension, decoding was entered at step 1 as decoding is requisite for the comprehension of written material; it accounted for 74.8% of the variance in reading comprehension for the HFASD sample and 82.6% of the variance for the non-ASD sample. Once decoding was entered at step 1 the ability of the remaining variables to independently account for any additional variance was explored with each variable entered separately at step 2 even if this resulted in a non-significant outcome. For the HFASD sample PA, semantics, and syntax accounted for a significant proportion of additional variance whilst for the non-ASD group full scale IQ, semantics, and syntax made additional unique contributions (see Table 5).

Table 5. Regression models for reading comprehension for the HFASD and non-ASD groups

	HFASD ($n = 39$)	Non-ASD ($n = 138$)
Variable entered	**Variance**	**Variance**
Decoding	74.8%	82.6%
Full scale IQ	<1% (ns)	4.5% (87%)
PA	4.2% (78.4%)	<1% (ns)
PM	<1% (ns)	<1% (ns)
RAN	<1% (ns)	<1% (ns)
Semantics	7.5% (81.9%)	3.1% (85.6%)
Syntax	4.4% (78.5%)	3.1% (85.6%)

Discussion

The first aim of this study was to examine language and literacy subtypes within young children diagnosed with a HFASD as previous research had identified a great deal of variability in language and reading skills within this population (Jones et al.

2009; Mayes & Calhoun 2008; Tager-Flusberg 2006; Rapin et al. 2009). Our results revealed that HFASD children presented with language and reading profiles that parallel those reported for non-ASD children. That is, specific reading disability (SRD), specific language impairment (SLI), deficits associated with both SLI and SRD, and average or above average language and reading abilities were found. Hence, language and reading skills of HFASD children in the early years of school are heterogenous, just as they are in the broader population of young children.

The second aim was to examine the predictors of literacy in children with HFASD as compared with non-ASD children. Full scale IQ and phonological awareness accounted for the majority of the variance in decoding scores for children with HFASD as well as children who did not have HFASD. Decoding accounted for almost all the variance in reading comprehension in both groups of children. Overall, there were few differences in predictors of reading between children with and without a diagnosis of HFASD.

Comparisons between the HFASD children with SLI versus the non-ASD children with SLI were particularly noteworthy considering the interest in specific language deficits that are present in some children diagnosed with an ASD (Kjelgaard & Tager-Flusberg 2001; Tager-Flusberg 2006; Whitehouse et al. 2007, 2008). In the present study HFASD children with SLI appeared to perform better than non-ASD children with SLI on syntax and phonological memory (which incorporated a nonword repetition task), two measures purported to specifically identify SLI. This finding may be in contrast with those of Tager-Flusberg (2006) and Whitehouse et al. (2008) who reported that there were no group differences between ASD children with SLI and non-ASD children with SLI. Two explanations are possible. First, the SLI participants in the current study most likely had lower structural language skills than SLI participants in the Tager-Flusberg (2006) and Whitehouse et al. (2008) studies due to differences in the definition of SLI used. Many researchers diagnose SLI on the basis of receptive or expressive or composite language scores of 1.0 or 1.25 *SD* below the mean (Catts et al. 2005; Fey 1986; Flax et al. 2003; Lee 1974; Paul 1995; Silva 1980). In our study children met diagnostic criteria that required language scores to be at least 2.0 *SD* below the mean. Hence, our children with SLI are likely to be more impaired than SLI children reported in many previous studies. We acknowledge that the sample sizes in some of our sub groups were modest and that the ratio of males to females and the proportion of those who spoke English as a second language varied across sub groups. It would be preferable for future research to address these concerns before any firm conclusions can be drawn.

Second, phonological memory has been linked to verbal IQ and language ability, in particular vocabulary (a measure of semantics) (Bishop et al. 2004; Tager-Flusberg 2006). In the present study, HFASD children with comorbid SLI had better semantic skills than non-ASD children diagnosed with SLI. Thus, the superior phonological memory abilities of the HFASD children compared with the SLI group parallels their superior semantic abilities. As such, our findings align with previous research showing that phonological memory is related to general verbal ability and differences may disappear if differences in language (in particular semantics) are controlled for (Kjelgaard & Tager-Flusberg 2001).

The children with HFASD and comorbid SLI did not differ from non-ASD children with SLI on pragmatics, even though pragmatic impairment is mandatory for a diagnosis of HFASD but not SLI. The similarity in pragmatic impairment may also be associated with the greater level of language impairment present in our SLI participants compared with children in previous SLI research. The similar level of pragmatic impairment is also consistent with problems in differential diagnosis between SLI and ASD children noted by others, especially in the early years (Howlin 1998; Stone et al. 1999).

Reading skills also did not differentiate between children with HFASD and comorbid SLI versus non-ASD children with SLI despite the better phonological memory (linked with decoding) and syntax (linked with reading comprehension) scores found for the HFASD children with SLI. However the non-ASD children with SLI performed better than the HFASD children with SLI on visual perception. Visual contextual clues are associated with word pattern recognition in the early stages of reading development (Frith 1995). The non-ASD children with SLI may be relying on visual rather than phonological skills for reading, which will become untenable as reading demands increase. Hence, the literacy abilities of children with HFASD and comorbid SLI may improve more than that of non-ASD children with SLI in the middle to upper primary school years. A longitudinal study could identify if this occurs.

With regard to literacy skills in children with HFASD we have demonstrated for the first time that literacy development parallels that found in the broader population of children in the early school years. Literacy development in young HFASD children may be typical, that is average to above average, or it may be impaired as found for children with a specific reading disability or children with a combined reading disability and language impairment. In particular, we have shown that decoding skills have similar underpinnings in HFASD as in other children and that decoding is of primary importance for reading comprehension in young children with HFASD as it is in other young children. This is consistent with research showing that children with HFASD may have poor decoding skills (Manjiviona 2003; Mayes & Calhoun 2008) and that decoding and reading comprehension vary from below to above average in ASD (Griswold et al. 2002). We found no evidence that visual-perceptual skills may underpin reading in children with HFASD as has been suggested by some researchers (Williams et al. 2006). Indeed it was only in the non-ASD SLI group that we found any evidence for visual-perceptual skills being important for early reading.

This is the first study to report on the predictors of literacy development in young children with HFASD as compared with children with a specific reading disability, a specific language impairment, or children who are typically developing. Future research could examine whether or not the variety of language and reading ability types identified for HFASD children within the early primary school years continue to be identified in the later primary school years, into the secondary school period, and then into adulthood. Longitudinal research is also required to identify whether or not stability exists with regard to ability group membership. Do HFASD children remain within the same language and reading ability group throughout their school years or does movement occur across the ability groups identified here with time? If movement occurs, which children show such movement would be important to identify as it may have implications for early intervention for language and literacy development. For example, in a study of 242 children diagnosed with SLI attending a language unit in the United Kingdom, Conti-Ramsden and Botting (1999) found that whilst the range of speech-language impairment subgroups identified in children with SLI remained stable across a one year period, between subgroup movement was notable with 45% of children changing subgroups. It is unclear if this will also occur in children with HFASD within the language and reading ability groups identified here.

Conclusions

The findings of our study demonstrate that young school-age children diagnosed with a HFASD are a heterogenous group with language and literacy skills that parallel the development found in other children in the same age range. The variables of IQ, visual-perception, and oral language predict early literacy development. For all children, full scale IQ and phonological awareness are the most important skills for the development of decoding skills, accounting for over 50% of the variance in decoding, while decoding accounts for 75% to 80% of the variance in early reading comprehension.

References

Adlof, S.M., Catts, H.W., & Little, T.D. (2006). Should the simple view of reading include a fluency component? *Reading and Writing, 19*, 933–958.

American Psychological Association. (2000). *The Diagnostic and Statistical Manual of Mental Disorders, Fourth Edition, Text Revision.* Washington, DC: Author.

Baddeley, A.D., Gathercole, S.E., & Papagno, C. (1998). The phonological loop as a language learning device. *Psychological Review, 105* (1), 158–173.

Beitchman, J.H., Nair, R., Clegg, M., Ferguson, B., & Patel, P.G. (1986). Prevalence of psychiatric disorders in children with speech and language disorders. *Journal of the American Academy of Child Psychiatry, 25*(4), 528–535.

Bishop, D.V.M., & Edmundson, A. (1987). Language impaired 4-year-old: Distinguishing transient from persistent impairment. *Journal of Speech and Hearing Disorders, 52*, 156–173.

Bishop, D.V.M., Mayberry, M., Maley, A., Wong, D., Hill, W., & Hallmayer, J. (2004). Using self-report to identify the broad phenotype in parents of children with autistic spectrum disorders: a study using the Autism-Spectrum Quotient. *Journal of Child Psychology and Psychiatry, 45*(8), 1431–1436.

Bishop, D.V.M., & Norbury, C.F. (2002). Exploring the borderlands of autistic disorder and specific language impairment: A study using standardised diagnostic instruments. *Journal of Child Psychology and Psychiatry, 43*(7), 917–929.

Catts, H.W., Adlof, S.M., Hogan, T.P., & Weismer, S.E. (2005). Are specific language impairment and dyslexia distinct disorders? *Journal of Speech, Language, and Hearing Research, 48*(6), 1378–1396.

Catts, H.W., & Kamhi, A.G. (2005). *Language and Reading Disabilities* (2nd ed.). Boston, MA: Allyn and Bacon.

Catts, H.W., Fey, M.E., Zhang, X., & Tomblin, J.B. (1999). Language basis of reading and reading disabilities: Evidence from a longitudinal investigation. *Scientific Studies of Reading, 3*(4), 331–361.

Church, C., Alisanski, S., & Amanullah, S. (2000). The social, behavioral, and academic experiences of children with Asperger syndrome. *Focus on Autism and Other Developmental Disabilities, 15*(1), 12–20.

Conti-Ramsden, G., & Botting, N. (1999). Classification of children with specific language impairment: Longitudinal considerations. *Journal of Speech, Language, and Hearing Research, 42*(5), 1195–1204.

Dewart, H., & Summers, S. (1995). *The pragmatics profile of everyday communication in school-aged children*. Windsor: NFER Nelson.

Dunn, L.M., & Dunn, L.C. (1997). *Examiners Manual for the Peabody Picture Vocabulary Test (PPVT)* (3rd ed.). Circle Pines, MN: American Guidance Service.

Ehri, L. (2002). Reading processes, acquisition, and instructional implications. In G. Reid & J. Wearmouth (Eds.), *Dyslexia and literacy: Theory and Practice* (pp. 167–185). West Sussex, UK: John Wiley and Sons.

Fey, M.E. (1986). *Language Interventions with Young Children*. San Diego, CA: College Hill Press.

Flax, J.F., Realpe-Bonilla, T., Hirsch, L.S., Brzustowicz, L.M., Bartlett, C.W., & Tallal, P. (2003). Specific language impairment in families: Evidence for co-occurrence with reading impairments. *Journal of Speech, Language, and Hearing Research, 46*(3), 530–543.

Frith, U. (1995). Dyslexia: Can we have a shared theoretical framework? *Educational and Child Psychology, 12*(1), 6–17.

Frith, U., & Snowling, M. (1983). Reading for meaning and reading for sound in autistic and dyslexic children. *British Journal of Developmental Psychology, 1*(4), 329–342.

Gabig, C.M. (2010). Phonological awareness and word recognition in reading by children with autism. *Communication Disorders Quarterly, 31*(2), 67–85.

Gardner, M.F. (1996). *Test of Visual-perceptual Skills (Non-motor) – Revised*. Hydesville, CA: Psychological and Educational Publications.

Gillon, G. (2004). *Phonological Awareness*. New York, NY: The Guilford Press.

Goldstein, G., Minshew, N.J., & Siegel, D.J. (1994). Age differences in academic achievement in high-functioning autistic individuals. *Journal of Clinical and Experimental Neuropsychology, 16* (5), 671–680.
Griswold, D.E., Barnhill, G.P., Myles, B.S., Hagiwara, T., & Simpson, R.L. (2002). Asperger syndrome and academic achievement. *Focus on Autism and Other Developmental Disabilities, 17*(2), 94–102.
Hooper, S.R., Poon, K.K., Marcus, L., & Fine, C. (2006). Neuropsychological characteristics of school-age children with high-functioning autism: Performance on the NEPSY. *Child Neuropsychology, 12*, 299–305.
Howell, D.C. (2007). *Fundamental Statistics for the Behavioural Sciences.* London: Wadsworth.
Howlin, P. (1998). Practitioner review: Psychological and educational treatments for autism. *Journal of Autism and Developmental Disorders, 39*(3), 307–322.
Howlin, P. (2003). Outcome in high-functioning adults with autism with and without early language delays: Implications for the differentiation between autism and Asperger syndrome. *Journal of Autism and Developmental Disorders, 33*(1), 3–13.
Jones, C.R.G., Happe, F., Golden, H., Marsden, A.J.S., Tegay, J., Simonoff, E., et al. (2009). Reading and arithmetic in adolescents with autism spectrum disorders: Peaks and dips in attainment. *Neuropsychology, 23*(6), 718–728.
Kjelgaard, M.M., & Tager-Flusberg, H. (2001). An investigation of language impairment in autism: Implications for genetic subgroups. *Language and Cognitive Processes. Special Issue: Language and Cognitive Processes in Developmental Disorders, 16*(2–3), 287–308.
Lee, L. (1974). *Developmental Sentence Analysis.* Evanston, IL: Northwestern University Press.
Lewis, F.M., Murdoch, B.E., & Woodyatt, G.C. (2007). Communicative competence and metalinguistic ability: Performance by children and adults with autism spectrum disorder. *Journal of Autism and Developmental Disorders, 37*, 1525–1538.
Leyfer, O.T., Tager-Flusberg, H., Dowd, M., Tomblin, J.B., & Folstein, S.E. (2008). Overlap between autism and specific language impairment: Comparison of autism diagnostic interview and autism diagnostic observation schedule scores. *Autism Research, 1*, 284–296.
Manjiviona, J. (2003). Assessment of specific learning difficulties. In M. Prior (Ed.), *Learning and Behavior Problems in Asperger Syndrome.* New York, NY: The Guilford Press.
Mayes, S.D., & Calhoun, S.L. (2008). WISC-IV and WIAT-II profiles in children with high-functioning autism. *Journal of Autism and Developmental Disorders, 38*, 428–439.
McArthur, G.M., Hogben, J.H., Edwards, V.T., Heath, S.M., & Mengler, E.D. (2000). On the "specifics" of specific reading disability and specific language impairment. *Journal of Child Psychology and Psychiatry, 41* (7), 869–874.
Minshew, N.J., Goldstein, G., Muenz, L.R., & Payton, J.B. (1992). Neuropsychological functioning nonmentally retarded autistic individuals. *Journal of Clinical and Experimental Neuropsychology, 14*(5), 749–761.
Meyer, M.S., Wood, F.B., Hart, L.A., & Felton, R.H. (1998). Selective predictive value of rapid automatized naming in poor readers. *Journal of Learning Disabilities, 31*(2), 106–117.
Minshew, N.J., Goldstein, G., & Siegel, D.J. (1995). Speech and language in high-functioning autistic individuals. *Neuropsychology, 9*(2), 255–261.
Neale, M.D. (1999). *Neale Analysis of Reading Ability* (3rd ed.). Melbourne: ACER Press.
Neilson, R. (1995). *Sutherland Phonological Awareness Test.* Jamberoo, NSW: Private publication.
Newman, T.M., Macomber, M., Naples, A.J., Babitz, T., Volkmar, F., & Grigorenko, E.L. (2006). Hyperlexia in children with autism spectrum disorders. *Journal of Autism and Developmental Disorders, 37*(4), 760–774.

Ozonoff, S., & Strayer, D.L. (2001). Further evidence of intact working memory in autism. *Journal of Autism and Developmental Disorders, 31*(3), 257–263.

Paul, R. (1995). *Language Disorders from Infancy Through Adolescence. Assessment and Interventions* (1st ed.). St Louis, MO: Mosby.

Rapin, I., Dunn, M., Allen, D.A., Stevens, M.C., & Fein, D. (2009). Subtypes of language disorders in school-aged children with autism. *Developmental Neuropsychology, 34*(1), 66–84.

Renfrew, C. (1995). *The Bus Story: A Test of Continuous Speech.* Bicester Oxon: Winslow.

Rumsey, J.M., & Hamburger, S.D. (1988). Neuropsychological findings in high-functioning men with infantile autism, residual state. *Journal of Clinical and Experimental Neuropsychology, 10*(2), 201–221.

Rutter, M., & Yule, W. (1975). The concept of specific reading retardation. *Journal of Child Psychology and Psychiatry, 16*, 181–197.

Saldana, D., Carreiras, M., & Frith, U. (2009). Orthographic and phonological pathways in hyperlexic readers with autism spectrum disorders. *Developmental Neuropsychology, 34*(3), 240–253.

Sattler, J.M. (2001). *Assessment of Children: Cognitive Applications.* San Diego, CA: Jerome M. Sattler.

Scarborough, H.S. (1998). Early identification of children at risk for reading disabilities. phonological awareness and some other promising predictors. In B.K. Shapiro, P.J. Accardo, & A.J. Capute (Eds.), *Specific Reading Disability. A View of the Spectrum* (pp. 75–119). Timonium, MD: New York Press.

Schopler, E., Reichler, R.J., & Renner, B.R. (1998). *Childhood autism rating scale.* Los Angeles, CA: Western Psychological Services.

Semel, E.M., Wiig, E.H., & Secord, W. (1995). *Clinical Evaluation of Language Fundamentals* (3rd ed.). San Antonio, TX: The Psychological Corporation.

Siegel, D.J., Minshew, N.J., & Goldstein, G. (1996). Wechsler IQ profiles of high-functioning autism. *Journal of Autism and Developmental Disabilities, 26*, 389–406.

Silva, P.A. (1980). The prevalence, stability, and significance of developmental language delay in preschool children. *Developmental Medicine and Child Neurology, 22*(6), 768–777.

Stone, W.L., Lee, E.B., Ashford, L., Brissie, J., Hepburn, S.L., Coonrod, E.E., et al. (1999). Can autism be diagnosed accurately in children under 3 years? *Journal of Child Psychology and Psychiatry, 40*(2), 219–226.

Stothard, S.E., & Hulme, C. (1992). Reading comprehension difficulties in children. The role of language comprehension and working memory skills. *Reading and Writing: An Interdisciplinary Journal, 4*, 245–256.

Swanson, H.L., Trainin, G., Necoechea, D.M., & Hammill, D.D. (2003). Rapid naming, phonological awareness, and reading: A meta-analysis of the correlation evidence. *Review of Educational Research, 73*(4), 407–440.

Tager-Flusberg, H. (1981). On the nature of linguistic functioning in early infantile autism. *Journal of Autism and Developmental Disorders, 11*(1), 45–56.

Tager-Flusberg, H. (2006). Defining language phenotypes in autism. *Clinical Neuroscience Research, 6*, 219–224.

Tager-Flusberg, H., Paul, R., & Lord, C. (2005). Language and communication in autism. In F. Volkmar, R. Paul, A. Klin, & D.J. Cohen (Eds.), *Handbook of Autism and Pervasive Developmental Disorders: Diagnosis, Development, Neurobiology, and Behavior* (3rd ed., Vol. 1, pp. 335–364). New York, NY: Wiley.

Torgesen, J.K., Wagner, R.K., & Rashotte, C.A. (1994). Longitudinal studies of phonological processing and reading. *Journal of Learning Disabilities, 27*(5), 276–286.

Tunmer, W.E., & Hoover, W.A. (1992). Cognitive and linguistic factors in learning to read. In P.B. Gough, L.C. Ehri & R. Treiman (Eds.), *Reading Acquisition* (pp. 175–214). Hillsdale, NJ: Lawrence Erlbaum Associates.

Vellutino, F.R. (1979). *Dyslexia. Theory and Research.* Cambridge, MA: The MIT Press.

Vellutino, F.R., Scanlon, D.M., & Lyon, G.R. (2000). Differentiating between difficult-to-remediate and readily remediated poor readers: More evidence against the IQ-achievement discrepancy definition of reading disability. *Journal of Learning Disabilities, 33,* 223–238.

Vickers, A.J. (2005). Parametric versus non-parametric statistics in the analysis of randomised trials with non-normally distributed data. *BMC Medical Research Methodology, 5,* 35–47.

Volden, J., Coolican, J., Garon, N., White, J., & Bryson, S. (2009). Brief report: Pragmatic language in autism spectrum disorder: Relationships to measures of ability and disability. *Journal of Autism and Developmental Disorders, 39,* 388–393.

Wagner, R.K., Torgesen, J.K., & Rashotte, C.A. (1999). *Comprehensive Test of Phonological Processing* (*CTOPP*). Austin, TX: PRO-ED.

Wahlberg, T., & Magliano, J.P. (2004). The ability of high function individuals with autism to comprehend written discourse. *Discourse Processes, 38*(1), 119–144.

Wechsler, D. (1991). *The Wechsler Intelligence Scale for Children, Third edition* (*WISC-III*). San Antonio, TX: Harcourt Assessment.

Wechsler, D. (1989). *The Wechsler Pre-school and Primary Scale of Intelligence – Revised* (*WPPSI-R*). San Antonio, TX: Harcourt Assessment.

Wechsler, D. (1999). *The Wechsler Abbrieviated Scale of Intelligence.* San Antonio, TX: Harcourt Assessment.

Whitehouse, A.J.A., Barry, J.G., & Bishop, D.V.M. (2007). The broader language phenotype of autism: A comparison with specific language impairment. *Journal of Child Psychology and Psychiatry, 48*(8), 822–830.

Whitehouse, A.J.A., Barry, J.G., & Bishop, D.V.M. (2008). Further defining the language impairment of autism: Is there a specific language impairment subtype? *Journal of Communication Disorders, 41,* 319–336.

Williams, T. (1997). *Expressive Vocabulary Test* (*EVT*). Circle Pines, MN: American Guidance Service.

Williams, D.L., Goldstein, G., & Minshew, N.J. (2006). The profile of memory function in children with autism. *Neuropsychology, 20*(1), 21–29.

Wolf, M., & Bowers, P.G. (1999). The double-deficit hypothesis for the developmental dyslexias. *Journal of Educational Psychology, 91*(3), 415–438.

Woodcock, R. (1987). *Woodcock Reading Mastery Tests – Revised.* Circle Pines, MN: American Guidance Services.

SECTION 4

Complex Language Skills

CHAPTER 8

The use of narrative in studying communication in Autism Spectrum Disorders

A review of methodologies and findings

Lesley Stirling[1], Susan Douglas[1], Susan Leekam[2] & Lucy Carey[3]
[1]The University of Melbourne / [2]Cardiff University / [3]Durham University

The construction and communication of narratives is a fundamental and distinctive aspect of our human experience. Investigation of narrative language has been used extensively in studying the impairments in language, communication and cognitive functioning associated with Autism Spectrum Disorders (ASDs). However the field has been characterized by a high degree of inconsistency in research findings and difficulty in drawing clear conclusions about narrative abilities in this diverse clinical population. For a range of measures, studies can be identified which have shown impairments in the narrative abilities of children with ASDs, while other studies show no significant differences when compared with neurotypical populations. In this article we critically review studies of language and communication in ASDs which include narrative data. We consider the range of methodologies used and some of the theoretical assumptions which have shaped these. We also review the findings from the studies and the potential impact that choice of methodological techniques may have had on these results. We address the kind of narrative data studied, the nature of the task used to elicit it, and the modality of presentation of stimulus materials. We provide a definitive picture of the state of play in narrative research on ASDs and propose directions for future research.

The purpose of this review is to survey and evaluate the ways in which narrative language data has been used in the study of language and communication in Autism Spectrum Disorders (ASDs),[1] and the claims which have consequently

1. In discussion of specific studies we use the terminology for diagnostic classification used by the authors. More generally, we speak of "Autism Spectrum Disorder(s)", abbreviated as "ASD(s)", to encompass the broad range of diagnostic classifications included in the review studies. See Section 2.

been made about the narrative abilities of individuals with these disorders. We thus consider both the use of narrative as a tool in studying autism and ASDs, and also the findings which have been reported to date concerning the profile of abilities and deficits which individuals with ASDs display.

The only previous review to take a similar focus was undertaken by Loveland and Tunali, whose 1993 article presented an appraisal of narrative language in autism from the perspective of the Theory of Mind hypothesis. At this time, Loveland and Tunali noted that there were very few studies of narrative in autism, stating that "It is difficult to draw conclusions from the existing studies relating to narrative in autism, because of the variety of methods, purposes and data examined" (p. 248–249). Almost twenty years later, we consider that it is instructive to properly survey the field once again. While it remains true to say that methodological variations make an evaluation of the research findings a complex business, in our view there is much to learn from a detailed investigation of these variations and the findings they have given rise to.

In the following section, we describe what we mean by "narrative", consider the specific contribution the study of narrative discourse can offer in clinical domains, and outline some of the ways in which narrative language data have been included in studies of ASDs, and indeed of other clinical populations. We then present a literature review of narrative in ASD, focusing in particular on the large body of studies that have elicited narratives using visual stimuli such as picture books. We consider methodological issues that could contribute to inconsistencies in the literature and attempt to draw out consistent themes across the studies. We also briefly consider other methods of narrative elicitation in studies of ASD before discussing the present state of the field and directions for future research.

What is narrative?

There are substantial bodies of literature on narrative and storytelling from a range of disciplinary perspectives, including literary studies, linguistics, and anthropological and sociological research. Here we take a linguistic approach. "Narrative" can be understood as a genre, or type of discourse, involving the relation of a sequence of events.[2] This broad definition allows for a range of sub-genres of narrative to be identified (Polanyi 1989).

2. On some definitions, "narrative" is equated with "story", while other researchers make distinctions in their usage of these terms. We use the two terms interchangeably in this article.

Loveland and Tunali (1993) divided narrative into the sub-genres of: (1) story narrative (either original or retellings); (2) script narrative (e.g. accounts of rituals, or routines); (3) informative/didactic narratives (e.g. giving directions); and (4) recitations/performances (e.g. reciting a learned piece of text). Then, as now, the most frequently investigated sub-genre has been the story narrative.

As a genre of discourse, narrative is usually considered to contrast with other major types of use of language, such as conversation or expository discourse. In particular, narrative monologue and naturally occurring conversational interaction are often contrasted as representing distinct types of language use, with potentially significant differences in the language phenomena they exhibit. However, "conversational narratives" do occur – that is, narratives arising within the flow of a conversational interaction, and potentially jointly constructed by the interactants.

A similarity between conversation and narrative is that both occur very early in children's language development. Many have argued for the ontogenetic and phylogenetic priority of face-to-face conversational interaction. Such interactions are the primary form of linguistic and communicative engagement, the first type of language to which children are exposed, universal across all linguistic communities, and the type of language which most of us use most frequently throughout our lives. However narrative too is considered to be a universal type of language use and it is one which children are generally exposed to and begin to engage in themselves at a very young age. In this regard, it is second only to conversational interaction in its linguistic and communicative primacy, supporting its widespread use in studies of language and communication. Neurotypical children begin to engage in narrative discourse at a very young age, although their narrative abilities continue to develop until at least the age of nine or ten (Berman 2009).

The construction and communication of narratives seems to be a fundamental aspect of our human experience. As individuals we construct our experience of the world as narration and we use narrative to communicate with others about the world (e.g. Bruner 1991). There are strong similarities across cultures with regard to the overall structure and character of narrative communication, despite some subtle differences such as the role of evaluative comments in the narrative and the organisation of the story (Scollon & Scollon 1981). Narrative competence is thus recognised as a key component of personal identity and social functioning in all human communities.

As an early and pervasive form of discourse, narrative enables researchers to take a global focus on linguistic development which moves beyond the scope of the single utterance in gathering language samples (Berman 2009; Miller & Sperry 1988; Ninio 1988). Narrative production tasks have been used extensively to collect samples of connected language for many different purposes within research contexts examining language and communication. They also form part of the expressive language sampling protocols in measures used by clinicians to test for language impairment and for disorders such as autism (e.g. Autism Diagnostic Observation Schedule; Comprehensive Evaluation of Language Fundamentals). In these cases, it is not the narrative form of the language produced which is in focus, rather narrative is used as a convenient vehicle for collecting relatively fluent and naturalistic language data from participants for subsequent evaluation. It has the added advantage that it can be subject to constraints which make the data collected more readily comparable across participants, for instance retelling of the same story stimulus. Conversational language has been used much less frequently for this purpose. There may be an assumption that monologic data will provide an optimally comprehensive sample of an individual's speech, uncomplicated by the interactional nature of conversational language, where relative contributions of subject and interlocutor (often experimenter or clinician) may be more difficult to control. Narrative also tends to offer a potentially complete and self-contained chunk of language data, in the form of a bounded story.

An important consideration when studying narrative in clinical populations is that it is a complex cognitive task. It is well understood that conversational interaction involves a complex range of skills and behaviours, including the most basic ability to coordinate turn-taking with the interlocutor, as well as control over sequential relevance of contributions made and topic maintenance, shift and coordination. Narrative, too, involves its own distinct complex cognitive and linguistic demands, varying in accordance with the type of narrative at issue (Hudson & Shapiro 1991). In all cases, the production of narrative discourse requires the ability to relate a set of events which are sequentially organised in time and space. Generally, a story world needs to be constructed and maintained including the different perspectives and psychological states of the story characters and potentially the narrator. Depending on the task, the narrator may also be required to:

a. remember a segment of personal autobiographical experience and construct a narrative based on this;
b. remember a previously heard/read and comprehended story and construct a narrative based on this;
c. construct a narrative based on an understanding of nonverbal, visual input: an image or sequence of images to which the narrator is or was exposed;
d. use imagination and intertextual resources from memory to construct a novel creative narrative, with varying degrees of additional constraint (e.g. provided by a topic, title or stem).

The expectation has been that the study of narratives will further our understanding of language and cognition and potentially inform the development of assessment tools and therapeutic interventions for children with atypical language (see Botting 2002). Indeed, narrative has been studied in a range of clinical populations including Specific Language Impairment (SLI) (reviewed in Liles 1993), Down Syndrome (e.g. Reilly, Klima & Bellugi 1990; Chapman et al. 1998) and Williams syndrome (Reilly et al. 1990; Stojanovik 2006). For these studies, narrative is not simply a convenient way to collect language samples, rather it is considered important that the language is elicited in narrative form precisely due to the specific cognitive and linguistic abilities associated with this genre. A number of these studies have provided evidence for the diagnostic and prognostic value of narrative over and above analysis of language generally. For example, in the literature on SLI, performance on the Renfrew Bus Story task has been argued to be predictive of persistent linguistic impairment (Bishop & Edmondson 1987; Stothard et al. 1998). Liles et al. (1989) showed that apparently recovered traumatic brain injury patients who scored well on standardized language tests might nevertheless have difficulties with coherent discourse production as measured by narrative elicitation tasks.

Why might narrative provide us with unique insights into ASDs? The core deficits of ASDs and the cognitive theories proposed to explain these lead us naturally to some specific hypotheses about expected profiles of narrative ability and deficit in this population. For example, narrative has been considered an ideal environment in which to test for Theory of Mind deficits. Competent narration requires abilities of character building and perspectivising (telling the story from the spatial and/or psychological viewpoint of a character or narrator), including the identification and description of psychological states and motives, and it also involves construction of the narrative in line with expectations about audience knowledge. These abilities have been assumed by researchers to presuppose an understanding that individuals may have differing beliefs and viewpoints consequential for social behaviour (cf. e.g. Astington 1990). From a different perspective, good narratives are usually assumed to have a coherent global structure and message which may be particularly demanding for people with ASDs if they have a cognitive preference for local over global processing. The requirements of coordinating and integrating information involved in many narrative production tasks might also cause specific difficulties for a group considered to have problems with executive functioning.

However, studies of narrative in ASDs have given rise to a wide variety of findings, some of which appear inconsistent. Furthermore, a persistent theme in work on narrative and autism is the idea that the narratives of children with autism are "different", but that it is hard to pin down what makes them so using the standard metrics and analyses. This is touched on as an aside in some published work and arises anecdotally in personal communication between researchers. Thus

Diehl et al. (2006) noted that, although researchers have described the narratives of children with autism as unusual and idiosyncratic, few quantitative differences have been found between the narratives of children with high-functioning ASDs and matched control groups (e.g. Bruner & Feldman 1993; Loveland et al. 1990; Loveland & Tunali 1993).

Scope and methodology of the review

In conducting this review we adopted an inclusive approach with regard to clinical populations and diagnostic categories, taking into account any study of children or adults with a Pervasive Developmental Disorder, including in particular diagnostic classifications of "autism" or "autism disorder", "autism spectrum disorder", and "Asperger syndrome". We speak generally of "ASDs".

A literature search was undertaken to identify all peer-reviewed articles or publically available research dissertations on narrative and ASDs which had been published up until the beginning of 2011. A keyword search was done of relevant databases including PsycINFO and Linguistics and Language Behavior Abstracts (LLBA) using the search string "*narrative* OR *story* AND *autis**". The resulting set of references was augmented with additional materials identified from other sources, including reference lists of included works.

While our search identified studies of both language comprehension and production, our focus in this article will be on production studies, or on the production findings from studies investigating both. However it is important to note that many narrative production tasks indirectly test for comprehension also, in that they make use of stimulus stories which participants are asked to understand, recall and retell. For this reason, findings concerning the profile of abilities and deficits in narrative comprehension among populations with ASDs are relevant to our interpretation of the findings from narrative production studies in these populations.

Just as narrative production involves a specific range of linguistic and cognitive skills, so too does narrative comprehension, and the focus of studies of narrative comprehension has generally been to test the ability of the participants, often children, to understand the global structure and import of a story and in particular the causal relationships and evaluative "point" or moral that it has. There is evidence from some of these studies that the approach of children with autism to narrative comprehension tasks differs from that of neurotypical children in ways yet to be fully understood. For example a study by Norbury and Bishop (2002) suggested that children with autism experience difficulty with the global structure of narratives which affects their ability to comprehend a story.

However, in keeping with the pattern we will observe for narrative production studies, narrative comprehension studies have shown conflicting results. For example, some studies have suggested that children with autism are impaired at recognising mental states as motivators for character actions (Begeer, Malle, Nieuwland & Keysar 2010; Jiao 2001; Losh & Capps 2003; Ruffman, Garnham & Rideout 2001). If children do not recognise motivations for character actions in stimulus stories, we might expect this to affect the quality of their story retellings. However, Grant, Boucher, Riggs and Grayson (2005) found that children with autism were as likely as the control groups to judge the culpability of protagonists in the stories on the basis of motive (although they noted that the justifications offered by the children with autism for their judgements were of poor quality and typically reiterated the story).

To further constrain the scope of this review, we exclude from consideration sub-areas of research on intervention studies, including a dynamic body of work using computational resources (Davis, Dautenhahn, Nehaniv & Powell 2004; Ho, Davis & Dautenhahn 2009; Tartaro & Cassell 2006), as well as research on narrative use in testing protocols, and work on social stories (Gray 2000).

Literature review of elicited narrative studies

Table 1 below summarises the main features which have been investigated in a core body of research on narrative production in ASDs, consisting of a corpus of twenty-three studies published since the early 1980s. These studies involve experimental elicitation of oral narratives from ASD groups matched with comparison groups, where the controlled elicitation environment is intended to facilitate comparison of the stories produced. The table indicates whether the features analysed were found to be significantly different in the ASD group as compared to control groups. More detail is provided in Table 2, in the Appendix, which summarises the characteristics of this corpus of studies in full detail, including the participant groups and the type of methodology used to elicit the narratives.

The features identified were examined in these studies with a view to investigating the language abilities and deficits and the general cognitive abilities, deficits and "style" of people with ASDs. We categorise the features in accordance with the way they are discussed in the papers reviewed. The three main categories of analyses have considered (1) the length and complexity (particularly grammatical complexity) of the stories; (2) a range of phenomena which have been seen as indicative of ability to create a cohesive text, such as reference tracking, use of time and tense marking, and overt indication of causal relations between elements of the story; and (3) a range of phenomena associated (depending on the study) with Theory of Mind abilities and/or abilities to present a perspective on the story events described. Use of causal language can be seen to fall under category (3) as well as (2) so we treat it separately here. A number of studies refer collectively to a group of linguistic features identified as 'Evaluation' and grouped together on the basis that they all encode aspects of the narrator's view on the action (cf. Labov & Waletzky 1967; Bamberg & Damrad-Frye 1991; Reilly et al. 1998). These include such features as representation of character speech and thought, indication of causality and motivation, and linguistic highlighting of the important parts of the story. Presence of such features has often been taken as indicative of Theory of Mind ability as well as of greater sophistication in narration more generally.

Table 1. Major features and findings from oral narrative production studies. Asterisks indicate studies where the comparison group was not neurotypical

Main features analysed	Not significantly different in ASD group	Significant differences found for ASD group
Length and complexity		
Story length	*Loveland et al. 1990 Tager-Flusberg & Sullivan 1995 Losh & Capps 2003 Norbury & Bishop 2003 Diehl et al. 2006 *Seung 2007	Thurber & Tager-Flusberg 1993 Tager-Flusberg 1995 Capps et al. 2000 Klin 2000
Complexity	Diehl et al. 2006	Tager-Flusberg 1995 Capps et al. 2000
Cohesion measures		
Referential cohesion	*Seung 2007	Norbury & Bishop 2003 Colle et al. 2008
Time and tense	Goldman 2008	*Seung 2007 Colle et al. 2008
Focus on minor details of story OR problems with global coherence/gist of story		Waterhouse & Fein 1982 *Loveland et al. 1990 Diehl et al. 2006 (in production)
Causal language		
Presence, frequency or type of causal language	Baron-Cohen et al. 1986 (presence) Tager-Flusberg & Sullivan 1995 Norbury & Bishop 2003 Colle et al. 2008	Tager-Flusberg 1995 (frequency) Capps et al. 2000 (type of) Losh & Capps 2003 (type of) Diehl at al. 2006 (in production) Beaumont & Newcombe 2006

(Continued)

Table 1. (Continued)

Main features analysed	Not significantly different in ASD group	Significant differences found for ASD group
Other features associated with Theory of Mind/ perspectivisation		
Use of mental state language	Tager-Flusberg & Sullivan 1995 Beaumont & Newcombe 2006 Colle et al. 2008 *Garcia-Perez et al. 2008	Baron-Cohen et al. 1986 Begeer et al. 2010
Use of emotion language	Tager-Flusberg & Sullivan 1995	Pearlman-Avnion & Eviatar 2002 Brown et al. 2012
Ability to shift perspectives		*Garcia-Perez et al. 2008
Use of character speech	Tager-Flusberg 1995	Capps et al. 2000
Use of sound effects or onomatopoiea	Tager-Flusberg 1995	Capps et al. 2000
Amount of 'evaluation' overall	Capps et al. 2000. Norbury & Bishop 2003	Losh & Capps 2003
Range or type of evaluative devices		Capps et al. 2000 Losh & Capps 2003
Other findings		
Accuracy of story recall		Gabig 2008 Estigarribia et al. 2011
Subjective evaluation of story qualities by raters	Waterhouse & Fein 1982	De Marchena & Eigsti 2010
Perseveration		Waterhouse & Fein 1982 (supported by Martin 2009, Stirling et al. 2007a)
Use of 'bizarre' language		*Loveland et al. 1990
Use of non-grammatical pauses		Thurber & Tager-Flusberg 1993

As indicated in Table 1, studies of narrative production in autism have given rise to a range of apparently contradictory findings. For more than half of the linguistic features analysed across the range of studies, one can identify both publications showing ASD groups to behave differently from comparison groups, and publications showing no significant differences between groups. Nevertheless, more detailed investigation of study design and methodology can throw some light on these differences. We now discuss this core body of studies in detail, focusing first on a number of methodological issues, and then describing the main themes emerging from the findings. Overwhelmingly, the studies captured by this literature review investigate oral narrative (re)tellings elicited on the basis of visual or visual plus verbal stimuli, and these will be the focus of our discussion. Later we also consider a smaller body of work using alternative methodologies including elicitation of autobiographical or imaginative narratives as well as written narratives, functional neuroimaging, and qualitative research on more naturalistic data.

Methodological issues

Characteristics of ASD groups

Almost all the studies considered in this review are characterised by relatively small group sizes, as is clear from Table 2 in the Appendix: ASD groups range in size from four to 34, with group sizes of 20 or more in only eight studies. Researchers frequently mention this as a limitation of the study and for some studies, results which approach but do not reach significance may have done so with more power (e.g. see the comments in Diehl et al. 2006). Given the known heterogeneity of the ASD population, our developing understanding of the phenotypes, and explicit indication of great variation in results within groups for many studies, this feature remains a potential explanation for the kinds of variation observable in Table 1 independent of any other factors. Only continuing work with larger sample sizes and further exploration of individual variance will address this concern.

A further issue for some studies has been coverage of a wide age range of participants. Diehl et al. (2006) point out that a broad range of participants in terms of age increases the heterogeneity of the group, especially when considering the long time course of narrative development and significant changes in narrative ability which occur in childhood and early adolescence in neurotypical children (citing Bamberg 1987 as a supporting reference).

Studies further differ somewhat in focal diagnostic group, although the constraint that participants need to have sufficient language to attempt a narrative puts a lower bound on level of functioning. Most of the studies surveyed (14 of them) explicitly consider High Functioning Autism and/or Asperger Syndrome. Three studies compare HFA and AS groups (Klin 2000; Seung 2007; Craig & Baron-Cohen 2000).

Comparison group

The majority of studies include a comparison group consisting of neurotypical individuals. Other comparison groups include groups identified as having SLI, Pragmatic Language Impairment (PLI), Down syndrome, Intellectual Disability,

Developmental Delay, or Williams syndrome, with a handful of studies including more than one comparison (e.g. Norbury & Bishop 2003).

There is a strong suggestion in the literature surveyed that more rigorous matching of comparison groups in later studies has resulted in fewer observed differences in narratives produced and a clearer picture of atypicalities which do seem to be more specifically linked to autism as distinct, for instance, from more general cognitive and learning difficulties. Diehl et al. (2006) comment that when groups are closely matched on language, differences on measures of narrative ability disappear (they cite Tager-Flusberg & Sullivan 1995 as an example). Losh and Capps (2003) observe that previous studies had examined narrative in groups with limited cognitive abilities and proposed that focusing on a high-functioning group evidenced a pattern of narrative performance more like that of neurotypical groups. In this regard, some researchers have advocated the importance of comparison with both neurotypical controls and other, non-autistic, clinical groups (Diehl et al. 2006), even as other writers have cautioned about the complexities of matched group designs (Jarrold & Brock 2004). While most studies do include a comparison group of neurotypical children or adults, observed patterns in autism groups might be more confidently attributable to this disorder if there were larger scale norming studies of the phenomena at issue within the typically developing population as a whole.

Task design differences

The potential effects of subtle and apparently irrelevant changes in methodology have long been a focus of attention in work on child language development generally (e.g. Crain & Thornton 1998 on felicity conditions in test protocols). In relation to narrative production, Berman (2004: 265) noted that "...the general pattern of development will be affected by the communicative and cognitive demands evoked in different settings of narrative text production. This means that children may reveal more knowledge of narrative structure and they will perform the act of storytelling better in some situations than in others". Given the wide range of methods used in studies of narrative in ASD, the contradictory pattern of results is perhaps unsurprising.

As noted above, the majority of studies reviewed here have elicited narratives via the presentation of visual stimuli such as picture books. However, there have been other approaches. For example, Craig and Baron-Cohen (2000) elicited an imaginary story and a reality-based story based on verbally presented themes, Goldman (2008) elicited personal autobiographical stories based on a bounded set of specific verbally given topics, and Brown et al. (2011) asked children to relate the earliest event they remember.

Even within the studies using visual stimuli, there are important methodological differences. One such difference is the nature of the visual stimulus. Three studies used single images to elicit stories (Beaumont & Newcombe 2006; Garcia-Perez et al. 2008; Waterhouse & Fein 1983). Others have used puppet shows (Loveland, McEvoy & Tunali 1990) or animations of interacting geometric figures (Klin 2000; Seung 2007). However, most of the studies considered here used some kind of picture sequence such as the wordless picture story books *Frog, Where Are You?* (Mayer 1969) and *Frog On His Own* (Mayer 1973). In these studies, participants were shown a series of pictures and were invited to tell a story to an experimenter based on these. The picture sequence was designed to be linked by and elicit an implicit narrative by virtue of the depiction of the same characters, related places, and action development considered to indicate causality and temporal progression. In providing a narrative based on the pictures, study participants had to be able to understand the pictures and recognise the need to provide a sequenced interpretation of them rather than a picture by picture description.

One major difference across studies is whether verbal input is provided in addition to the visual stimulus. In some cases the verbal input available was in the form of a structured story. For example, the Renfrew Bus Story (Cowley & Glasgow 1994), used in two studies, involves a sequence of twelve pictures accompanied by a story read to the participants by the researchers. Inclusion of a verbal model of the story changes the task to involve remembering or re-constructing a previously heard/read and comprehended story. In other cases, the narrative was (apparently) derivable in a more complex way from verbal interactions between characters in dramatised stories.

Another potentially important aspect of task design may be the children's understanding of the knowledge state of their audience. Elicitation protocols for retelling of stories vary as to whether the children are asked to tell the story to the same experimenter who had originally shown them the book (Capps et al. 2000; Losh & Capps 2003; Norbury & Bishop 2003), or to another experimenter who they believe to be unfamiliar with the book (Loveland et al. 1990; Tager-Flusberg 1995; Thurber & Tager-Flusberg 1993). Such differences might be expected to affect aspects of "recipient design". For example, one study where the child could assume the experimenter knew the stimulus story (Capps et al. 2000) reported reduced use of evaluative devices such as character speech and sound effects by the autism group as compared with the typically developing children. However, otherwise similar methodologies using a task design assuming an unfamiliar audience found no group differences on these measures (Tager-Flusberg 1995; Thurber & Tager-Flusberg 1993), plausibly revealing different assumptions made by the comparison groups depending on this aspect of the context of interaction.

Application of analytical measures

In some cases group comparisons are made on the basis of composite scores using quantification of heterogeneous collections of linguistic features, thus increasing the danger that they may not be applied consistently across studies; this is the case for the concept of 'Evaluation'. For other linguistic phenomena, such as causal language, comparison across studies is complicated by differences in the ways these are measured. Losh and Capps (2003) and Diehl et al. (2006) found differences between ASD and typical groups on causal connections in narratives, whereas Tager-Flusberg and Sullivan (1995) along with others found no such differences. However, different metrics were used to investigate causality in these studies. Tager-Flusberg and Sullivan (1995) used a metric based on identified instances of use of lexical items with causal meaning, such as *so* and *because*, whereas the two later studies both used more elaborated metrics involving number and type of causal connections or nature of causal explanations. Furthermore, the often-assumed relationship between quantitative analysis of linguistic features (such as counts of mental state verbs) and cognitive abilities (such as "Theory of Mind") remains to be properly articulated and grounded at a theoretical level.

Emerging themes

Length and complexity of narratives

In Tager-Flusberg's (1995) study, children with autism and control groups of children with Down syndrome and neurotypical children were asked to tell the story of *Frog, Where Are You?* to an experimenter who had not previously seen it, with minimal supporting prompts. Tager-Flusberg (1995) found that the narratives produced by the children with autism were shorter and less complex than both control groups. Capps, Losh and Thurber (2000) used the related story *Frog On His Own* to examine the narrative skills of children with autism and control groups of children with developmental delays and neurotypical children matched on language ability and IQ. The children with autism produced shorter narratives than the typically developing children, and the stories of both clinical groups contained a greater proportion of morphological errors and less complex syntax than the neurotypical children's stories. Similar results were reported by Klin (2000) using the Social Attribution Task (Heider & Simmel 1944) in which participants watch a short video containing geometric figures enacting a social plot, then produce a narrative describing the events depicted in the video. Klin found that the adults with high functioning autism and Asperger Syndrome produced considerably shorter narratives than the control group of neurotypical adults.

However, other studies have failed to find group differences in length or complexity of narratives (Losh & Capps 2003; Norbury & Bishop 2003; see also Loveland et al. 1990). Diehl, Bennetto and Young (2006) suggested that while some of the studies finding differences may have done so because they included wide age ranges and ability levels, some of those studies which failed to differentiate between autism and control groups provided a higher degree of cognitive scaffolding in the design of the task, such as allowing children to look at the picture book while producing their narratives. They deliberately chose a different mode of stimulus presentation in their study – the participants listened to an audiotaped verbal narration of the *Frog, Where Are You?* story while looking through the book. In a further departure from previous studies, the participants were required to tell the story to the experimenter without the aid of the picture book. Despite the methodological changes, the results of their study revealed no differences between groups in terms of story length and complexity and no difference in the use of story gist (essential events of the story) to aid recall or in sensitivity to the importance of story events.

Coherence and cohesion of narratives

A more consistent theme within these studies is that individuals with ASD have difficulty maintaining the coherence of narratives. Waterhouse and Fein (1982) reported that, although experienced teachers could not readily discriminate between the narratives produced by different groups, those produced by children with autism tended to focus on the minor details of the story. Similarly, Loveland et al. (1990) noted that, when recalling a puppet show or film clip, some of the participants with autism seemed to experience difficulty in recognising the story as a set of meaningful events (similar to Peng's (1988) study of Japanese children with autism).

Further evidence comes from studies using the *"Frog"* picture books. Norbury and Bishop (2003) found no differences between children with autism, Specific Language Impairment, Pragmatic Language Impairment, and typically developing children, in terms of their use of causal connectives such as *so* and *because* (see also findings for causal language in Baron-Cohen et al. 1986; Tager-Flusberg 1995; and Tager-Flusberg & Sullivan 1989). However, participants with ASD were significantly more impaired in the referential cohesion of their narratives, demonstrating poor use of anaphora. Diehl, Bennetto and Young (2006) found no difference between typically developing and autistic children in their recall of gist (main) events of the story. However, in contrast to control participants, the overall connectedness of the stories by the children with ASDs was not significantly correlated with their recall of gist events. Colle, Baron-Cohen, Wheelwright and van der Lely (2008) found that adults with autism or Asperger Syndrome produced less cohesive stories than the control group of typically developing adults, reflected in more ambiguous use of pronouns and limited use of temporal expressions.

Mental state language

Finally, a range of studies have looked for evidence of differential Theory of Mind abilities in the type of language used in participants' narratives. Baron-Cohen, Leslie, and Frith (1986) tested children with autism on a picture sequencing task in which participants had to arrange a set of pictures in order and then tell a story based on the sequence. Compared with control groups of Down syndrome and typically developing children, those with autism had difficulty with sequences that involved mental states. Furthermore, while they used causal language in their narratives (e.g. *because* clauses, explicit mention of agency, causative constructions such as "made X happen"), they very rarely used mental state language.

The finding of reduced mental state language was replicated in a study by Pearlman-Avnion and Eviatar (2002), who found children with autism included fewer emotional elements than children with Williams syndrome and typically developing controls. However, other studies have failed to find significant group differences on measures of mental state language (Beaumont & Newcombe 2006; Colle et al. 2008; Norbury & Bishop 2003). For example, Tager-Flusberg and Sullivan (1995) found no differences in use of emotion or mental state related words between children with autism and typically developing or intellectually disabled control children.

Begeer, Malle, Nieuwland and Keysar (2010) suggested that the lack of significant results in some of these studies reflects a ceiling effect. They endeavoured to construct richer and more demanding task conditions on which competent performance required use of mental state language. Participants listened to a narrative about interaction and then retold it, without the support of any visual stimulus during the retell, arguably placing a greater cognitive load on the participants. Adolescents and adults with autism produced fewer mental state terms in their narratives when compared with the typically developing controls.

Two studies by Capps and colleagues have employed more sophisticated indices of mental state use in narratives. In the first study (Capps, Losh & Thurber 2000), children with autism were less likely than typically developing children to embed emotion descriptions within a causal frame and more likely to focus on character *behaviour* (although the same was also true of non-autistic children with developmental delay). Moreover, narrative ability in the autism group was correlated with Theory of Mind abilities (see also Tager-Flusberg & Sullivan 1995). The second study revealed a subtly different pattern of results

(Losh & Capps 2003). Children with high functioning autism or Asperger syndrome displayed limited use of causal language for both internal states *and* character behaviour, and narrative ability was associated with performance on measures of emotional understanding rather than Theory of Mind ability (see also Slaughter, Peterson & Mackintosh 2007).

Finally, García-Pérez, Hobson and Lee (2008) adopted Feffer's (1970) role-taking task in which participants are required to tell and re-tell stories from the perspectives of different protagonists using a single picture stimulus. Participants with autism (mean age 13;04) performed similarly to a control group of children without autism (mean age 14;02 matched on language) in the use of mental state language. However, their ability to adopt the different protagonists' perspectives and to navigate between the various viewpoints was significantly poorer.

Alternative methodologies

The studies considered in detail in the previous section provided visual or visual plus verbal stimuli to elicit roughly comparable sets of oral story (re)constructions or retellings from ASD and comparison groups (narrative Types b and c listed in the introduction). We next consider a number of alternative approaches.

Imaginative narratives

Craig and Baron-Cohen (2000) provided an imaginary theme (condition 1) and a reality-based theme (condition 2) to children with autism, children with Asperger Syndrome and control groups of neurotypical children and children with intellectual disabilities, and asked them to tell a story. The children with autism and Asperger Syndrome were less likely to include imaginative elements in their reality-based stories and the children with autism experienced more difficulty than the other groups in producing an imaginative narrative, leading the authors to conclude that the results of their study supported a theory of imaginative impairment in storytelling by children on the autism spectrum.

Personal experience narratives and autobiographical memory

A small but growing area of research ties an interest in narrative production to autobiographical memory of individuals with ASDs. This type of narrative requires participants to "remember a segment of personal autobiographical experience and construct a narrative based on this" (Type a listed in the introduction). Capps et al. (2000) and Losh and Capps (2003) both included one condition of this type and other studies focusing on autobiographical narrative include Capps et al. (1998),

Ehlers (2008), Goldman (2008) and Brown et al. (2012). All of these studies found differences in the personal experience narratives produced by individuals with ASDs centred on the sophistication of narratives with regard to features such as narrative high-point, psychological state terms and character reference.

Qualitative ethnographic research on naturalistic narratives

A few research projects have collected audio or video-recorded communicative interactions involving individuals with ASDs in more naturalistic settings than those represented in Tables 1 and 2, which all used purposive elicitation of narrative (see Solomon 2008). Prominent among these is the large study undertaken by Ochs and colleagues in Los Angeles, where conversational interactions involving children with ASDs in family and school settings were recorded (see Ochs & Solomon 2004). Soloman (2004) reports results of a study of the conversational narratives that arise in these data and finds that, while the children with autism did participate in conversational storytelling, and exhibited competence in introducing narratives into the interaction, they had difficulty in global organisation of the narrative co-telling. Sirota (2010a, b) used naturalistic audio- and video-taped data from the same study to discuss everyday narratives of personal experience as offering vehicles for children's subjective and intersubjective participation in family life. The children with autism displayed socio-communicative difficulties which were evident in their narratives, for example sometimes exhibiting delayed or absent responses when encouraged to engage in interactive narrative activity, and needing painstaking scaffolding from their parents in order to employ personal narrative for the purposes of self-reflection, as might typically occur in family dinner table conversation.

Written narratives

In their review of narrative research in autism, Loveland and Tunali commented that "It is unusual to encounter written narratives by autistic people" (p. 254), and research studies considering the written modality remain underrepresented compared to oral modality production studies. This is despite a growing body of autobiographical writing by adults with ASDs, which arguably provides a corpus of spontaneously produced material for further study: in a survey of these writings, Rose (2008) cited a web source indicating that there are more than 50 autistic autobiographies in print. One of the earliest research articles on written narrative production by people with autism does in fact draw on such sources: Happé (1992) examined three pieces of autobiographical writing by higher functioning adults with autism or Asperger syndrome and suggested that even these very able adults show some elements of style and content characteristic of their disorder, although the writings are also indicative of a range of abilities in social and communicative skill. Other reports on first-hand accounts of the experience of having an ASD are presented in Volkmar and Cohen (1985), Wallace (2000), and Prince (2010).

There is also a growing body of research on non-autobiographical written narrative in ASD. Carey (2007) investigated the narrative structure of written stories by high-functioning children with ASDs, in the context of an intervention study. She used Labov's (1997) framework of analysis to code the structure of the narratives: this defines six functional elements of narrative including Abstract (the précis of the story), Orientation (the setting), Complicating Action (the sequence of events), Resolution (the denouement), Evaluation (commentary or highlighting) and the Coda (taking us back to the real world). Carey found some impairments in the structure of the stories by children with ASDs, in particular in the proportional use of these elements of narrative, with a lower proportion of Orientation and Evaluation clauses and a higher proportion of Complicating Action clauses.

Stirling and colleagues investigated a small corpus of spontaneous written story retellings by one child with autism (Stirling & Barrington 2007; Stirling, Barrington & Douglas 2007a, b). The retellings were found to exhibit sophisticated episodic structure and the use of a range of devices for managing perspective, but were unusual in the way in which relative knowledge states of story participants and narrator were presented. Preliminary results from an on-going follow-up study of written narrative (Stirling, Barrington, Douglas & Delves 2009a, b) indicate some differences in the way reported speech and thought is represented in the story retellings of children with autism compared to a typical group.

Brown and Klein (2011) considered written compositions by adults with high-functioning ASDs in the context of Theory of Mind, and looked at both narrative and expository text genres. On a range of measures including narrative length they found that the adults with ASDs performed more poorly. In particular, performance according to a "quality" of writing composite was found both to differ significantly across groups and to correlate with Theory of Mind abilities as measured by performance on the Social Attribution Task. This quality composite consisted of the following measures: presence of essential structural elements, amount of background information and elaboration, how enjoyable the text was to read, global coherence, local coherence across adjacent sentences and complexity of representation of internal worlds of characters.

Functional neuroimaging

There is a growing body of neuroimaging research addressing processing of narrative discourse. However, at the time of review, a single published neuroimaging study of ASDs used narrative tasks in its methodology (Mason, Williams,

Kana, Minshew, and Just (2008; see Mason & Just 2009 for theoretical discussion). The researchers asked participants with High Functioning Autism and neurotypical participants to read narrative passages that required inferences based on either physical causality, emotional states or intentions. Functional magnetic resonance imaging of brain responses revealed two main findings. First, Right Hemisphere activation was greater for all conditions in the autism group compared with the control group. Second, a "Theory of Mind network" postulated based on a body of earlier studies was appropriately recruited in the control group only for the intention inference condition, but was active in all conditions for the autism group.

Conclusions

We have endeavoured in this review to explore why it is interesting to look at narrative in the context of autism; to summarise what we know so far about the narrative abilities and deficits of individuals with ASDs; and to reflect on the state of the art in terms of what we know regarding how best to use narrative in this research domain.

What can we glean from the body of research so far on narrative and ASDs? Whether or not robust differences in abilities specific to narrative construction exist between people with ASD and neurotypical people remains somewhat equivocal. Some researchers have argued that any differences observed can be accounted for entirely by broader linguistic deficits rather than by specific difficulties with narrative (cf. Norbury & Bishop 2003: 252), in contrast to some early hypotheses that saw narrative as a domain of specific difficulty for people with ASDs (e.g. Bruner & Feldman 1993). From the studies available so far, we can make the following observations.

At least some individuals with ASDs, in at least some conditions, are capable of producing narratives not readily distinguishable in length, complexity, structure and other characteristics from those of neurotypical individuals. All the studies surveyed show at least some differences between the ASD and comparison groups. However, a number of researchers commented on how similar performance across groups was, with studies such as Tager-Flusberg and Sullivan (1995) and Diehl et al. (2006) showing only minor and focused significant differences.

Many studies show no apparent differences in the ability of individuals with ASDs to use internal state language and other features which have typically been taken as indicative of perspectivising abilities (e.g. Tager-Flusberg & Sullivan 1995; Beaumont & Newcombe 2006; Colle et al. 2008). However, individuals with ASDs may have a lesser ability or propensity to describe internal states of characters or to move between character perspectives especially in contexts with a complex focus on these matters (Garcia-Perez et al. 2008; Begeer et al. 2010 and for explicit correlation with Theory of Mind testing, Tager-Flusberg 1995; Capps et al. 2000; though not Losh & Capps 2003).

One domain where there does seem to be a definite tendency for people with ASDs to perform more poorly in narrative production is in the establishment of global coherence through use of causal language. While numerous studies have confirmed that causal language is used by this group, others have shown group differences in its frequency and/or sophistication (Tager-Flusberg 1995; Capps et al. 2000; Losh & Capps 2003).

Research has come a long way with respect to understanding the range of possible abilities and deficits in narrative production which may be exhibited by people with ASDs. A major outcome is the recognition that "narrative" is not a monolithic concept. Yet, at this stage we have only the haziest idea of what the children involved in these studies consciously and/or unconsciously perceive to be the task(s) they are being asked to perform. We know that there is great variation in narrative ability within the ASD population, and some of this variation appears to correlate with other measures such as general linguistic ability or Theory of Mind status.

We conclude our review with some recommendations for on-going study of ASD and narrative. Firstly, researchers need to be sensitive to the potential effect on results of even small changes in task methodology (presentational format, presence of the experimenter) and analytical protocols. Certain techniques including adult scaffolding, schema-based retelling and written and computer-based story production compared with oral formats, may lead to a reduction in the cognitive load and social demands of the task; this may have the advantage of allowing participants with ASDs to perform to their maximal ability. Only three studies have compared more than one type of narrative task, with the two largest finding discrepant results across tasks (e.g. Losh & Capps 2003; Craig & Baron-Cohen 2000). A greater understanding of the cognitive demands of different tasks would aid such comparison. Ideally, explicit comparisons of task design parameters will be undertaken in future research.

Secondly, areas of focus for further work can be identified. More work on different (sub)genres of discourse across the same population is desirable, as initiated in existing studies by Losh and Capps, and Ehlers. There is great scope and on-going need for further comparison between ASD groups and other clinical groups. We have also identified gaps in the current research literature which could be pursued. One of these is longitudinal work on narrative development in autism. In pursuing these areas of research we advocate awareness of the potential relative value of a range of study designs, including case-study as well as group-based designs, data-driven as well as theory-driven studies, and qualitative as well as quantitative analyses. Norbury and Bishop (2003) called for better normative data and this plus further exploration of individual variation in performance within and across groups and over time would likely improve our understanding of the high degree of variance within groups and overlap in group comparisons.

Finally, the use of analytical concepts such as 'evaluation' or 'causal connection', their operationalisation in related metrics of measurement, and the way in which these linguistic observations reflect cognitive abilities is in need of clarification. This will lead to greater transparency of research findings and enable better comparison between and replicability of future studies.

Narrative is an important, universal, early-acquired genre of language which involves a range of complex cognitive skills. However narrative is also a complex discourse genre, and our study of narrative needs to respect this complexity. The study of narrative abilities and deficits of clinical populations continues to show promise in illuminating our understanding of these disorders, and, more broadly, the nature of the narrative task.

References

Astington, J. (1990). Narrative and the child's Theory of Mind. In B. Britton & A. Pelligrini (Eds.), *Narrative Thought and Narrative Language* (pp. 151–171). Hillsdale, NJ: Lawrence Erlbaum Associates.

Bamberg, M. (Ed.). (1987). *Narrative Development: Six Approaches.* Mahwah, NJ: Lawrence Erlbaum Associates.

Bamberg, M., & Damrad-Frye, R. (1991). On the ability to provide evaluative comments: Further explorations of children's narrative competencies. *Journal of Child Language, 18*, 689–710.

Baron-Cohen, S., Leslie, A.M., & Frith, U. (1986). Mechanical, behavioural and intentional understanding of picture stories in autistic children. *British Journal of Developmental Psychology, 4*, 113–125.

Beaumont, R., & Newcombe, P. (2006). Theory of mind and central coherence in adults with high-functioning autism or Asperger syndrome. *Autism, 10*(4), 365–382.

Begeer, S., Malle, B., Nieuwland, M., & Keysar, B. (2010). Using theory of mind to represent and take part in social interactions: Comparing individuals with high-functioning autism and typically developing controls. *European Journal of Developmental Psychology, 7*(1), 104–122.

Berman, R. (2004). *Language Development across Childhood and Adolescence* (Trends in Language Acquisition Research 3). Amsterdam: John Benjamins.

Berman, R. (2009). Language development in narrative contexts. In E. Bavin (Ed.), *Cambridge Handbook of Child Language* (pp. 354–375). Cambridge: CUP.

Bishop, D., & Edmundson, A. (1987). Specific language impairment as a maturational lag: Evidence from longitudinal data on language and motor development. *Developmental Medicine and Child Neurology, 29*, 442–459.

Botting, N. (2002). Narrative as a tool for the assessment of linguistic and pragmatic impairments. *Child Language Teaching and Therapy, 18*(1), 1–22.

Brown, H., & Klein, P. (2011). Writing, Asperger Syndrome and theory of mind. *Journal of Autism and Developmental Disorders, 41*(11), 1464–1474.

Brown, B., Morris, G., Nida, R., & Baker-Ward, L. (2012). Brief report: Making experience personal: Internal states language in the memory narratives of children with and without Asperger's Disorder. *Journal of Autism and Developmental Disorders, 41*(11), 441–446.

Bruner, J. (1991). The narrative construction of reality. *Critical Inquiry, 18*, 1–21.

Bruner, J., & Feldman, C. (1993). Theories of mind and the problem of autism. In S. Baron-Cohen, H. Tager-Flusberg, & D. Cohen (Eds.), *Understanding Other Minds: Perspectives from Autism* (pp. 267–291). Oxford: OUP.

Capps, L., Kehres, J., & Sigman, M. (1998). Conversational abilities among children with Autism and children with developmental delays. *Autism, 2*(4), 325–244.

Capps, L., Losh, M., & Thurber, C. (2000). "The frog ate the bug and made his mouth sad": Narrative competence in children with autism. *Journal of Abnormal Child Psychology, 28*(2), 193–204.

Carey, L. (2007). *Structural Narrative Analysis: Assessing Language Abilities in Autism.* Unpublished doctoral dissertation. University of Durham.

Chapman, R., Seung, H., Schwartz, S., & Kay-Raining Bird, E. (1998). Language skills of children and adolescents with Down Syndrome, II: Production deficits. *Journal of Speech, Language and Hearing Research, 41*, 861–873.

Colle, L., Baron-Cohen, S., Wheelwright, S., & van der Lely, H. (2008). Narrative discourse in adults with high-functioning autism or Asperger Syndrome. *Journal of Autism and Developmental Disorders, 38*, 28–40.

Cowley, J., & Glasgow, C. (1994). *The Renfrew Bus Story: Language Screening by Narrative Recall.* Circle Pines, MN: American Guidance.

Craig, J. & Baron-Cohen, S. (2000). Story-telling ability in children with autism or Asperger syndrome: A window into the imagination. *Israel Journal of Psychiatry and Related Sciences, 37*(1), 64–70.

Crain, S., & Thornton, R. (1998). *Investigations in Universal Grammar.* Cambridge, MA: The MIT Press.

Davis, M., Dautenhahn, K., Nehaniv, C., & Powell, S. (2004). Towards an interactive system facilitating therapeutic narrative elicitation in Autism. *Proceedings of the* 3rd *International Conference on Narrative and Interactive Learning Environments* (NILE (2004)).

De Marchena, A., & Eigsti, I-M. (2010). Conversational gestures in Autism Spectrum Disorders: Asynchrony but not decreased frequency. *Autism Research, 3*, 311–322.

Diehl, J., Bennetto, L., & Young, E. (2006). Story recall and narrative coherence of high-functioning children with Autism Spectrum Disorders. *Journal of Abnormal Child Psychology, 34*(1), 87–102.

Ehlers, C. (2008). *Effects of Listener and Context on the Spoken Stories of Children with ASD and TD Children.* Unpublished Master's thesis. University of Vermont.

Estigarribia, B., Martin, G., Roberts, J., Spencer, A., Gucwa, A., & Sideris, J. (2011). Narrative skill in boys with fragile X syndrome with and without autism spectrum disorder. *Applied Psycholinguistics, 32*, 359–388.

Feffer, M. (1970). Role-taking behaviour in the mentally retarded. ERIC Report to the Bureau of Education for the Handicapped, U.S. Office of Education, Department of Health and Social Welfare.
Gabig, C.S. (2008). Verbal working memory and story retelling in school-age children with autism. *Language, Speech, and Hearing Services in Schools, 39*, 498–511.
Garcia-Perez, R.M., Hobson, R.P. & Lee, A. (2008). Narrative role-taking in autism. *Journal of Autism and Developmental Disorders, 38*, 156–168.
Goldman, S. (2008). Brief Report: Narratives of personal events in children with autism and developmental language disorders: Unshared memories. *Journal of Autism and Developmental Disorders, 38*, 1982–1988.
Grant, C., Boucher, J., Riggs, K. & Grayson, A. (2005). Moral understanding in children with autism. *Autism, 9*(3), 317–331.
Gray, C. (2000). *The New Social Story Book: Illustrated Edition*. Arlington, TX: Future Horizons.
Happé, F. (1992). The autobiographical writings of three Asperger syndrome adults: Problems of interpretation and implications for theory. In U. Frith (Ed.) *Autism and Asperger syndrome* (pp. 207–242). Cambridge: Cambridge University Press.
Heider, F., & Simmel, M. (1944). An experimental study of apparent behavior. *American Journal of Psychology, 57*, 243–259.
Ho, W.C., Davis, M., & Dautenhahn, K. (2009). Supporting narrative understanding of children with autism: A story interface with autonomous autobiographic agents. IEEE Int. Conf. on Rehabilitation Robotics 2009, ICORR 2009 (pp. 905–911).
Hudson, J.A., & Shapiro, L.R. (1991). From knowing to telling: The development of children's scripts, stories, and personal narratives. In A. McCabe & C. Peterson (Eds.), *Developing Narrative Structure* (pp. 89–136). Hillsdale, NJ: Lawrence Erlbaum Associates.
Jarrold, C., & Brock, J. (2004). To match or not to match? Methodological issues in autism-related research. *Journal of Autism and Developmental Disorders, 34*(1), 81–86.
Jiao, Q. (2001). Research on theory of mind in autism. *Chinese Mental Health Journal, 15*(1), 60–62.
Klin, A. (2000). Attributing social meaning to ambiguous visual stimuli in higher-functioning autism and Asperger syndrome: The Social Attribution Task. *Journal of Child Psychology and Psychiatry, 41*(7), 831–846.
Labov, W., & Waletzky, J. (1967). Narrative analysis: Oral versions of personal experience. In J. Helm (Ed.), *Essays on the Verbal and Visual Arts* (pp. 12–44). Seattle, WA: University of Washington Press.
Labov, W. (1997). Some further steps in narrative analysis. *Journal of Narrative and Life History, 7*, 395–415.
Landa, R. (2000). Social language use in Asperger Syndrome and High-Functioning Autism. In A. Klin, F. Volkmar, & S. Sparrow (Eds.), *Asperger Syndrome* (pp. 125–158). New York, NY: The Guildford Press.
Landa, R., Martin, M., Minshew, N., & Goldstein, G. (1995). Discourse and abstract language ability in non-retarded individuals with autism. Paper presented at the Society for Research in Child Development, Indianapolis.
Liles, B. (1993). Narrative discourse in children with language disorders and children with normal language: A critical review. *Journal of Speech Hearing Research, 36*, 868–882.
Liles, B., Coelho, C., Duffy, R., & Zalagens, M. (1989). Effects of elicitation procedures on the narratives of normal and closed head-injured adults. *Journal of Speech and Hearing Disorders, 54*, 356–366.

Losh, M., & Capps, L. (2003). Narrative ability in High-Functioning children with Autism or Asperger's Syndrome. *Journal of Autism and Developmental Disorders, 33*(3), 239–251.
Loveland, K., McEvoy, R., & Tunali, B. (1990). Narrative story telling in autism and Down's syndrome. *British Journal of Developmental Psychology, 8*(1), 9–23.
Loveland, K., & Tunali, B. (1993). Narrative language in autism and the theory of mind hypothesis: A wider perspective. In S. Baron-Cohen, H. Tager-Flusberg, & D. Cohen (Eds.), *Understanding Other Minds: Perspectives from Autism* (pp. 247–266). Oxford: OUP.
Manolitsi, M., & Botting, N. (2011). Language abilities in children with autism and language impairment: using narrative as an additional source of clinical information. *Child Language Teaching and Therapy, 27*(1), 39–55.
Martin, G.E. (2009). *Verbal Perseveration in Boys with Fragile X Syndrome with and Without Autism Compared to Boys with Down Syndrome*. Unpublished Doctoral dissertation. University of North Carolina.
Mason, R.A., Williams, D.L., Kana, R.K., Minshew, N. & Just, M.A. (2008). Theory of Mind disruption and recruitment of the right hemisphere during narrative comprehension in autism. *Neuropsychologia, 46*, 269–280.
Mason, R.A., & Just, M.A. (2009). The role of the Theory-of-Mind cortical network in the comprehension of narratives. *Language and Linguistics Compass, 3*(1), 157–174.
Mayer, M. (1969). *Frog, Where Are You?* New York, NY: Puffin.
Mayer, M. (1973). *Frog on his Own*. New York, NY: Puffin.
Miller, P.J., & Sperry, L.L. (1988). Early talk about the past: The origins of conversational stories about personal experience. *Journal of Child Language, 15*, 293–315.
Ninio, A. (1988). On formal grammatical categories in early child language. In Y. Levy, I. Schlesinger, & M.D.S. Braine (Eds.), *Categories and Processes in Language Acquisition* (pp. 99–119). Hillsdale, NJ: Lawrence Erlbaum Associates.
Norbury, C.F., & Bishop, D.V.M. (2002). Inferential processing and story recall in children with communication problems: A comparison of specific language impairment, pragmatic language impairment and high-functioning autism. *International Journal of Language and Communication Disorders, 37*(3), 227–251.
Norbury, C.F., & Bishop, D.V.M. (2003). Narrative skills of children with communication impairments. *International Journal of Language and Communication Disorders, 38*(3), 287–313.
Ochs, E., & Solomon, O. (2004). Introduction: Discourse and autism. *Discourse Studies, 6*, 139–146.
Peng, F.C.C. (1988). On the acquisition of discourse among autistic children. *Language Sciences, 10*(1), 193–224.
Pearlman-Avnion, S., & Eviatar, Z. (2002). Narrative analysis in developmental social and linguistic pathologies: Dissociation between emotional and informational language use. *Brain and Cognition, 48*(2–3), 494–499.
Polanyi, L. (1989). *Telling the American Story: A structural and cultural analysis of conversational storytelling*. Cambridge, MA: The MIT Press.
Prince, D.E. (2010). An exceptional path: An ethnographic narrative reflecting on autistic parenthood from evolutionary, cultural, and spiritual perspectives. *Ethos, 38*(1), 56–68.
Reilly, J., Bates, E., & Marchman, V. (1998). Narrative discourse in children with early focal brain injury. *Brain and Language, 61*, 335–375.
Reilly, J., Klima, E., & Bellugi, U. (1990). Once more with feeling: Affect and language in atypical populations. *Development and Psychopathology, 2*, 367–391.
Rose, I. (2008). Autistic autobiography or autistic life narrative? *Journal of Literary Disability, 2*(1), 44–54.

Ruffman, T., Garnham, W., & Rideout, P. (2001). Social understanding in autism: Eye gaze as a measure of core insights. *Journal of Child Psychology and Psychiatry, 42*(8), 1083–1094.

Scollon, R., & Scollon, S. (1981). *Narrative, Literacy and Face in Interethnic Communication* (Advances in Discourse Processes). Norwood, NJ: Ablex.

Seung, H.K. (2007). Linguistic characteristics of individuals with high functioning autism and Asperger syndrome. *Clinical Linguistics and Phonetics, 21*(4), 247–259.

Sirota, K.G. (2010a). Narratives of transformation: Family discourse, autism and trajectories of hope. *Discourse and Society, 21*(5), 544–564.

Sirota, K.G. (2010b). Narratives of distinction: Personal life narrative as a technology of the self in the everyday lives and relational worlds of children with autism. *Ethos, 38*(1), 93–115.

Slaughter, V., Peterson, C.C. & Mackintosh, E. (2007). Mind what mother says: Narrative input and Theory of Mind in typical children and those on the autism spectrum. *Child Development, 78*(3), 839–858.

Solomon, O. (2004). Narrative introductions: Discourse competence of children with autistic spectrum disorders. *Discourse Studies, 6*(2), 253–76.

Solomon, O. (2008). Language, autism, and childhood: An ethnographic perspective. *Annual Review of Applied Linguistics, 28*, 150–169.

Stirling, L., & Barrington, G. (2007). "Then I'll huff & I'll puff or I'll go on the roff!" thinks the wolf: Spontaneous written narratives by a child with autism. In A. Schalley & D. Khlentzos (Eds.), *Mental States: Language and Cognitive Structure* (pp. 133–172). Amsterdam: John Benjamins.

Stirling, L., Barrington, G., & Douglas, S. (2007a). Two times three little pigs: Dysfluency, cognitive complexity and autism. *Proceedings of the 2006 Australian Linguistic Society Conference,* Brisbane, 7–9 July (2006).

Stirling, L., Barrington, G., & Douglas, S. (2007b). Progression in narrative ability: A case study comparing successive written and oral retellings of 'The Three Little Pigs' by a child with autism. AWN Research Report-2-07, School of Languages and Linguistics, The University of Melbourne. (Originally presented at The Biennial National Autism Conference, The Gold Coast, 14–16 March 2007.)

Stirling, L., Barrington, G., Douglas, S., & Delves, K. (2009a). Analysis of perspective management and reported interaction in story retellings by children with ASD and typically developing children. *Electronic Journal of Applied Psychology, 5*(1), 31–38. Special issue on *Innovations in Autism.*

Stirling, L., Barrington, G., Douglas, S., & Delves, K. (2009b). The developmental profile of editing and repair strategies in narrative structure: A cross-sectional study of primary school children. In *The Proceedings of the 33rd Annual Boston University Conference on Language Development* (Vol. 2, pp. 504–515). Somerville, MA: Cascadilla Press.

Stojanovik, V. (2006). Social interaction deficits and conversational inadequacy in Williams syndrome. *Journal of Neurolinguistics, 19*, 157–173

Stothard, S., Snowling, M., Bishop, D., Chipcase, B., & Kaplan, C. (1998). Language-impaired preschoolers: A follow-up into adolescence. *Journal of Speech, Language, and Hearing Research, 41*, 407–418.

Tager-Flusberg, H. (1995). "Once upon a ribbit": Stories narrated by autistic children. *British Journal of Developmental Psychology, 13*(1), 45–59.

Tager-Flusberg, H., & Sullivan, K. (1995). Attributing mental states to story characters: A comparison of narratives produced by autistic and mentally retarded individuals. *Applied Psycholinguistics, 16*(3), 241–256.

Tartaro, A., & Cassell, J. (2006). Using virtual peer technology as an intervention for children with Autism. In J. Lazar (Ed.) *Universal Usability: Designing Computer Interfaces for Diverse User Populations* (pp. 231–262). New York, NY: John Wiley and Sons.

Thurber, C., & Tager-Flusberg, H. (1993). Pauses in the narratives produced by autistic, mentally retarded, and normal children as an index of cognitive demand. *Journal of Autism and Developmental Disorders, 23*(2), 309–322.

Volkmar, F.R., & Cohen, D.J. (1985). The experience of infantile autism: A first-person account by Tony W. *Journal of Autism and Developmental Disorders, 15*, 47–54.

Wallace, J. (2000). Walter. In A. Klin, F. Volkmar, & S. Sparrow (Eds.), *Asperger Syndrome* (pp. 434–462). New York, NY: The Guildford Press.

Waterhouse, L., & Fein, D. (1982). Language skills in developmentally disabled children. *Brain and Language, 15*(2), 307–333.

Table 2. Experimental oral narrative production studies

Study	Yr	Elicitation method/task	Type of narrative and cognitive requirements	ASD participants	Comparison groups	Focus of study	Results: Nsig. diffs	Results: Sig. diffs
Waterhouse & Fein.	1982	(1) **Stimulus:** sequence of 4 cartoon pictures (animals in social interactions) presented 2 at a time. **Task:** produce a narrative based on the picture sequence. (2) Stimulus: A scene and the start of a story about it. **Task:** complete the story.	Comprehension of implicit narrative depicted by picture sequence. Construction/ Retelling of non-verbally presented stimulus story.	Group of 83 children prev. diagnosed as 'psychotic', aged 5–15; a subgroup of 33 were classified as having autism. Minimal language requirements.	3 groups of TD children (total 234 matches), matched respectively on chron. age, MLU and visual perception. Other diagnostic subgroups from the 'psychotic' group were 'childhood scizophrenia' – overlapping with autism group – and 'other severe disturbance'.	Differentiation of subgroups of developmentally disabled children and comparison to typical children on a range of language measures.	**NSig**. In a subjective rating study by experienced special ed. and early childhood teachers, they could not discriminate between narrative from the clinical and control groups, when these were matched for MLU and story length, except when particularly marked by features to right. No language differences between diagnostic subgroups.	**Sig**. Abnormal perseveration (repetition of same words, themes or grammatical forms), and a focus on the minor details of the story.

(*Continued*)

Table 2. (Continued)

Study	Yr	Elicitation method/task	Type of narrative and cognitive requirements	ASD participants	Comparison groups	Focus of study	Results: Nsig. diffs	Results: Sig. diffs
Baron-Cohen et al.	1986	**Stimulus:** sequences of 4 pictures in 3 conditions – causal-mechanical; descriptive-behavioural; psychological-intentional. **Task:** arrange the pictures into a preferred story sequence then tell the story.	Comprehension of implicit narrative depicted by picture sequence. Construction/ Retelling of non-verbally presented stimulus story.	21 children with HFA (10 provided verbal stories); aged 6–16 with mean Chron. age 12;4	27 NT pre-school children aged 3–5; mean 4;5 (stories gathered from random 1/3). 15 children with Down Syndrome aged 6–17; mean 10;5 (7 provided verbal stories).	Ability to identify sequences of events based on increasingly more abstract reasoning. Theory of Mind hypothesis.	**NSig**. Presence of causal and descriptive language in the narratives.	**Sig**. Very rarely used mental state language; HFA group performed worse than both NT and DS groups. (Results for narrative task were in line with results for picture sequencing task and a previous ToM task.)

Loveland et al	1990	**Stimulus:** short puppet show or video sketch (depending on level of maturity) depicting a main character and a thief who tries but fails to steal something from the main character. **Task:** retell the story to an experimenter who was not present for the stimulus presentation.	Comprehension of acted play. Construction/ Retelling of stimulus story (presented with both verbal and visual input) to audience unfamiliar with it.	16 individuals with HFA (aged 5–27; mean 13;5)	16 with Down Syndrome individually matched on composite verbal age; NVIQ and chronological age kept similar. [NOTE: no NT controls]	Ability of participants to tell a story to a listener. Are there narrative deficits specific to autism vs. other clinical groups? Context of Theory of Mind hypothesis.	**Nsig.** Story length (on a range of measures) and language use generally.	**Sig.** Greater tendency to produce bizarre language and to see the story characters (puppets or actors) as objects rather than characters; some seemed to have difficulty recognising the story as a set of meaningful events. DS subjects produced more communicative gestures.
Thurber & Tager-Flusberg	1993	**Stimulus:** wordless picture book *Frog Where Are You?*. **Task:** tell story based on book to an experimenter who had not been previously seen it while original experimenter turned pages & prompted.	Comprehension of implicit narrative depicted by picture sequence. Construction/ Retelling of non-verbally presented stimulus story to audience unfamiliar with it.	10 children with autism, mean age 12;1; 'relatively high functioning'	10 NT children; mean age 7;9. 10 Children with ID; mean age 11;3. Matched on verbal mental age.	Investigated pauses & repairs as index of cognitive demand and engagement.	**NSig.** Story length in TNW; syntactic complexity; number of repetitions, false starts & grammatical pauses.	**Sig.** Fewer 'nongrammatical' pauses (taken as index of cognitive demand/ engagement). Shorter less complex stories on MLU, number of propositions, NDW.

(*Continued*)

Table 2. (Continued)

Study	Yr	Elicitation method/task	Type of narrative and cognitive requirements	ASD participants	Comparison groups	Focus of study	Results: Nsig. diffs	Results: Sig. diffs
Tager-Flusberg	1995	**Stimulus:** wordless picture book *Frog Where Are You?*. **Task:** tell story based on book – to an experimenter who had not looked through the book with them and could not see the pictures.	Comprehension of implicit narrative depicted by picture sequence. Construction/ Retelling of non-verbally presented stimulus story to audience unfamiliar with it, who cannot see pictures.	10 children with autism, mean age 12;1; 'relatively high functioning'	10 NT children; mean age 7;9. 10 Children with ID; mean age 11;3. Matched on verbal mental age	Investigate a range of linguistic and social-cognitive aspects including Theory of Mind.	**NSig.** Use of character speech and sound effects; use of mental state language.	**Sig.** Story length (shorter); Fewer causal statements, less complex syntactically – than both comparison groups. While freq. of use of affective evaluative devices nsig., were sig. diffs. in number of children to use sound effects as well as causal language.

Tager-Flusberg & Sullivan.	1995	**Stimulus:** wordless picture book *Frog On His Own.* **Task:** tell story based on book to new experimenter.	Comprehension of implicit narrative depicted by picture sequence. Construction/ Retelling of non-verbally presented stimulus story to audience unfamiliar with it.	27 subjects with autism or PDD-NOS, aged 6–22; mean 16;8	17 NT children aged 7–10. 27 subjects with ID aged 7–17. Matched on measures of language comprehension & production	Narrative abilities and relation to Theory of Mind.	**NSig.** Story length, lexical cohesion (incl. causal connectives), use of emotion and mental state terms (lacking in all groups).	**Sig.** Narrative performance of children with autism sig. correlated with performance on ToM task. When asked comprehension questions, were less accurate in labeling emotions and gave fewer appropriate causal explanations.
Landa et al. (reported in Landa 2000)	1995	**Stimulus**: story beginning. **Task**: complete story.	Construction of novel narrative constrained by provision of a story stem.	Adolescents and adults with HFA	NT controls matched on age, IQ and gender	Focus on episodic structure of stories.	**NSig.** Story length (in number of independent clauses) but HFA participants had much greater variability in length. Many produced conventionally structured stories.	**Sig.** Generation of complete vs. incomplete episode structures; irrelevant information; presuppositional errors; rated as less coherent with linking left out.

(*Continued*)

Table 2. (Continued)

Study	Yr	Elicitation method/task	Type of narrative and cognitive requirements	ASD participants	Comparison groups	Focus of study	Results: Nsig. diffs	Results: Sig. diffs
Capps et al.	1998	A 6 minute long informal, semi-structured conversation on specific topics.	Inter alia, construction of personal experience narratives in a pseudo-conversational setting.	15 children with autism; mean age 11;9	15 children with developmental delays; mean age 9;4. Matched on language age and mental age	Involvement of children with autism in conversation.		**Sig.** Produced fewer narratives of personal experience. Observed qualitative differences in length, relevance, personal nature ("impoverished").

Capps et al.	2000	(1) **Stimulus:** wordless picture book *Frog On His Own.* **Task:** tell story based on wordless picture book – to experimenter who had shown them the book. (2) An informal, semi-structured conversation on various topics.	Comprehension of implicit narrative depicted by picture sequence. Construction/ Retelling of non-verbally presented stimulus story – to familiar audience. Inter alia, construction of personal experience narratives in a pseudo-conversational setting.	13 children with autism, mean age 12;6	13 NT children, mean age 6. 13 children with developmental delays, mean age 9;8. Matched on IQ and language ability	Replicate and expand on previous research using *Frog* story to elicit narratives. Relate narrative ability to Theory of Mind and conversational ability.	**NSig.** Amount of evaluation; use of causal language; use of internal state terms.	**Sig.** Story length (shorter) vs. TD group; stories of both clinical groups contained less complex syntax, and made use of more restricted range of evaluative devices – esp. causal explanations provided, more likely to focus on character behaviour vs. NT children who were more likely to embed emotion descriptions within a causal frame. Narrative ability of autism group correlated with ToM abilities. NT group provided more character speech and sound effects.

(*Continued*)

Table 2. (Continued)

Study	Yr	Elicitation method/task	Type of narrative and cognitive requirements	ASD participants	Comparison groups	Focus of study	Results: Nsig. diffs	Results: Sig. diffs
Craig & Baron-Cohen	2000	**Stimulus:** story themes (one imaginary and one reality based). **Task:** to construct a story based on the themes.	Story construction to fit a theme.	13 children with autism and 14 children with AS (both with mean age 12;9); children with autism not as high-functioning	14 NT children (mean age 5;3). 15 children with moderate learning difficulties (mean age 12;4). Matched on verbal mental age	Ability to produce imaginative stories compared with ability to produce stories based on a reality based theme.		**Sig.** Autism & AS: less likely to include imaginative elements in their reality-based stories. Autism: more difficulty in producing an imaginative narrative than AS or controls.

Klin	2000	**Stimulus:** short video containing geometric figures enacting a social plot (part of the Social Attribution Task). **Task:** produce a narrative describing the depicted events.	Understanding of geometric figures as animate actors. Comprehension of acted play. Construction/ Retelling of non-verbally presented stimulus story.	20 adolescents & adults with HFA (mean age 20;5) & 20 with AS (mean age 18;9)	20 NT adolescents and adults (mean age 20;2)	Theory of Mind and attribution of social meaning.		**Sig.** Shorter stories [and performed less well on SAT measures assessing social cognition]; the stories themselves indicated social deficits – fewer social elements mentioned; attributions irrelevant to the social plot made; ToM terms used infrequently.
Pearlman-Avnion & Eviatar.	2002	**Stimulus:** A 27 slide show depicting a story with accompanying verbal component. **Task**: retell the story to the experimenter.	Comprehension of implicit narrative depicted by slide sequence. Construction/ Retelling of non-verbally presented stimulus story to familiar experimenter.	13 children & adolescents with HFA (aged 8–16)	TD children (2 groups of 13 at different ages – mean 7.36 and 11.5). 13 Children & adolescents with Williams Syndrome (aged 8–21).	To examine use of emotional and informational aspects of language in 2 clinical populations.		**Sig**. Included fewer emotional elements than either comparison group. Both clinical groups produced fewer informational elements than NT controls.

(*Continued*)

Table 2. (Continued)

Study	Yr	Elicitation method/task	Type of narrative and cognitive requirements	ASD participants	Comparison groups	Focus of study	Results: Nsig. diffs	Results: Sig. diffs
Losh & Capps	2003	(1) **Stimulus**: wordless picture book *Frog Where Are You?*. **Task**: tell story based on wordless picture book – to experimenter who had shown them the book. (2) Children were engaged in semi-structured conversational storytelling during which personal narratives were elicited by questions.	Comprehension of implicit narrative depicted by picture sequence. Construction/ Retelling of non-verbally presented stimulus story. Memory for autobiographical events. Construction of a retell of remembered events.	28 children with HFA / AS, aged 8–14; mean 11;3	22 NT children, matched for chronological age and VIQ	Two types of story telling.	**NSig.** Story length, plus both groups told longer stories in the personal narrative condition. Few differences in wordless picture book condition. No differences in number of personal narratives and few in range of topics.	**Sig.** ASD groups had more difficulties with the personal experience narratives, for which they had less complex syntax, less evaluation, less diverse range of evaluation, produced more bizarre/irrelevant comments. In both conditions, limited use of causal language for internal states and explanations of character behaviour. Narrative ability associated with performance on measures of emotional understanding vs. ToM ability. ASD groups required more prompts for clarification.

Norbury & Bishop.	2003	**Stimulus:** wordless picture book *Frog Where Are You?*. **Task:** tell story based on wordless picture book – to same experimenter who had shown them through the book.	Comprehension of implicit narrative depicted by picture sequence. Construction/ Retelling of non-verbally presented stimulus story – for familiar audience.	12 children with HFA; age range 6–10 for all groups	17 children with SLI. 21 children with PLI. 18 NT children.	How language and pragmatic ability impact on narrative competence in different groups of children with communication impairments.	**NSig.** Story length; global structure; evaluation (incl. causal connectives)	**Sig.** Poorer referential cohesion, poor use of anaphora. More syntactic errors.
Beaumont & Newcombe.	2006	**Stimulus:** 6 cards from the Thematic Apperception Test depicting realistic, dramatic scenes. **Task:** provide a narrative account for each card, explaining what happened before, during and after the depicted event & describing characters thoughts and feelings.	Comprehension of scene depicted by picture. Construction of story based on non-verbally presented stimulus.	20 young adults with HFA (n = 4) or AS (n = 16), mean age 27;7.	20 NT adults matched on IQ, age and gender	Theory of Mind and central coherence in adults with ASDs.	**NSig.** Story length in total number of propositions. Number of mental state words. Proportion of explanations for non-mental state phenomena (action causal statements).	**Sig.** Proportion of mental state causal statements: less inclined to provide explanations for characters' mental states.

(*Continued*)

Table 2. (Continued)

Study	Yr	Elicitation method/task	Type of narrative and cognitive requirements	ASD participants	Comparison groups	Focus of study	Results: Nsig. diffs	Results: Sig. diffs
Diehl et al.	2006	**Stimulus:** *Frog Where Are You?* wordless picture book with audiorecorded telling of the story. **Task:** retell story (without access to picturebook) to an experimenter who had left the room during story.	Comprehension of implicit narrative depicted by picture sequence. Construction/ Retelling of non-verbally presented stimulus story – to experimenter unfamiliar with it.	17 children with HFA, mean age 8.8	17 NT children, matched on age, gender, language ability and cognitive ability (mean age 9.4)	Story recall and narrative coherence.	**NSig.** Story length, complexity, proportion of story elements recalled; no difference in likelihood to recall gist events than details; no difference in causality or in sensitivity to importance of story events (both more likely to recall causally more connected events).	**Sig.** Less coherent narratives; less likely to use the gist of the story to enhance the coherence of their narratives; more cases of inappropriate storytelling; lower causal connections per unit.

Seung	2007	**Stimulus:** short silent video containing geometric figures enacting a social plot (part of the Social Attribution Task). **Task:** produce a narrative describing the depicted events.	Understanding of geometric figures as animate actors. Comprehension of acted play. Construction/ Retelling of non-verbally presented stimulus story.	children and adults with HFA. children and adults with AS. 10 participants matched on gender, chronological age, IQ, age range 11-49	[comparison was between HFA and AS groups]	Language ability differences between autism and AS.	**NSig.** Story length and narrative cohesion (=number of ambiguous pronouns).	**Sig.** AS: used verb past tense more appropriately as a narrative device.
Colle et al.	2008	**Stimulus:** wordless picture book *Frog Where Are You?* which participants looked through on their own. **Task**: tell story based on book to an experimenter they were told had not seen the book and who could not see the pictures.	Comprehension of implicit narrative depicted by picture sequence. Construction/ Retelling of non-verbally presented stimulus story.	12 adults with HFA/AS (10 with AS), mean age 27;5.	12 NT adults matched on IQ, chronological age	Use of temporal and anaphoric referential expressions to assess pragmatic skills.	**NSig.** TNW, number of episodes, syntactic complexity, number of references overall. Use of causal or mental state expressions.	**Sig.** Less cohesive stories i.e. more ambiguous use of pronouns and limited use of temporal expressions. Lower proportion of pronouns used overall to maintain reference.

(*Continued*)

Table 2. (Continued)

Study	Yr	Elicitation method/task	Type of narrative and cognitive requirements	ASD participants	Comparison groups	Focus of study	Results: Nsig. diffs	Results: Sig. diffs
Gabig.	2008	**Stimulus:** Renfrew Bus Story; script read by experimenter while subjects see series of 12 pictures. **Task:** Retell the story with the aid of the pictures.	Comprehension of verbally and pictorially presented story. Retelling of stimulus story.	15 children with autism, mean age 6;6	10 TD children, age matched (mean, 6;8)	Verbal working memory and story retelling.		**Sig.** Story recall much poorer (i.e. less close match between retold story and stimulus story in % of propositions recalled); lower 'longest utterance length'.
Garcia-Perez et al.	2008	**Stimulus:** single pictures of background scenes plus cut-out figures. **Task:** tell and re-tell stories based on scenes and selected figures, from perspectives of different protagonists (3 versions for each of 2 stories).	Parsing of single scene. Story construction based on scene and character figures. Retelling of same story.	15 participants with ASD, mean age 13;04	15 participants with ID but not autism, matched on chronological age and verbal ability. [no NT controls]	ToM and beyond: Perspectivisation; social cognition.	**Nsig.** Use of mental state terms. Understanding of task and ability to adjust narrative for alternative viewpoints.	**Sig.** Poorer ability to adopt different perspectives & shift between them. However wide variation in ability.

Goldman	2008	**Stimulus**: personal events elicited based on given topics. **Task:** describe personal experiences from autobiographical memory to unfamiliar audience based on given topic.	Memory for autobiographical events. Construction of a retell of remembered events.	14 children with HFA, aged 9–13; mean 11;3	12 children with developmental language disorder. 12 NT children. Matched for chronological age and NVIQ	Narrative analysis of personal event stories.	**NSig.** Basic knowledge of conversational narrative format; situated story in time.	**Sig.** Produced fewer proper narratives and needed more support. Off-topic answers from some. Consistent lack of 'high point'; fewer persons or resolutions in story elements; lacked coherence; failed to specify goals; seemed not to understand why we tell stories. Few interpretations of behaviours.

(*Continued*)

Table 2. (Continued)

Study	Yr	Elicitation method/task	Type of narrative and cognitive requirements	ASD participants	Comparison groups	Focus of study	Results: Nsig. diffs	Results: Sig. diffs
Ehlers	2008	**3 types of narrative:** (1) generated from wordless picture book *Frog On His Own*; (2) retell of a wordless short film *Frog Goes to Dinner*; (3) personal experience narratives elicited through conversation with topic suggestions. Each told to both peer and adult audiences.	Comprehension of implicit narrative depicted by picture sequence or enacted in video dramatization. Construction/ Retelling of non-verbally presented stimulus stories. Memory for autobiographical events. Construction of a retell of remembered events.	4 children with ASD (AS and PDD-NOS), 8–11; average or above NVIQ	4 NT children, language-age matched	Comparison of narrative ability across different types of narratives and to different types of audience.	**NSig.** Length, mention of internal states, irrelevant information, prompts. No sig. diffs. in narratives told across various contexts and listeners.	**Sig.** Less likely to include causal statements in story retell and picture book narratives told to adults & more likely to use inaccurate or ambiguous references to characters in personal narratives told to adults. Used more correct character references to adults than to peers.

Begeer et al.	2010	**Stimulus:** read a short story about an interaction in a domestic context; included no explicit mental state terms but provided clues about mental state. **Task:** retell it. [they also took part in a communication game requiring taking into account another's perspective].	Comprehension of heard narrative. Retelling of verbally-presented stimulus story.	34 adolescents & adults with ASDs, mean age 16;7	34 NT adolescents & adults, matched on chronological age and cognitive abilities	Theory of Mind.	**Nsig.** Same level of performance in the communication game.	**Sig.** Fewer mental state terms in description of people's behaviour in narrative task.
De Marchena & Eigsti	2010	**Stimulus:** 6 drawings on cards, depicting a story. **Task:** examine the picture cards one at a time, then stand and tell the story to the experimenter without access to the cards.	Comprehension of implicit narrative depicted by picture sequence. Construction/ Retelling of non-verbally presented stimulus stories.	15 adolescents with HFA, age 12–17, mean 15;0	15 NT adolescents matched on age, gender & IQ	Spontaneous production of gesture during storytelling and ratings of story quality.	**NSig.** Utterance and gesture rates.	**Sig.** Naive observers rated ASD stories as less clear and engaging and ratings correlated with ASD symptom severity scores. Gestures were less closely synchronised with speech. Story ratings were associated with gesture count in TD group but not in ASD group.

(*Continued*)

Table 2. (Continued)

Study	Yr	Elicitation method/task	Type of narrative and cognitive requirements	ASD participants	Comparison groups	Focus of study	Results: Nsig. diffs	Results: Sig. diffs
Estigarribia et al.	2011	**Stimulus:** Bus story language test: 12 pictures with a story script read by an experimenter. **Task:** retell the story while looking at the pictures.	Comprehension of verbally and pictorially presented story. Retelling of stimulus story.	28 boys with Fragile-X syndrome and ASD (not high-functioning), age 6–15, mean 10;9	29 boys with Fragile-X syndrome and without ASD, age 6–15, mean 11;7. 33 Boys with Down Syndrome, age 6–15, mean 9;10. 39 NT boys, age 3–7, mean 5;1. Minimal language requirements for all clinical groups	Narrative recall ability and its correlation with caregiver characteristics.	**Nsig.** Basics of story structure. Number of narrative elements relating to human characters and character motivations. Internal response difficult for all groups. No sig. differences between the two FX groups (w/ out ASD). No correlation of narrative skill with syntactic ability.	**Sig.** ASD had lower overall story grammar scores than NT. Both FX groups mention fewer attempts and actions than NT and DS. Some specific observations relating to mentions of the anthropomorphised bus and its driver.

Brown et al.	2012	In an interview context, children were asked to retell their earliest memories and one positive and one negative emotional experience.	Memory for autobiographical events. Construction of a retell of remembered events.	30 children with AS aged 6–14	20 NT children, matched for age	Autobiographical narratives and internal state reports.	**NSig.** All children provided at least one narrative (exc. 1 NT child).	**Sig.** Fewer emotional, cognitive and perceptual terms.
Manolitsi & Botting	2011	**Stimulus:** experimenter narrated a story accompanied by a picture book (*Peter and the cat*). **Task:** retell the story using the same picture book.	Comprehension of verbally and pictorially presented story. Retelling of stimulus story.	13 Greek children with ASD, age 4;2–13;0	13 Greek children with SLI, age 5;0–13;0	Investigating tools for distinguishing ASD and SLI.	**NSig.** Some narrative measures.	**Sig.** While standardised language tests showed ASD to be more impaired in receptive vs. expressive language, some narrative measures showed poorer ASD performance in expressive skills: involving wider story-telling skill, esp. referencing.

CHAPTER 9

Using conversational structure as an interactional resource

Children with Asperger's syndrome and their conversational partners

Johanna Rendle-Short
The Australian National University

One of the diagnostic criteria for children with Asperger's Syndrome (AS) is pragmatic impairment. Yet, minimal interactional research has been carried out on what exactly 'pragmatic impairment' might mean. What do children with AS do (or not do) when interacting? What do they find interactionally 'difficult'? What do the conversational partners do to manage social and pragmatic difficulties as they emerge, moment by moment, in interaction? Using a conversation analytic framework, this paper explores some of the ways in which two pragmatically impaired children with AS, aged 8 years, interact with four different conversational partners. Using a competence model, it examines the conversational partners' use of adjacency pairs as a scaffolding device enabling the children with AS to make contributions to the talk-in-interaction in a safe, predictable environment. It also examines the different strategies used by the children with AS in environments in which the talk is less well-scaffolded, such as when initiating new topics or repair sequences. The analysis highlights the need for further research into how interaction is collaboratively managed by children with AS and their interactional partners.

Previous research has shown that children with High Functioning Autism (HFA) and Asperger's Syndrome (AS) find social interaction difficult (e.g. Attwood 2000; Fine, Bartolucci, Szatmari & Ginsberg 1994; Gillberg & Gillberg 1989; Minshew, Goldstein & Siegel 1995; Rendle-Short 2003; Tager-Flusberg & Anderson 1991; Wing 1981; Wootton 2003). Yet social interaction is of utmost importance, especially for developing peer relationships and in forming friendships (Erwin 1993; Margalit 1994). Being able to make and keep friends is important for *all* children, including those who have been diagnosed with AS. Friendship offers long-term benefits for school adjustment, improves self-esteem and personal well-being, and reduces loneliness and the possibility of depression (Diehl, Lemerise, Caverly, Ramsay & Roberts 1998; Dunn 2004; Erwin 1993; Margalit 1994). Yet Koning and Magill-Evans (2001) reported that within a group of twenty-one adolescent boys with AS nearly half of them reported having no friends.

In order for children to show friendship through displayed feelings of belonging based on shared concerns, interests or other activities, and to voluntarily show mutual respect for each other (Margalit 1994), they require the necessary interpersonal skills and the ability to understand the reciprocal nature of social interaction. For example, they need to know how to initiate a conversation, how to be a 'good listener', and how to let their conversational partner (a potential friend) know that they are listening, through gaze or minimal response tokens. They need to realise not to ask inappropriate questions or not to talk repeatedly about the same idea, especially if their conversational partner is not interested in what they are talking about. They need to learn to moderate the volume of their voice. Yet these are the sort of difficulties experienced by children with AS (Knott, Dunlop & Mackay 2006).

So it is not surprising that children with AS who lack the fine interactional control required for successful social interaction find friendships difficult (e.g. Attwood 2000; Bauminger & Kasari 2000). Even though they might *want* to make friends with other children, they tend to approach the other child in a clumsy and not very successful way (Prior et al. 1998). They may also find it difficult to maintain the quality of the friendship as they are not skilled at reciprocal play and talking about things in common (Bauminger & Kasari 2000). As a result of such difficulty in forming individual friendships, they are less likely to be included in larger friendship groups, resulting in further social isolation (Margalit 1994). So even though children with AS might want more social interaction with peers (Bauminger & Kasari 2000), because they are less able than their similar aged cohort to engage in social interaction, they experience difficulty in forming friendships (Attwood 2000; Koning & Magill-Evans 2001) and strong peer relationships.

Although we might have an intuitive understanding of some of the pragmatic difficulties experienced by children with AS, we are only beginning to appreciate what it is that children with AS do, or do not do, when interacting with others and how this might impact on their ability to form friendships. One of the reasons for the lack of social interaction research within the field of autism is due to the context-specific nature of interaction. Quantification may show that children with autism generally initiate fewer bids for interactions, comment less often and respond less often to family member communication bids (e.g. Jones & Schwartz 2009), but it is only through detailed analyses of how participants behave in real time that we can begin to understand the interactional difficulties for this group of children, including, how they organise structural aspects of interaction (e.g. Kremer-Sadlik 2004;

Ochs & Solomon 2004; Ochs, Kremer-Sadlik, Gainer Sirota & Solomon 2004; Rendle-Short 2003), how they manage repair (e.g. Stribling, Rae & Dickerson 2007; Volden 2004) and how they display mutual understanding or intersubjectivity (e.g. Sterponi & Fasulo 2010).

Previous research into the interactions of neurotypical children has demonstrated the children's interactional competency across a range of settings. Focus has been given to how their talk is designed and received within the unfolding organization of social interaction, foregrounding the competencies that children demonstrate, whether talking to peers (e.g. Blum-Kulka & Snow 2004; Church 2009; Cobb-Moore, Danby & Farrell 2009; Danby & Baker 1998b; Goodwin 1990; Sheldon 1992, 1996), or adults (e.g. Filipi 2009; Forrester & Reason 2006), including interactions within specific institutional settings, such as medical settings (e.g. Cahill 2010; Silverman 1987), child counselling (e.g. Hutchby & Moran-Ellis 2001; Hutchby 2002, 2010), or parent-teacher interviews (e.g. Silverman, Baker & Keogh 1998).[1] Particular emphasis has been given to young children's display of mutual understanding or intersubjectivity (Filipi 2009; Gardner & Forrester 2010; Jones & Zimmerman 2003; Sidnell 2010) through use of repair and questioning repeats (e.g. Corrin 2010; Filipi 2009; Forrester 2008; Jones & Zimmerman 2003; Laakso 2010; Pike 2010; Salonen & Laakso 2009; Sidnell 2010; Wootton 2007), use of gaze as social control (Kidwell 2005), and use of interactional devices to co-construct and maintain social order (e.g. Cobb-Moore, Danby & Farrell 2009; Danby & Baker 1998a, 2000, 2001; Goodwin & Kyratzis 2007; Kyratzis 2007).

Overwhelmingly, the research demonstrates that as children go about their everyday mundane tasks of interacting with parents, siblings, teachers, and doctors they are competent manipulators of verbal and interactional resources (e.g. Bruner 1983; Cromdal 2009; Ervin Tripp 1979; Forrester 2008; Garvey 1984; Keenan 1974; McTear 1985; Ochs 1988; Ochs & Schieffelin 1979, 1983; Salonen & Laakso 2009; Schieffelin 1990; Sidnell 2010; Wells 1981; Wootton 1994, 2006, 2007).

Against this background of the interactional competencies displayed by children in general, it is important to examine how children with AS cope within a neuorotypical world. This paper, therefore, focuses on the interactional competencies of two 8-year-old children with AS as they interact in naturally-occurring situations. Such detailed interactional analysis is in response to recent calls in the autism literature for fine grained micro-level analyses of social behaviour in naturalistic settings (e.g. Geils & Knoetze 2008; Macintosh & Dissanayake 2006; Muller & Schuler 2006).

1. For an overview, see Hutchby 2005.

Pragmatic and social difficulties for children with AS

Overwhelmingly, as indicated in the diagnostic criteria (American Psychiatric Association ([DSM-IV-TR] 2000)) and as described in the literature, children with AS find social interaction more difficult than their typically developing peers. Attwood (2000: p. 85–86) lists the most conspicuous characteristics of social difficulty, including lack of reciprocity; little appreciation of social cues; failure to share enjoyment, interests or achievements with other people; an inability or lack of desire to interact with their peers or a failure to develop peer relationships appropriate to the child's developmental level; a failure to adequately use eye gaze, facial expressions, body posture and gesture to regulate social interaction; socially and emotionally inappropriate behaviour, and difficulty reading emotion from facial expressions.

Cognitive explanations for why children with AS have difficulty with social skills have highlighted executive dysfunction, weak central coherence, and difficulties in engaging and shifting attention (see for example, Barry et al. 2003: p. 686), including an impairment in the fundamental ability to 'mind read' (Baron-Cohen 1995). Whereas typically developing children understand (from the age of around 4 years) that other people have thoughts, knowledge, beliefs and desires that influence and explain other's behaviour, many children with AS may have considerable difficulty conceptualizing and appreciating the thoughts and feelings of others. As Attwood (2000: p. 87) says, they are not able to 'think about thoughts'. This makes social reasoning much more difficult as they are not able to understand or 'read' what it is that the other person is doing. Such children are often uncertain as to whether the other person is just doing something accidentally (for example, just happening to look at them at that particular moment) or whether there is some intentionality involved (for example, the other person looked at them because they expected a response to a question or comment). Not being able to work out what is behind someone's talk or non-verbal cues, or not being able to 'read' the interaction, results in confusion concerning what the other person might be saying/doing (or not saying/doing).

In terms of their interactive and discourse ability, one area of difficulty for children with AS is that they do not seem to intuitively understand how to link ideas together (Wing 1981). Fine et al. (1994), for example, found that children with AS made unclear references, showing an inability to design their talk for their interlocutor or conversational partner. In another study examining how autistic children maintain and develop topics of conversation, Tager-Flusberg & Anderson (1991) showed that the clearest difference between the high functioning autistic children in their study and the controls (children with Down's syndrome) was that the children with autism failed to develop categories of discourse that added new information to the topic of discourse. In an analysis of narratives, Solomon

(2001, cited in Ochs et al. 2004: p. 150) found that high functioning children with autism spectrum disorders atypically used connective markers such as 'and', 'but' and 'so' to link topically disjunctive propositions. Such lack of cohesion, combined with the tendency for children with AS to monopolise the conversation through perseveration of their favourite topics of interest (Wing 1981), can make it difficult for conversational partners to keep the conversation 'on track' by following the expected conversational rules and structuring principles.

Interactional scaffolding

Interaction is a jointly constructed activity that requires both participants to make appropriate and timely contributions to the progression of talk (Sacks, Schegloff & Jefferson 1974). If one of the interactional participants is pragmatically impaired then it may fall to the other person, the conversational partner, to interactionally manage the conversation as it emerges, moment by moment. This interactional management of the conversation can be likened to the process of scaffolding, whereby a child can be assisted in solving a problem, carrying out a task or achieving a goal which may be beyond his or her unassisted efforts (Wood, Bruner & Ross 1976). Kirchner (1991) has utilized this notion of scaffolding when facilitating conversational participation in children with language impairment. The scaffolding process enables the more competent interactant (generally an adult) to control "those elements of the task that are initially beyond the learner's capacity, thus permitting him *[sic]* to concentrate upon and complete only those elements that are within his range of competence." (Wood, Bruner & Ross: p. 90).

Given the structural organization of naturally-occurring conversation (Sacks et al. 1974), more competent interlocutors can use conversational structure as a scaffolding device. One possible interactional scaffolding device is the adjacency pair. The adjacency pair is made up of an action initiating first pair part (FPP), sometimes simply called a 'first', and a second pair part (SPP), or 'second', that completes the action initiated by the first (Sacks et al. 1974). Classic adjacency pair sequences are question and answer sequences, in which there is a clear expectation of 'conditional relevance', such that given a first, the second is the socially expected next action. As argued by Schegloff (1968: p. 1083), the strength of the conditional relevance is such that if the second does not occur it can be heard as being 'officially absent' and therefore accountable in the ensuing talk. For example, a missing SPP may be commented upon or the FPP may be asked again in a reformulated form. Adjacency pairs in which FPPs are routinely followed, with minimal gap and minimal overlap, by SPPs are therefore both predictable and stable (Ochs et al. 2004: p. 158; Sacks et al. 1974).

Adjacency pairs and children with autism spectrum disorders

Research from ethnographic and discourse analytic studies show that individuals with autism spectrum disorders experience difficulty responding to questions (Kremer-Sadlik 2004). This may be due to the complexity of the question or their inability to take the interlocutor's perspective into account. For example, young adults with autism do better on short simple questions compared to questions that draw inferences (Hewitt 1998) and, in a single case study, it was shown that an 8-year-old girl with AS was most successful at answering yes/no questions (Rendle-Short 2003).

In addition, an ethnographic study (Kremer-Sadlik 2004) examining the conversational skills of 8–12-year-old children with HFA or AS showed that when interacting with family members at home, the 16 children who participated in the study demonstrated a strong knowledge of the socio-cultural norms of providing an answer when asked a question: they answered 85% of the questions, and only ignored 15% of them. Kremer-Sadlik (2004) argued that this high response rate may have been due to the fact that the children were in a familiar environment with lots of scaffolding by the conversational partners.

Furthermore, Dobbinson, Perkins and Boucher (1998) showed that children and adults with autism spectrum disorders have longer pauses both within turns and between one turn and the next when answering questions. For example, in the context of an adjacency pair, such as a question and answer sequence (Sacks et al. 1974), it has been shown that children with autism spectrum disorders may delay responding to the question (e.g. Rendle-Short 2003; Ochs et al. 2004). Whereas an adult or a typically developing older child would respond immediately with minimal gap (Sacks et al. 1974) and if there was a short pause, it would be less than a second (Jefferson 1989), for children with AS they may take longer than a second to respond to a question (Rendle-Short 2003; Ochs et al. 2004). Providing an explanation for such pauses is not easy. One explanation is that children with AS have an impairment in information processing (Bauminger 2002) which means that they may not be able to react fast enough to the presence of social cues in the conversation, so that they do not 'keep up with' what is happening. However, as pointed out by Ochs et al. (2004 p. 162) longer pauses may just reflect a desire to withdraw from the interaction at hand.

This paper contributes to our understanding of social interaction for children with AS in two key ways. First, it examines whether conversational predictability, through interactional sequences such as adjacency pairs, provides scaffolding opportunities for children with AS and their conversational partners. It contrasts interactions with conversational predictability in which children with AS are able to make a contribution to the talk-in-interaction in a safe, predictable environment, with interactions which are not so predictable, such as when initiating new topics or repair sequences. Second, using a competence model, it examines the specific conversational skills and interactional strategies that children with AS use in these less predictable environments.

Data and methodology

This paper uses the methodological framework of conversation analysis to analyse the way in which two 8-year-old children with AS talk to their conversational partners. Conversation analysis (CA) arises from ethnomethodology (Garfinkel 1967; Garfinkel & Sacks 1970) and is based on the premise that talk is orderly and organised (Sacks 1984; Sacks 1992). Sacks et al. (1974) demonstrate orderliness through ideas fundamental to CA including the 'turn construction unit' (TCU) as the basic unit of talk and the 'transition relevance place' (TRP) as the point in interaction where speaker change becomes interactionally 'relevant'. TCUs can be complete sentences, phrases or even single words. A speaker beginning a turn of talk has the right to produce a single TCU, although speakers often produce turns composed of more than one TCU. In determining possible completion points of a TCU (in other words, the point at which speaker change *could* occur), next speakers orient to the grammar, intonation and pragmatics of the current speaker's emerging talk (Sacks et al. 1974).

One of the advantages of using the methodology of conversation analysis is that it provides a powerful lens for examining social activity through its rigorous and finely-tuned analysis of ordinary conversations in naturally-occurring settings. Such fine-grained analysis is important given the subtle social and pragmatic difficulties experienced by children with AS. A second advantage relates to the fact that conversation analysis works from the premise that any claims made *about* the data must be demonstrable *in* the data. Instead of drawing on abstract theories or pre-determined analytical constructs, conversation analysts treat the data as the participants' phenomena, as evidence of how the participants themselves understood and acted upon each others' contributions. A third advantage arises from the way in which the methodology of conversation analysis encourages analysts to apply a competence model with emphasis placed on what it is that children with AS *can do* rather than adopting a deficit model that emphasises the children's poor social interaction skills.

The naturally-occurring conversational data analysed in this paper is taken from a larger data set of children with AS interacting with friends and family. The data under consideration in this paper consists of two case studies of two 8-year-old children each talking to two different conversational partners. Both children have diagnoses of Asperger's Syndrome. The conversational partners are either family members or close friends. In the first case study, Jancis (pseudonym) was audio recorded during a telephone conversation in which she rang her friend, Tyffany (pseudonym), after she had not been at school one day. She initially talked to her friend's mother and then she talked to Tyffany herself (also aged 8 years old). It was just before Easter, and Jancis rang her friend to ask if she had brought back her decorated boiled egg from the classroom. In the second case study, Will (pseudonym) was video recorded while talking at home in the living room. First of all, Will is talking to his mother on the couch and then to his slightly older brother (aged 10 years).

The first case study consists of 4.4 minutes of data with a total of 104 TCUs: 29 TCUs were spoken by Jancis; 57 TCUs were spoken by her friend, Tyffany; 18 TCUs were spoken by her friend's mother. The second case study consists of 12.8 mins of Will talking to his mother (with a total of 266 TCUs: 137 TCUs were spoken by Will;129 TCUs were spoken by his mother) and 12.3 mins of Will talking to his brother (with a total of 297 TCUs: 171 TCUs were spoken by Will;126 TCUs were spoken by his brother). The complete data sets were transcribed using CA transcription conventions (see Appendix).

The following analysis is based on 9 representative extracts from the data sets that most clearly demonstrate the phenomenon under discussion. As with any micro-level analysis of a limited data set, the following analysis is not intended to be generalised to all cases. Rather, the aim of the analysis is to utilise the principles of conversation analysis to highlight the interactional complexity of naturally-occurring conversations and to highlight the interactional work done by both the child with AS and their conversational partners. The more we understand about how individual children with AS interact, the more we will be able to understand the broader population of children with AS.

Analysis

The following will show how the two children with AS under analysis are, on the one hand, very skilled interactionists who at times may appear to behave like many of their unaffected friends or peers. However, it will also show how the children can be vulnerable to pragmatic language challenges that may result in the interaction not proceeding as anticipated. The first two sections of the following analysis demonstrate the structured predictability to the interaction when responding to an action initiated by a conversational partner. Initially the focus is on how conversational partners use the adjacency pair structure as a scaffolding device enabling the two children with AS to make contributions to the talk-in-interaction in a safe, predictable environment. It builds on a comment by Ochs et al. (2004: p. 158) that adjacency pairs exhibit a 'conventional interactional implicature' that is both predictable and stable. This is followed by analysis of how the second child with AS, Will, responds with an extended turn to a query about his day. Providing a telling requires the child to structure the talk so that it is coherent and makes sense to the listener. This contrasts with the different scenario whereby the child might have to initiate a new action themselves. The third and fourth sections of the analysis focus on why the children might find it difficult to move from the predictable position of responding to the prior talk, to the more challenging role of initiating a new topic or repairing some aspect of the prior talk. In the discussion section, the paper returns to a consideration of the implications of the findings for understanding the role played by conversational partners. It discusses the children's vulnerability to pragmatic language challenges that may result in the interaction not always proceeding as anticipated.

Predictability: Responding within the adjacency pair format

Overwhelmingly in the conversations under analysis, and in accordance with the findings by Jones and Schwartz (2009), conversational partners were much more likely to use FPPs to initiate actions compared to the children with AS. Such first pair parts (FPPs) with their 'conventional interactional implicature' (Ochs et al. 2004: p. 158) provide a high level of orderliness and structure to the conversation, and more specifically to turn-taking. As a result, the children only have to provide an appropriate SPP of the same pair type.

The following extract shows the mother of Will asking a series of questions while they are sitting on the couch together.

(1) [Will and mother]

1. M: where did you get that one from.
2. W: huh huh. the fair.
3. at Saint Thomas.
4. M: yeah?
5. W: I got it from trash and treasure.
6. M: you did. didn't ya.
7. you're lucky you found some treasure.
8. W: yeah.
9. M: do you remember how you found it?
10. (1.0)
11. W: in a little bit of a ugh ugh ugh like that.
12. wasn't it. ((nonverbal action and noises of pushing))

The adjacency pair sequences in the above extract provide a structured predictability to the interaction. The mother asks the questions and the child provides the answers. But the child is doing more than just showing that he is able to answer questions – he demonstrates his interactional ability in a number of different ways. In line 2, in response to the question asking where he got the book from, he initially laughs before providing the necessary information. The laughter contextualises the response, demonstrating his appreciation of the event as funny. In line 5, he appropriately treats the mother's rising intonation 'yeah' in line 4 as a request for additional information. In line 8, he appropriately provides an agreement token to his mother's comment about being lucky to find some treasure. Finally in line 11 he resorts to a nonverbal response when he is not able to explain how he found the book at the trash and treasure.

Initial evidence that this 'do you remember' question might be more difficult is provided through the pause in line 10. Normally, there is a minimal gap between a FPP and SPP (Sacks et al. 1974) and if there is inter-turn silence the maximum length of silence in adult conversations would generally be between 0.8 – 1.2 seconds (Jefferson 1989). So although this 1.0 second silence (line 10) is within the expected maximum length of pauses between turns (Jefferson), the silence indicates potential difficulty in answering the question (Pomerantz 1984; Schegloff 2007). During this silence the mother looks at the child, but does not assist him by rephrasing the question or by providing a candidate answer. Instead, she waits and in line 11, Will non-verbally shows his mother what happened and how he and another child had 'a little bit of a' push as they both tried to get the same book. He accompanies his pushing gestures with appropriate noises to illustrate the action.

Sometimes, however, the child with AS does not respond to the FPP. If a question is not 'appropriately' responded to, the conversational partner has choices as to whether they rephrase the question (extract 2) or pursue an adequate response through a slightly different question type (extract 3).

(2) [Will and brother]

12. W: and then we went to Kmart,
13. and shopped for my clo::thes.
14. Br: and what did you ge::t.
15. (1.0)
16. W: NOTHING NICE.
17. Br: and what did you get.
18. (1.0)
19. W: coloured (clothes).
20. Br: what colours
21. W: green, yellow, blue, and navy.

(3) [Will and mother]

17. M: but that was- =you found that book
18. before then. didn't ya?

19. W: yeah I did.
20. M: where did you find that one.
21. W: I found it when I was looking for books.
22. (1.2)
23. M: mhm.
24. do you want to tell me about it?

In extract 2, the conversational partner (the brother) does not accept Will's SPP in line 16 as an adequate response to the 'what did you get' question. Already the inter-turn gap in line 15 indicates that there may be a problem in providing a SPP. Then the louder than expected statement 'NOTHING NICE' (line 16) marks the response as being in some way different from expected. So although Will demonstrates his understanding of the requirements of the adjacency pair format and that an SPP is expected, his brother does not accept this louder SPP and he re-asks the question in exactly the same form (line 17). Will again delays 1.0 second before providing a response to the second question. But this second time, he does provide the information, as asked, although in a minimal form.

In contrast, in Extract 3, the response to 'where did you find that one' (line 20) is not a type conforming response in that the answer indicates 'when he found it' not 'where he found it'. However, the conversational partner (mother) does not comment on the inappropriate response. Instead there is a 1.2 second pause (as possible indication of trouble associated with an inappropriate response), an acknowledgement of the SPP ('mhm.' in line 23), followed by another FPP. This telling-request FPP opens up a space for Will to answer the question about finding the books in his own way.

If there is no response to a question, then the conversational partner might pursue a response as shown in extract 4 when Jancis is talking on the phone to her friend's mother (M).

(4) [Jancis and friend's mother]

3. M: hello Jancis,=did you just call
4. a minute ago an' then hang up?
5. (1.6)
6. J: y:es:, hh
7. M: wh:y did you do that.
8. (4.0)
9. M: ↑yoo hoo::,↓
10. J: he he.hh
11. M: are ya there?
12. J: ye::s, hhh
13. M: what happened.
14. J: heh heh

In this extract, the mother asks 'why did you do that' (line 7) in order to find out why the child rang a few minutes ago and then hung up. This is a difficult question for the child to answer and she pauses for 4.0 seconds. However, the conditional relevance of the FPP is evident through the mother's pursuit of a response. In other words, it is not sufficient that no SPP is provided. The mother initially checks that the child is still on the phone (line 9). When the child responds by laughing, she checks again that Jancis is there (line 11). The mother then returns to the original question of why she rang a few minutes ago and hung up, although this time she reframes the 'why' question as a 'what happened' question.

Responding to an action initiated by the conversational partner provides a straightforward predictable context for the child with AS to demonstrate their conversational abilities. Following the interactional expectation that talk is structured through adjacency pairs (Sacks et al. 1974) with an initiated action only being completed once the action initiating turn (FPP) has been responded to by the SPP, children with AS only need display their ability to provide a SPP in response to the initiating turn. If their SPP is missing or insufficient the conversational partner can then ask a second FPP as a way of clarifying or obtaining additional information. This interactional scaffolding was provided in a range of ways in the above extracts: asking FPPs; refraining from talking during inter-turn silences; reframing FPPs; checking recipiency. The scaffolding provides an interactional structure or framework for the children as well as providing them with an opportunity to learn what counts as legitimate responses or different ways in which interactive contributions are responded to.

Predictability: Providing a telling

Responding to questions about your day, such as 'how was your day' or 'what did you do today' are slightly more complex as they require the child with AS to order the talk into a coherent telling. In the following extract, Will and his brother were talking on the couch.[2]

(5) [Will and brother]

1. Br: hello Will.
2. W: HELLO. James.
3. Br: how was your da::y.
4. W: goo::d,

---

2. The beginning of this interaction highlights the difficulty of obtaining recordings of children with AS within naturally occurring settings – the brother begins the recorded interaction with 'hello Will' as if he were starting a conversation on the telephone.

5. Br: what didya do.
6. W: we we:::nt
7. (0.2)
8. Br: what did you do first.
9. W: we took you-
10. we went to the dentist,
11. and we took you to sch:ool,
12. and then we went to Kmart,
13. and shopped for my clo::thes.
14. Br: and what did you ge::t.
15. (1.0)
16. W: NOTHING NICE.
17. Br: and what did you get.
18. (1.0)
19. W: coloured (clothes.)
20. Br: what colours
21. W: green, yellow, blue, and navy.
22. and.hh (.) and then we went ho::me,
23. and I played on the computer
24. for a little while.

Understanding what is required interactionally may not always be clear, and in this extract Will requires some prompting. In response to the initial question 'what didya do' (line 5), Will begins a turn at talk (TCU) with an elongated 'we we:::nt', followed by a short pause. The brother interprets this incomplete TCU as evidence of difficulty in providing the telling. The brother then limits the scope of the question by asking, 'what did you do first' (line 8). Although breaking the question down into smaller components, facilitates the likelihood of the child with AS providing an appropriate response, Will is still not able to start a coherent account straight away. Again he stops talking before completing his first turn at talk. However, once he recommences his telling, the temporal ordering of his account gives the story a clear predictability and ordered structure. As shown in the previous extracts, the conversational partner provides the interactional scaffolding in a range of ways: by limiting the scope of the request for a telling (line 8); through repeated questions if the response is not satisfactory (in line 17 and as we saw in extract 2 above); and through requests for clarification (line 20).

But although the brother provided a clear context for the telling to encourage Will to tell him what happened during the day, the next bit of interaction shows that even with such scaffolding and high predictability, a child with AS can find it difficult to provide a coherent account.

(6) [Will and brother]

22. W: and.hh (.) and then we went ho::me,
23. and I played on the computer
24. for a little while.
25. but I decided to have fr- (.)
26. some time off playing.
27. so I- (.) do you know what I looked at?
28. Br: what.
29. W: the rug rats.
30. Br: good.
31. W: then I played the rug rats
32. on the pla:y sta:tion,
33. and d'you know what Emby said?
34. Br: what.-
35. W: there's no-one playing it.
36. and do you know how I- (.)
37. there's always time to pick you up
38. when I come a:t
39. Br: so.
40. W: and so we went to the library,
41. and d' you know what we-
42. and I jumped-
43. had time to borrow two books,
44. and then we went out of the library,
45. to pick you up,
46. and then we went to gym.
47. Br: so what did you do at gym.

One challenge for any storyteller is to order their talk using multi-TCU turns, to link subsequent ideas to prior ideas, and to have a story resolution. The extract shows Will continuing with the chronologically ordered telling with 'and' prefaced linking devices (lines 22 – 24). In line 27, however, Will breaks off a potential resolution 'so I-' to change the trajectory of the storytelling by asking a story-related question. Such a technique enables Will to shift the sequential ordering of the interaction while still talking about his day. It is an effective strategy to ensure smooth and continuing progression of the telling.

Will uses this technique again in line 33, 'and d' you know what Emby said'. Both times his 'do you know x' question receives a 'what' questioning response from his brother, thus allowing him to initiate an action in the form of a question while at the same time limiting the scope of the question. As a strategy for maintaining coherence it is very successful. It enables Will to provide additional information in response to his own question. It also works well in terms of ensuring predictability, as the brother responds both times with 'what'.[3]

However, the next two times Will tries to use the 'do you know' strategy, it is less successful. Both times he doesn't complete the 'do you know' TCU and so the strategy of initiating an action and receiving a 'what' question in return doesn't work. In the first of these unsuccessful attempts, Will says 'and do you know how I-' (line 36), cutting off the end of the TCU before making it clear what he wants to say. In the second of these unsuccessful attempts, he similarly says 'and do you know what we-' (line 41), again cutting off the end of the TCU before making it clear what he wants to say. On each occasion the next TCU is incoherent. In the first instance, he says a partially incomplete 'there's always time to pick you up when I come at' (lines 36 – 38). In the second instance he says 'and I jumped-' (line 42) which doesn't fit the logic and temporal coherence of the telling.

So the data clearly shows that when Will completes his 'do you know' question, as in lines 27 and 33, it is a very effective strategy. However, when he doesn't complete the 'do you know' question, as in lines 36 and 41, the coherence is lost. The subsequent talk on both of these latter occasions consists of an incomplete TCU. Evidence of the lack of coherence is given by the brother who asks 'so' in line 39. The fact that the subsequent talk doesn't follow the logic of the question and is not complete, thus making the telling sound incoherent, contrasts strongly with the effectiveness of the strategy when it is provided in full.

So far the analysis has shown Will and Jancis' contributions to talk in fairly predictable environments, answering questions or talking about their day. In such contexts, they were responding to actions initiated by the other party and so there was an inbuilt predictability to the interaction. The FPP (such as 'where did you get that one from' or 'how was your day') limits the type of SPP, although when telling a story, it still requires the child to structure the talk so that it is coherent and makes sense to the listener. However, talking in less predictable environments is more complex. The second part of the analysis focuses on the way in which the two children deal with the more challenging task of initiating new topics or repairing the prior talk.

Reduced predictability: Initiating actions

Initiating an action rather than responding to an action requires participants to think about the sequential ordering of the interaction in a different way. There is a

3. The effectiveness of this interactional strategy has been provided in terms of sequential analysis. It may also be that Will is legitimately asking for information as to whether the brother 'knows x'. In other words, he may be checking what is known and not known.

predictability about providing a response that completes the action initiated by the first, both in terms of what is required (a type conforming response) and in terms of when it is required (within the maximum permissible time span).

In contrast, when initiating an action the speaker has to work out where in the conversation as a whole they should introduce this initiating talk. It is not possible to initiate a new action by, for example, asking a question or introducing a new topic just anywhere in the conversation; it needs to be sequentially relevant. An interactant might need to think about whether there is a lull in the conversation or whether other topics are still being talked about. The following example shows how even if a child might work out where a new topic might be sequentially relevant, they need to be able to execute it in a timely manner to ensure smooth transition of the information to the other person.

(7) [Jancis and friend]

1.	T:	are you still there?
2.	J:	yes.
3.	T:	good.
4.		(1.2)
5.	J:	I wanted t'a::sk, hh (1.2)
6.	T:	Jancis guess what you missed.
7.	J:	wha'
8.	T:	a big easter egg 'cos
9.		you brought all your homework in.
10.		an' a li'le one too.
11.		(1.0)
12.	T:	but [never mind.] you'll get i- them=
13.	J:	[( )]
14.	T:	= on the first day back.
15.		(0.8)
16.	T:	heh heh
17.	J:	hh.hh ((sniffing))
18.	T:	yeah.=what did you want me [to a::?-what] do=
19.	J:	[uhm hh]
20	T:	=you want t' ask?
21.	J:	did you bring back my boiled e:gg?

Jancis chooses an appropriate place to initiate her new topic, following a short checking sequence in lines 1–3 and a 1.2 second silence. She commences her new topic with 'I wanted to ask' (line 5) which demonstrates an orientation to her reason for calling her friend. However, although the turn beginning indicates that a question is going to follow, there is a vulnerability of execution highlighted by the slow delivery and long intra-turn pause of 1.2 seconds. The vulnerability becomes a reality when the friend Tyffany highjacks the turn by asking her own question in line 6. Tyffany orients to her question being 'out of place' in two ways. First, she uses an address term at the beginning of her turn in line 6, marking her turn as being different and maybe out of place. Second, she orients to the still relevant, yet unasked, question in line 17 when she says 'what did you want me to a::?- what do you want t' ask?'

So although Jancis does eventually get an opportunity to ask her question, this extract highlights how progressivity of the talk can be delayed due to the way in which Jancis chose to introduce the new topic into the conversation. Jancis' opportunity to ask her question only comes after Tyffany has told her own story about the Easter egg. Being able to finally ask her question also relied on her conversational partner remembering that the question was outstanding and that she still didn't know what Jancis was going to say. So although Jancis successfully chose a sequentially appropriate position to launch her reason for call, her delayed execution meant that the talk did not progress as anticipated and eventually it relied on her conversational partner to re-introduce the new topic. Once again, Jancis found herself in the more predictable position of responding to an action rather than successfully initiating her own action.

Announcing what you are going to do next is another useful way of letting your conversational partner know that you want to initiate a new topic.

(8) [Will and brother]

1. W: there's one last thing I need to talk about.
2. Br: okay?
3. W: <o::h I don't have to start,>
4. (1.5)
5. a::nd, (2.0)
6. the first of all the people you need
7. to know about Asperger's Syndrome,
8. that we enjoy TALKING ABOUT,
9. is that (1.5) even if it's a disability
10. and you don't have any strong (or),
11. it's just (1.0) you don't have to go
12. around the world complaining about it,
13. Br: yes. they are very special.
14. W: [AND]
15. Br: [so]
16. (2.0)
17. Br: I think I might go and watch:
18. some TV so [I'll
19. W: [but there's one more thing

20.		I meant to say.
21.	Br:	okay.
22.	M:	you can go now
23.	Br:	no. you can s [ay. [me
24.	W:	[I:: [I:::
25.	Br:	talk to me.=
26.	W:	=me and many other people in the world
27.		about 300 or something (2.0)
28.		have ASPERGER'S SYNDROME.
29.		see ya.

As in the previous extract in which Jancis set up her question with 'I wanted to ask', so too Will introduces the new topic with 'there's one last thing I need to talk about' (line 1). But once he has been given the go ahead in line 2, his hesitancy is evident and he even tries to delay initiating a new topic (even though he had set it up). In spite of the uncertain beginning (line 3), elongated pauses (lines 4 and 5), unclear grammar (lines 6–12), and intra-turn pauses (lines 9 and 11), the first part of his extended turn is heard to the end. It receives agreement and an assessment that people with Asperger's Syndrome are 'very special'. However, in spite of having said 'first of all' to show that there will be two parts to his talk, the second part isn't forthcoming. Will does say a louder 'AND' to foreshadow the second part at the end of his brother's assessment in line 13, but this is said in overlap with his brother's talk. Eventually, Will overtly says, 'but there's one more thing I meant to say' (line 19 and 20) in order to foreshadow that he has more to say.

Again, therefore, this extract demonstrates how difficult it can be for a child with AS to initiate a new topic and to ensure that there is enough interactional space to present their ideas. As with Jancis, although Will correctly chose an appropriate sequential environment to initiate his new topic, actually getting his ideas out is not straightforward, once again delaying the progressivity of the talk. As with Jancis, it relies on the conversational partner providing the necessary interactional scaffolding to ensure that the topic is eventually 'on the table'. Again, as with Jancis, Will found himself in the more predictable recipient role responding to the instruction 'talk to me' (line 25). So although metapragmatically, Will is able to show a sophisticated understanding of how to ensure that his talk is heard as intended, its execution is difficult and progressivity of the interaction is delayed.

Reduced predictability: Initiating repair

An interactionally more complex environment occurs when the conversational partner says something that is not correct. One possibility is that the child with AS could choose to ignore the incorrect statement; alternatively, they could tell the other person that they have said something that is not correct by initiating a repair sequence (Schegloff 1992). Interactionally, this requires the child to initially recognise that the statement is not correct, and then to let the other person know that it is not correct. Difficulties for a child with AS are threefold. First, possible trouble sources can appear anywhere in the interaction and so interactants have to be alert to the possibility of the potential for repair. Second, repairing a trouble source needs to be done quickly, as close as possible to the trouble source (Schegloff 1992); yet repairing a trouble source in the next turn might be difficult for a child with AS due to their slowness in executive function (Barry et al. 2003). Third, initiating a repair can be difficult as it is very unlikely that a repair initiator will be the sequentially relevant next action.

Mistakes can occur at any point in the interaction and so the possibility that a repair is required is a potentiality that interactants have to take into consideration. The following extract, taken from the end of the telephone conversation between Jancis and her friend, Tyffany, highlights the unpredictable nature of talk.

(9) [Jancis and friend]

5.	T:	heheh so (0.2) bye,
6.		I'll see you::.hh in 300 days
7.		time. right?
8.		(1.8)
9.	T:	you [still there?]
10.	J:	[no. hh]
11.	T:	alright by::e.
12.	J:	by:e.
13.	T:	bye. hang up.
14.		(0.6)
15.	J:	I'll see you at Annie's party.

In line 5 Tyffany says 'bye' as a move toward closure of the conversation. The closing implicative environment consists of an arrangement to see each other 'in 300 days time'. But the fictitious arrangement of '300 days' is problematic for Jancis. She delays for 1.8 seconds before saying 'no' in line 10, in overlap with her friend checking that she is still on the phone (line 9). Eventually Jancis provides a different arrangement for when they will next see each other, by saying 'I'll see you at Annie's party' (line 15). Although the repair of '300 days' is successful in that Jancis correctly reminds Tyffany of Annie's party and that they will see each other at the party (in a week's time), the conversation is very nearly terminated (at line 14) before the repair is executed.

Between the trouble source (line 6) and the repaired arrangement (line 15), a number of different things happen – Tyffany asks if Jancis is still on the phone (line 9); Jancis already says 'bye' (line 12); Tyffany instructs Jancis to hang up (line 13). Why was it difficult to carry out the repair? One difficulty was due to the delayed and overlapping 'no' in line 10. Jancis did not make it clear enough that there was a problem, and she didn't do it soon enough. She delayed so long (and much more than the maximum possible of 1.2 seconds), that the conversation moved onto checking if Jancis was still on the line (line 9) and then moved to closure (lines 11 – 13) before Jancis was able to let her friend know that the 300 days statement was, from her point of view, not correct. As a result, the 'no' repair initiation was lost in overlap. Had it been more explicit, it may have been noted. But as it was, the conversation moved on and Jancis lost her opportunity to repair the statement.

Tyffany may not have been aware that the 300 days was problematic for Jancis. Even when Jancis does say that she will see Tyffany at Annie's party, she does it in the form of an embedded repair, by framing the corrected arrangement within the same syntactic structure "I'll see you x", rather than overtly saying that the '300 days' time frame is incorrect. In addition, the embedded repair occurs following the terminal sequence (that would normally lead to closure) which is a difficult sequential environment to introduce more information – it runs the risk that it may not be heard as her friend may have already put down the phone.

So, although Jancis' repair of the 300 days was eventually heard and responded to (the following talk is not shown in the extract), it was not smoothly executed. The conversation faltered delaying progressivity and it may have moved to closure before any talk about Annie's party was forthcoming. Extract 9 therefore demonstrates the difficulties and the risks involved in trying to do more than simply respond to actions initiated by the other person. In this instance, trying to repair the conversational partner's talk was very nearly unsuccessful and very nearly led to the breakdown of the interaction. Having said that, utilising an embedded repair to repair another person's talk without giving offence was an excellent interactional strategy that eventually enabled Jancis to achieve a successful outcome.

Concluding discussion

Conversations involving a child with AS can be quite variable. Sometimes the children appear to interact quite well enabling a smooth turn-by-turn flow of conversation with minimal silence between turns, minimal repetition of ideas and coherent topic development. But at other times, they do not cope so well – their responses may be delayed; they may not be able to express themselves grammatically; they may find it difficult to initiate new topics, and their talk may not always be coherent. This means that for frequent and familiar conversational partners there is an accumulated sense that, at times, the interaction may not seem 'quite right'. The question that this paper has been trying to focus on is what is the nature of this accumulated sense of things being 'not quite right'.

Interaction is not like grammaticality in which there is a clear sense of whether an utterance is syntactically correct or not. Interaction emerges moment by moment and each person needs to listen carefully to what is said (and not said). Have the interactants understood what was just said or what just happened? Do they have an expectation of what might be done next or said next? Do they know what they themselves need to do next? Interactants have to listen carefully to what is going on so that they can appropriately respond to, and locally manage, the talk (Sacks et al. 1974). It is this *contextualised* nature of talk that makes it difficult to identify context-free norms of interaction against which one can assess the communicative abilities of children with AS. As a result, within a conversation analytic framework, any analysis of the interaction of children with AS needs to be situated within the local context of the talk – what the individual children and conversational partners are doing as they talk together at this particular moment in time. Through analysis of the next turn it is possible to see how the interactants themselves, at that moment in time, responded to a particular contribution to talk. For example, the next speaker will tell us, as analysts, if they understood the prior talk or if they needed more information. We saw this when Will was talking to his brother and the brother clarified questions (extracts 2 and 5) or when the brother tried to find a resolution to the telling (extract 6). We saw it when Jancis was talking to her friend's mother and the mother treated the silence as indicative of trouble – the mother asked whether the child was still on the phone (extract 4). We also saw it when Jancis was talking to her friend and her friend didn't realise that Jancis said 'no' because she thought that seeing each other in '300 days' was not correct (extract 9).

In terms of their competencies, the above analysis has shown that the two children are able to use specific conversational skills and a range of interactional strategies. For example, Will used the 'do you know' strategy to shift the sequential organization of the talk so that he could maintain interactional coherence. Although we saw that this interactional strategy did not always work, when it *did* work it was very effective. Similarly, Jancis used the strategy of saying 'I wanted to say' so that she could tell her friend why she made the phone call. Even though Jancis was not successful in immediately initiating the new topic of talk, she was eventually able to tell her friend what the call was about. So although these children may find it interactionally 'easier' to respond to FPP due to the structured nature of adjacency pairs, they were still able to ensure that their contributions to talk were successfully responded to by their conversational partner. However, as the analysis demonstrated, the interaction often had the potential to be delayed and often depended on the conversational partner and their ability to provide the necessary interactional scaffolding.

One way in which the above conversations appear less polished or not quite as smooth as might be expected relates to the institutional, or tightly constrained feel, inherent in some of the conversations. Because children with AS are less skilled at initiating topics (e.g. Jones & Scwartz 2009), they tend to sit back and allow their conversational partner to take the lead. Wootton (2003), in a broader discussion of the 'pragmatically unusual', similarly showed that young children with autism, AS and pragmatic impairment find it difficult to initiate interaction. Additionally, even if they do provide a SPP or a response, the above data show that the children with AS found it difficult to develop the topic in sophisticated ways. For example, they did not add more information to the topic, challenge the ideas of the topic, or introduce related topics. This may be because they tend not to take the listener's perspective into account which affects their ability to engage in conversations in a sustained or meaningful way (Hale & Tager-Flusberg 2005).

The above analysis has shown that conversational predictability provides a structural framework for the ensuing interaction with it being easier for the children to respond to a FPP rather than initiating their own FPPs. However, when thinking about how such children would cope interactionally when talking to friends or peers at school, it is clear that if the conversational partner is not able, or willing, to manage the interaction by providing the necessary interactional scaffolding, then the children with AS may find it difficult to initiate and sustain a conversation. The above extracts showed how all 4 conversational partners scaffolded the conversations by re-asking and re-framing questions, limiting the scope of the questions, refraining from talking during inter-turn silences, checking recipiency, requesting clarification, creating the interactional space for the child with AS to initiate a new topic. Similar aged peers who may not know that these children find social interaction difficult, may not be able, or willing, to do this sort of interactional work. As a result, ongoing difficulty in peer talk and conversations may make it difficult for children with AS to make friends and develop peer relationships.

So although this paper has shown that the two children with AS are, on the one hand, very skilled interactionists who may appear to behave like many of their unaffected friends or peers, it has also shown how they are vulnerable to pragmatic language challenges which might mean that at times the interaction does not progress as anticipated. The above analysis has shown how such challenges can be minimised through interactional scaffolding provided by conversational partners. Of course *any* interaction is locally managed and so *anyone*, including adults and children with no impairment, can also utilise such scaffolding techniques. But it seems that the children with AS themselves tend not to do the scaffolding work and tend not to utilise interactional scaffolding strategies when resolving interactional difficulties. Instead, they rely on others, their conversational partners, to re-ask and re-frame questions, to limit the scope of questions, to check whether someone is listening, and to request clarification. Additional research into the nature of this interactional scaffolding, who uses the scaffolding, and how it provides greater stability and predictability to the interaction is required as we begin to understand in more detail the nature of pragmatic impairment for children with AS.

References

American Psychiatric Association. (2000). *Diagnostic and Statistical Manual of Mental Disorders (4th ed.) (DSM-IV-TR)*. Washington, DC: American Psychiatric Association.

Atkinson, J.M., & Heritage, J. (Eds.) (1984). *Structures of Social Interaction: Studies in Conversational Analysis*. Cambridge: CUP.

Attwood, T. (2000). Strategies for improving the social integration of children with Asperger Syndrome. *Autism, 4*, 85–100.

Baron-Cohen, S. (1995). *Mindblindness: An Essay on Autism and Theory of Mind*. Cambridge, MA: The MIT Press.

Barry, T.D., Klinger, L.G., Lee, J.M., Palardy, N., Gilmore, T., & Bodin, S.D. (2003). Examining the effectiveness of an outpatient clinic based social skills group for High Functioning children with autism. *Journal of Autism and Developmental Disorders, 33*, 685–701.

Bauminger, N. (2002). The facilitation of social-emotional understanding and social interaction in High-Functioning children with autism: Intervention outcomes. *Journal of Autism and Developmental Disorders, 32*, 283–298.

Bauminger, N., & Kasari, C. (2000). Loneliness and friendship in high-functioning children with autism. *Child Development, 71*, 447 – 456.

Blum-Kulka, S., & Snow, C. (2004). Introduction: the potential of peer talk. *Discourse Studies*, 6(3), 291–306.

Bruner, J. (1983). The acquisition of pragmatic commitments. In R.M. Golinkoff (Ed.), *The Transition from Prelinguistic to Linguistic Communication* (pp. 27–42). Hillsdale, NJ: Lawrence Erlbaum Associates.

Cahill, P. (2010). Children's participation in their primary consultations. In H. Gardner & M. Forrester (Eds.), *Analysing Interaction in Childhood: Insights from Conversation Analysis* (pp. 128–145). Chichester: Wiley-Blackwell.

Church, A. (2009). *Preference Organisation and Peer Disputes: How Young Children Resolve Conflict*. Aldershot: Ashgate.

Cobb-Moore, C., Danby, S., & Farrell, A. (2009). Young children as rule makers. *Journal of Pragmatics, 41*, 1477–1492.

Corrin, J. (2010). 'Hm? What?': Maternal repair and early child talk. In H. Gardner & M. Forrester (Eds.), *Analysing Interaction in Childhood: Insights from Conversation Analysis* (pp. 23–41). Chichester: Wiley-Blackwell.

Cromdal, J. (2009). Childhood and social interaction in everyday life: Introduction to the special issue. *Journal of Pragmatics, 41*, 1473–1476.

Danby, S., & Baker, C. (1998a). "What's the problem?" Restoring social order in the preschool classroom. In I. Hutchby & J. Moran-Ellis (Eds.), *Children and Social Competence: Arenas of Action* (pp. 157–186). London: Falmer Press.

Danby, S., & Baker, C. (1998b). How to be masculine in the block area. *Childhood, 5*, 151–175.

Danby, S., & Baker, C. (2000). Unravelling the fabric of social order in block area. In S. Hester & D. Francis (Eds.), *Local Educational Order Ethnomethodological Studies of Knowledge in Action* (pp. 91–140). Amsterdam: John Benjamins.

Danby, S., & Baker, C. (2001). Escalating terror: Communicative strategies in a preschool classroom dispute. *Early Education and Development, 12*(3), 343–358.

Diehl, D.S., Lemerise, E.A., Caverly, S.L., Ramsay, S., & Roberts, J. (1998). Peer relations and school adjustment in ungraded primary children. *Journal of Educational Psychology, 90*, 506–515.

Dobbinson, S., Perkins, M.R., & Boucher, J. (1998). Structural patterns in conversation with a woman who has autism. *Journal of Communication Disorders, 14*, 383–394.

Dunn, J. (2004). *Children's Friendships: The Beginnings of Intimacy*. Malden, MA: Blackwell.

Ervin-Tripp, S. (1979). Children's verbal turn-taking. In E. Ochs & B. Schieffelin (Eds.), *Developmental Pragmatics* (pp. 391–414). New York, NY: Academic Press.

Erwin, P. (1993). *Friendship and Peer Relations in Children.* New York, NY: John Wiley & Sons.

Filipi, A. (2009). *Toddler and Parent Interaction: The Organisation of Gaze, Pointing and Vocalisation.* Amsterdam: John Benjamins.

Fine, J., Bartolucci, G., Szatmari, P., & Ginsberg, G. 1994. Cohesive discourse in pervasive developmental disorders. *Journal of Autism and Developmental Disorders, 24*, 315–329.

Forrester, M. (2008). The emergence of self-repair: A case study of one child during the early preschool years. *Research on Language and Social Interaction, 41*(1), 99–128.

Forrester, M., & Reason, D. (2006). Competency and participation in acquiring mastery of language: A reconsideration of the idea of membership. *The Sociological Review, 54*(3), 446–466.

Gardner, H., & Forrester, M. (2010). Introduction. In H. Gardner & M. Forrester (Eds.), *Analysing Interaction in Childhood: Insights from Conversation Analysis* (pp. ix–xvi). Chichester: Wiley-Blackwell.

Garfinkel, H. (1967). *Studies in Ethnomethodology*. Englewood Cliffs NJ: Prentice-Hall.

Garfinkel, H., & Sacks, H. (1970). On formal structures of practical action. In J.C. McKinney, & E.A. Tiryakian (Eds.), *Theoretical Sociology: Perspectives and Developments* (pp. 338–366). New York, NY: Appleton-Century-Crofts.

Garvey, C. (1984). *Children's Talk*. Cambridge: CUP.

Geils, C., & Knoetze, J. (2008). Conversations with Barney: A conversation analysis of interactions with a child with autism. *South African Journal of Psychology, 38*(1), 200–224.

Gillberg, C., & Gillberg, C. (1989). Asperger Syndrome. Some epidemiological considerations: A research note. *Journal of Child Psychology and Psychiatry, 30*, 631–638.

Goodwin, M. (1990). *He-Said-She-Said: Talk as Social Organization among Black Children.* Bloomington, IN: Indiana University Press.

Goodwin, M., & Kyratzis, A. (2007). Children socializing children: Practices for negotiating the social order among peers. *Research on Language and Social Interaction, 40*(4), 279–289.

Hale, C., & Tager-Flusberg, H. (2005). Social communication in children with autism: The relationship between theory of mind and discourse development. *Autism, 9*, 157 – 178.

Hewitt, L.E. (1998). Influence of question type on response adequacy in young adults with autism. *Journal of Communication Disorders, 31*, 135–152.
Hutchby, I. (2002). Resisting the incitement to talk in child counselling: Aspects of the utterance 'I don't know'. *Discourse Studies 4*(2), 147–168.
Hutchby, I. (2005). Children's talk and social competence. *Children and Society, 19*(1), 66–73.
Hutchby, I. (2010). Feelings-talk and therapeutic vision in child-counsellor interaction. In H. Gardner & M. Forrester (Eds.), *Analysing Interaction in Childhood: Insights from Conversation Analysis* (pp. 146–162). Chichester: Wiley-Blackwell.
Hutchby, I., & Moran-Ellis, J. (2001). Introduction: Relating children, technology and culture. In I. Hutchby & J. Moran-Ellis (Eds.), *Children and Social Competence: Arenas of Action* (pp. 1–10). London: Falmer Press.
Jefferson, G. (1989). Preliminary notes on a possible metric which provides for a 'standard maximum' silence of approximately one second in conversation. In D. Roger, P. Roger, & P. Bull (Eds.), *Conversation: An Interdisciplinary Perspective,* (pp. 166–196). Clevedon: Multilingual Matters.
Jefferson, G. (2004). Glossary of transcript symbols with an introduction. In G.H. Lerner (Ed.), *Conversation Analysis: Studies from the First Generation* (pp. 13–31). Amsterdam: John Benjamins.
Jones, C.D., & Schwartz, I.S. (2009). When asking questions is not enough: An observational study of social communication differences in high functioning children with autism. *Journal of Autism Developmental Disorders, 39*, 432–443.
Jones, S., & Zimmerman, D. (2003). 'A child's point and the achievement of intentionality'. *Gesture, 3*, 155–185.
Keenan, O.E. (1974). Conversational competence in children. *Journal of Child Language, 1*(2),163–183.
Kidwell, M. (2005). Gaze as social control: How very young children differentiate "the look" from a "mere look" by their adult caregivers. *Research on Language and Social Interaction, 38*(4), 417–449.
Kirchner, D. (1991). Using verbal scaffolding to facilitate conversational participation and language acquisition in children with pervasive developmental disorders. *Communication Disorders Quarterly, 14*, 81–98.
Knott, F., Dunlop, A., & Mackay, T. (2006). Living with ASD: How do children and their parents assess their difficulties with social interaction and understanding? *Autism, 10*, 609–617.
Koning, C., & Magill-Evans, J. (2001). Social and language skills in adolescent boys with Asperger syndrome. *Autism, 5*, 23–36.
Kremer-Sadlik, T. (2004). How children with autism and Asperger Syndrome respond to questions: A 'naturalistic' theory of mind task. *Discourse Studies, 6*, 185–206.
Kyratzis, A. (2007). Using the social organizational affordances of pretend play in American preschool girls' interactions. *Research on Language and Social Interaction, 40*(4), 321–352.
Laakso, M. (2010). Children's emerging and developing self-repair. In H. Gardner & M. Forrester (Eds.), *Analysing Interaction in Childhood: Insights from Conversation Analysis* (pp. 75–99). Chichester: Wiley-Blackwell.
Macintosh, K., & Dissanayake, C. (2006). A comparative study of the spontaneous social interactions of children with high-functioning autism and children with Asperger's disorder. *Autism, 10*(2), 199–220.
Margalit, M. (1994). *Loneliness among Children with Special Needs.* New York, NY: Springer.

McTear, M. (1985). *Children's Conversations*. Oxford: Basil Blackwell.

Minshew, N., Goldstein, G., & Siegel, D. (1995). Speech and language in high-functioning autistic individuals. *Neuropsychology, 9*, 255–261.

Muller, E., & Schuler, A. (2006). Verbal marking of affect by children with Asperger Syndrome and High Functioning Autism during spontaneous interactions with family members. *Journal of Autism and Developmental Disorders, 36*, 1089–1100.

Ochs, E., (1988). *Culture and Language Development: Language Acquisition and Language Socialization in a Samoan village*. Cambridge: CUP.

Ochs, E., & Schieffelin, B.B. (Eds.) (1979). *Developmental Pragmatics*. New York, NY: Academic Press.

Ochs, E. & Schieffelin, B.B. (1983). *Acquiring Conversational Competence*. Boston, MA: Routledge Kegan Paul.

Ochs. E., & Solomon. O. (2004). Introduction: Discourse and autism. *Discourse Studies, 6*, 139 – 146.

Ochs, E., Kremer-Sadlik, T., Gainer Sirota, K., & Solomon, O. (2004). Autism and the social world: An anthropological perspective. *Discourse Studies, 6*, 147–183.

Pike, C., (2010). Intersubjectivity and misunderstanding in adult-child learning conversations. In H. Gardner & M. Forrester (Eds.), *Analysing Interaction in Childhood: Insights from Conversation Analysis* (pp. 163–182). Chichester: Wiley-Blackwell.

Pomerantz, A. (1984). Agreeing and disagreeing with Assessments: Some features of preferred/dispreferred turn shapes. In M. Atkinson, & J. Heritage (Eds.), *Structures of Social Action: Studies in Conversation Analysis* (pp. 57–101). Cambridge: CUP.

Prior, M., Leekman, S., Ong, B., Eisenmajer, R., Wing, L., Gould, J., & Dowe, D. (1998). Are there sub-groups within the Autistic Spectrum? A cluster analysis of a group of children with Autistic Spectrum Disorder. *Journal of Child Psychology and Psychiatry, 39*, 893–902.

Rendle Short, J. (2003). Managing interaction: A conversation analytic approach to the management of interaction by an 8 year-old girl with Asperger's Syndrome. *Issues in Applied Linguistics, 13*, 161–186.

Sacks, H. (1984). Notes on methodology. In M. Atkinson, & J. Heritage (Eds.), *Structures of Social Action: Studies in Conversation Analysis* (pp. 2–27). Cambridge: CUP.

Sacks, H. (1992). *Lectures on Conversation, 2 vols*. G. Jefferson, (Ed.) Oxford: Basil Blackwell.

Sacks, H., Schegloff, E., & Jefferson, G. (1974). A simplest systematics for the organization of turn-taking for conversation. *Language, 50*, 696–735.

Salonen, T., & Laakso, M. (2009). Self-repair of speech by four-year-old Finnish children. *Journal of Child Language, 36*, 855–882.

Schegloff, E.A. (1968). Sequencing in conversational openings. *American Anthropologist, 70*, 1075–1095.

Schegloff, E.A. (1992). Repair after next turn: The last structurally provided defense of intersubjectivity in conversation. *American Journal of Sociology, 97*, 1295–1345.

Schegloff, E. (2007). *Sequence Organization in Interaction: A Primer in Conversation Analysis, Vol 1*. Cambridge: CUP.

Sheldon, A. (1992). Conflict talk: Sociolinguistic challenges to self-assertion and how young girls meet them. *Merrill-Palmer Quarterly, 38*(1), 95–117.

Sheldon, A. (1996). You can be the baby brother but you aren't born yet: Preschool girls' negotiation for power and access in pretend play. *Research on Language and Social interaction, 29*(1), 57–80.

Schieffelin, B.B. (1990). *The Give and Take of Everyday Life: Language Socialization of Kaluli Children*. Cambridge: CUP.

Sidnell, J. (2010). Questioning repeats in the talk of four-year-old children. In H. Gardner & M. Forrester (Eds.), *Analysing Interaction in Childhood: Insights from Conversation Analysis* (pp. 103–107). Chichester: Wiley-Blackwell.

Silverman, D. (1987). *Communication and Medical Practice*. London: Sage.

Silverman, D., Baker, C., & Keogh, J. (1998). Advice giving and advice reception in parent-teacher interviews. In I. Hutchby & J. Moran-Ellis (Eds.), *Children and Social Competence: Arenas of Action* (pp. 220–240). London: Falmer Press.

Sterponi, L., & Fasulo, A. (2010). "How to go on": Intersubjectivity and progressivity in the communication of a child with autism. *Ethos, 38*, 116–142.

Stribling, P., Rae, J., & Dickerson, P. (2007). Two forms of spoken repetition in a girl with autism. *International Journal of Language and Communication Disorders, 42*, 427–444.

Tager-Flusberg, H., & Anderson, M. (1991). The development of contingent discourse ability in autistic children. *Journal of Child Psychology and Psychiatry, 32*, 1123–1134.

Volden, J. (2004). Conversational repair in speakers with autism spectrum disorder. *International Journal of Language and Communication Disorders, 39*, 171–189.

Wells, G. (1981). *Learning through Interaction: The Study of Language Development*. Cambridge: CUP.

Wing, L. (1981). Asperger's Syndrome: A clinical account. *Psychological Medicine, 11*, 115–129.

Wood, D., Bruner, J., & Ross, G. (1976). The role of tutoring in problem solving. *Journal of Child Psychology and Psychiatry, 17*(2), 89–100.

Wootton, A.J. (1994). Object transfer, intersubjectivity and third position repair: Early developmental observations of one child. *Journal of Child Language, 21*, 543–564.

Wootton, A.J. (2003). Interactional contrasts between typically developing children and those with autism, Asperger's Syndrome, and pragmatic impairment. *Issues in Applied Linguistics, 13*, 133–160.

Wootton, A.J. (2006). Children's practices and their connections with "mind". *Discourse Studies, 8*, 191–198.

Wootton, A.J. (2007). A puzzle about please: Repair, increments, and related matters in the speech of a young child. *Research on Language and Social Interaction, 40*(2),171–198.

Appendix

Transcription conventions are based on Gail Jefferson's notation (presented in Atkinson & Heritage (1984) and Jefferson (2004)). The principal notions are as follows:

hello.	falling terminal intonation
hello,	slight rising intonation
hello¿	rising intonation, weaker than that indicated by a question mark
hello?	strongly rising terminal intonation
hel-	talk that is cut off
>hello<	talk is faster than surrounding talk
<hello>	talk is slower than surrounding talk
HELLO	talk is louder than surrounding talk

°hello°	talk is quieter than surrounding talk
he::llo	an extension of a sound or syllable
hello	emphasised talk
(1.0)	timed intervals
(.)	short untimed pause
.hh	audible inhalations
hh	audible exhalations
=	latched talk
[ ]	overlapping talk
( )	transcriber uncertainty

SECTION 6

Distal Causes of Language Impairment

CHAPTER 10

Atypical cerebral lateralisation and language impairment in autism

Is fetal testosterone the linking mechanism?

Lauren P. Hollier, Murray T. Maybery &
Andrew J.O. Whitehouse
University of Western Australia

Autism is among the most severe, prevalent and heritable of all neurodevelopmental disorders. However, the factors causing autism are still unclear. Language difficulties are at the core of autism, and any aetiological theory must incorporate a plausible explanation of this symptom. The development of cerebral lateralisation has long been theorised to be associated with language impairment. This chapter reviews the empirical evidence linking cerebral lateralisation and language impairment in both typical and atypical development, with a particular focus on the communication difficulties characteristic of autism. Potential causal pathways are also considered, such as fetal testosterone exposure. Finally, methodological limitations in this area and future avenues for research are discussed.

Atypical cerebral lateralisation and language impairment in autism: Is fetal testosterone the linking mechanism?

Autism is among the most severe, prevalent and heritable of all neurodevelopmental disorders. However, despite greater understanding of the clinical phenotype, and extraordinary growth in the amount of research on the disorder, the exact biological mechanisms contributing to autism remain unclear.

Language difficulties are a hallmark of autism. However, the exact communicative profile differs greatly between individuals. A number of studies have focused on the pragmatic deficits apparent within the autism population (Baltaxe 1977; Capps, Kehres & Sigman 1998; Eales 1993; Surian 1996; Tager-Flusberg 1981). Research in this area has found that individuals with autism exhibit a restricted range of speech acts (Loveland, Landry, Hughes, Hall & McEvoy 1988; Wetherby

1986) and impaired conversational and narrative skills (Loveland & Tunali 1993; Tager-Flusberg & Sullivan 1995). In addition to these communicative deficits, individuals with autism may also suffer deficits in vocabulary, grammatical knowledge, and articulation skills (Lord & Paul 1997). Accumulating research has investigated the biological mechanisms that may subserve the language difficulties observed within the autism population. One such proposed mechanism is atypical cerebral lateralisation.

This chapter reviews studies that have investigated a relationship between cerebral lateralisation and language impairment, as well as the evidence for a possible biological mechanism linking the autism and language impairment phenotypes: fetal testosterone exposure.

Atypical cerebral lateralisation and language impairment

It has long been speculated that developmental language difficulties may reflect failure to develop typical cerebral lateralisation (Orton 1929). Functional differences between the two cerebral hemispheres are among the most replicated findings in all of neuropsychology (Whitehouse & Bishop 2009). Typically, the most crucial areas involved in language production are found in the left hemisphere, while the right hemisphere is more specialized for visuospatial functions.

The bulk of research in this area has investigated behavioural measures that are thought to index the direction and degree of cerebral lateralisation, such as handedness and dichotic listening. The majority of right-handed people are left-hemisphere dominant for language, whereas left-handers are more likely to have mixed patterns of hemispheric dominance (Pujol, Deus, Losilla & Capdevila 1999; Whitehouse & Bishop 2009). While population-based studies suggest that handedness does not tend to co-vary with language ability within the normal range of variation, there is some evidence to suggest that extreme left handedness (indicating reduced cerebral lateralisation for language) is over-represented in children with early language difficulties (Natsopoulos, Koutselini, Kiosseoglou & Koundouris 2002), such as language delay associated with autism.

Colby and Parkinson (1977) provided the first systematic examination of handedness in individuals with autism. Over half of the 20 children with autism investigated were found to be either left or mixed-handed (13/20, 65%), which was a significantly higher proportion than that observed in the typically developing control group (3/25, 12%). While several subsequent studies have also reported an increased proportion of non-right handedness among children with autism (Dane & Balci 2007; Escalante-Mead, Minshew & Sweeney 2003; Lewin, Kohen & Mathew 1993; Soper et al. 1986), there have been a number of notable failures to replicate (Barry & James 1978; Cornish & McManus 1996; Markoulakis, Scharoun, Bryden & Fletcher 2012).

Dichotic listening tasks involve the simultaneous presentation of different auditory stimuli to the two ears. Participants are asked to repeat which stimuli they heard more clearly. The task is argued to be sensitive to whether the left or right cerebral hemisphere is dominant for language, with a right ear advantage (i.e. selecting the stimuli presented to the right ear more often than the one presented to the left ear; REA) representing left-hemispheric dominance for language, and vice versa for a left ear advantage (LEA; Kimura 1961). This theory stems from animal studies that illustrated that the crossed neural pathways from the ear to auditory cortex predominate over the uncrossed pathways (Rosenzweig 1951; Tunturi 1946). Kimura (1961) observed a REA among human participants and proposed that the crossed pathways were more effective than the uncrossed pathways.

Studies of dichotic listening in children with autism have revealed inconsistent findings. Prior and Bradshaw (1979) observed a lack of REA among 23 individuals with autism, aged between 8 and 13 years, on a task using pairs of single syllable words. However, Arnold and Schwartz (1984) found a clear REA among 6- to 14-year-old children with autism for stop consonants. Another study showed that children with autism had a LEA for speech sounds, while typically developing children showed the typical REA (Blackstock 1978). The inconsistent findings in this area may be due to the poor validity and/or reliability of the dichotic listening methodology; neuroimaging studies have found that dichotic listening indices correlate weakly with other indices of cerebral dominance, such as functional magnetic resonance imaging (fMRI) (Jäncke & Shah 2002). However, other studies have found good within-subjects agreement between dichotic listening and Wada tests results (Hugdahl, Carlsson Uvebrant & Lundervold (1997). Furthermore, numerous neuroimaging studies have confirmed the anatomical basis for the REA effect as originating from the left persylvian region, including the superior temporal gurus and planum temporale areas (Brancucci et al. 2004; Brancucci et al. 2005; Hugdahl et al. 1999; Jung et al. 2003; van den Noort, Specht, Rimol, Ersland & Hugdahl 2008).

Neuroimaging techniques have been utilised to provide a more direct investigation of the possible relationships between atypical cerebral lateralisation and language difficulties. Takeuchi et al. (2004) used functional magnetic resonance imaging (fMRI) to examine the cerebral activation of children with autism and controls matched for age (mean age 10 years), handedness, gender and IQ while they read a passage and silently answered questions about it. While the typically developing group exhibited greater left- than right- frontal lobe activation during task completion, the reverse was true for the autism group. This finding was replicated by Redcay and Courchesne (2008) again using fMRI, who found that

23 toddlers, aged between 2 and 3 years, with autism exhibited significantly more activity in right-hemisphere frontal and parietal regions in response to speech compared with typically developing control toddlers.

Three studies have used fMRI to investigate cerebral dominance for language in adolescents with autism. Knaus et al. (2008) found that adolescents with autism, aged between 11 and 19 years, were less likely to exhibit left-hemisphere lateralisation during a response naming task than typically developing controls. However, a further fMRI study by this group, examining the same age range, revealed no significant differences in cerebral dominance for adolescent males with autism during a rapid naming task compared to typically developing controls (Knaus et al. 2010). Another study examined cerebral activation during letter and category fluency tasks. Relative to controls, males with autism displayed significantly less left-hemisphere activation during the letter-fluency task, but there was no significant group difference in activation during the category fluency task (Kleinhans, Müller, Cohen & Courchesne 2008).

The findings from the five fMRI studies reviewed here appear to indicate that atypical cerebral lateralisation is present in individuals with autism across the developmental life span, as shown by a number of different language tasks.

A range of other neuroimaging techniques have been used to investigate cerebral lateralisation in children with autism. Using electroencephalography (EEG), Dawson, Warrenburg and Fuller (1982) measured the neural responses of children with autism to a series of verbal and non-verbal tasks. The boys with autism exhibited significantly greater right-hemisphere dominance during the verbal tasks compared to age-matched controls. No differences were found for the non-verbal tasks. This finding was supported in a later study by this same research group (Dawson, Finley, Phillips & Galpert 1986), who investigated event related potentials (ERP) for auditory stimuli and revealed that children with autism exhibit significantly reversed cerebral asymmetry compared to typically developing controls.

Flagg, Oram Cardy, Roberts and Roberts (2005) assessed language lateralisation in children with autism and typically developing children using magnetoencephalography (MEG) recordings taken as the children listened to vowels. The children with autism showed a significant trajectory towards right hemisphere dominance with increasing age, whereas the typically developing children showed a significant trajectory towards left hemisphere dominance with increasing age.

Using positron emission tomography (PET), Mueller et al. (1998) found that young adults with autism exhibited significantly less left-hemisphere dominance than typically developing comparison participants when both listening to and generating sentences. There was no significant group difference in lateralisation for a repeating-sentences task. A further study by this research group also found that young adults with autism exhibited reduced left-hemisphere dominance compared to typical controls, when listening to sentences. In contrast, sentence generation was associated with normal left-hemisphere dominance for the individuals with autism (Müller et al. 1999). The results from these two studies indicate that individuals with autism exhibit atypical asymmetry for tasks that involve language reception, whereas the evidence on asymmetry for language expression is more ambiguous.

Boddaert et al. (2003) also reported differences in PET activation for adults with autism and typically developing controls, this time as participants passively listened to speech-like sounds. Individuals with autism exhibited right-bias asymmetry, whereas typically developing controls exhibited left-biased asymmetry in PET activation. Using similar methodology, Boddaert et al. (2004) found that typically developing children exhibited left-biased asymmetry when passively listening to the speech-like sounds, but this bias was not observed in children with autism. The findings from these two studies support those from the fMRI studies reviewed earlier, with atypical cerebral lateralisation in autism present across development.

Finally, Herbert et al. (2002) used MRI to investigate structural cortical asymmetry in boys with autism. Larger right frontal language areas were identified in boys with autism compared to typically developing controls. A further study by this research group found similar patterns of rightward shifts in cerebral asymmetry in boys with autism compared to age-matched typically developing boys (Herbert et al. 2005). Another study used MRI scans to compare structural cortical asymmetry in boys with autism, with and without language impairment, and typically developing boys. The boys with autism and language impairment exhibited a reversed (rightward) asymmetry, while the boys with autism without language impairment exhibited normal leftward asymmetry. This finding suggests that abnormal asymmetry in autism may be more closely associated with structural language impairments than with an autism diagnosis (De Fossé et al. 2004). However, a more recent study using functional Transcranial Doppler[1] found no difference between autistic adults with language impairment and typically developing controls in cerebral dominance for language (Whitehouse & Bishop 2008). Furthermore, using diffusion tensor imaging (DTI),[2] Verhoeven et al. (2011) found no significant differences between children with autism and age-matched typically

1. Functional Transcranial Doppler (fTCD) uses ultrasound to measure event-related changes blood-flow velocity in the left and right middle cerebral arteries. The fTCD is based on the premise that increases in neural activity leads to greater glucose and oxygen consumption that much be replenished via enhanced blood flow to the area (Lohman, Ringelstein & Knecht 2006).

2. Diffusion Tensor Imaging is a radiological technique by which the non-random movement of water molecules through white matter provides an image of white matter neural tracts (Li Behan et al. 2001).

developing controls, for the amount of white matter measured in the superior longitudinal fascicle (SLF). In addition, there were no significant differences between the left and right SLF for both children with autism and the control group.

From the literature reviewed above, we conclude that there is a large body of evidence which suggests there are increased rates of atypical cerebral lateralisation for language in children and adults with autism. This finding holds across development and over a variety of language tasks, indicating that the language impairment that characterises autism may be caused by atypical language lateralisation. However, it is still important to interpret these findings with caution. Most studies in this area do not make a distinction between individuals with autism with and without language impairment, although they still report atypical cerebral lateralisation (Williams, Botting & Boucher 2008). An important area of future research is to determine whether atypical cerebral lateralisation in autism is observed only in those individuals with structural language difficulties, or whether this lateralisation pattern is related to the autism diagnosis more broadly.

Fetal testosterone and atypical cerebral lateralisation

From the literature reviewed, there appears to be some evidence for a relationship between atypical cerebral lateralisation and language impairment in autism. However, it is still unclear what the biological mechanism linking atypical cerebral lateralisation and language impairment may be. In this review, we discuss one possibility: prenatal exposure to testosterone.

Two prominent theories address the influence of fetal testosterone exposure on cerebral lateralisation. The theories differ as to the biological mechanism proposed and the nature of the purported effects on lateralisation. Geschwind and Galaburda (1987) proposed that testosterone acts during critical periods of prenatal neurodevelopment to slow the growth of certain cortical areas of the left hemisphere. Exposure to significantly higher than normal levels of testosterone may cause sufficient growth retardation in the left-hemisphere to shift the development of some functions, such as language and handedness, predominantly to the right hemisphere. A second theory, the callosal hypothesis put forward by Witelson and colleagues (Witelson 1991; Witelson & Nowakowski 1991), is that exposure to higher concentrations of fetal testosterone increases axonal pruning in the corpus callosum. The callosal hypothesis is based on the finding that, in males, the corpus collosum is smaller in right-handed compared with non right-handed individuals (Witelson 1985, 1989). This finding stimulated the proposal that higher concentrations of fetal testosterone increase axonal pruning, which leads to a more pronounced form of the typical lateralisation of functions. This section will review the evidence for the relationship between fetal testosterone and atypical cerebral lateralisation.

Natural experiments of children exposed to elevated levels of testosterone *in utero* have provided one means of examining this link. Congenital Adrenal Hyperplasia (CAH) is a genetic condition occurring in 1 in 15,000 live births and is characterized by impairment of the enzyme that leads to cortisol biosynthesis. This results in an *in utero* pattern of adrenal cortisol deficiency and excess testosterone production (Mueller et al. 2008), which is present as early as week five of gestation (Mathews et al. 2004). Because testosterone is secreted by the testes during normal pregnancies, males with CAH are not exposed to higher than typical concentrations of testosterone (Knickmeyer et al. 2006). In contrast, female fetuses with CAH are exposed to significantly higher concentrations of testosterone than is the case for normal pregnancies (Merke & Bornstein 2005) and therefore provide an opportunity to examine the postnatal effects of exposure to varying levels of fetal testosterone.

Two studies have reported a higher proportion of left- and mixed-handedness in females with CAH, when compared with female siblings (Nass et al. 1987) and with unrelated age- and gender-matched control participants (Kelso, Nicholls, Warne & Zacharin 2000). However, atypical handedness in CAH has not always been identified. For example, Helleday, Siwers, Ritzen, and Hugdahl (1994) found no differences between females with CAH and age- and gender-matched controls in patterns of handedness based on the Edinburgh Handedness Inventory (EHI). Helleday et al. (1994) also investigated dichotic listening performance and reported no differences between the CAH and control females for REA. These findings were replicated by Mathews, Fane, Pasterski, Conway, Brook and Hines (2004), who also found no differences between girls with CAH and age-matched unaffected relatives on dichotic listening or handedness (EHI) measures.

Twins provide a further method for investigating the effects of exposure to fetal testosterone. According to the twin transfer hypothesis, testosterone may transfer between fetuses by diffusing across fetal membranes (Even & Vom Saal 1992; Ryan & Vandenbergh 2002). Therefore fetuses gestated with a male co-twin will be 'masculinised' compared with fetuses gestated with a female co-twin. The primary evidence for this position comes from animal studies (e.g. studies of rodents and pigs), which have shown that females gestated between two males demonstrate increases in male-typical characteristics, including aggression, terroritorality and male sexual behaviour (e.g. mounting), compared with females gestated between two females (Clark, Tucker & Galef 1992; Clark, vom Saal & Galef Jr 1992; Ryan & Vandenbergh 2002). Although evidence is lacking for a biological mechanism that promotes hormone transfer between human twins, considerable research has compared indices of laterality between opposite- and same-sex twins (Tapp, Maybery & Whitehouse 2011).

Elkadi, Nicholls and Clode (1999) investigated handedness in opposite- and same-sex dizygotic twins, and found no significant differences in hand preference between the two types of twins for either sex. Two studies examining a large cohort of twins found no differences in the prevalence of left-handedness between same- and opposite-sex twins for either sex (Medland et al. 2009; Medland, Loehlin & Martin 2008). Dichotic listening preferences have also been investigated for the two twin-types. Cohen-Bendahan, Buitelaar, van Goozen, and Cohen-Kettenis (2004) found that females with a male twin demonstrated a greater REA than did females with a twin of the same sex. This finding is indicative of increased left-hemisphere lateralisation in the former group, which is consistent with the callosal hypothesis.

A number of studies have also examined the relationship between adult testosterone levels and patterns of cerebral lateralisation for various functions. Moffat and Hampson (2000) obtained saliva samples from men and women in early adulthood, and analysed these for testosterone concentration. Cerebral lateralisation was indexed using a variety of handedness measures as well as dichotic listening and tachistoscopic (mental rotation) tasks. Among left-handers, participants with a LEA for the dichotic listening task had significantly higher testosterone levels than those with a REA, in both men and women. Among right-handers, there were no significant differences in testosterone levels between participants with a REA and those with a LEA. A further finding was that those who exhibited a left visual field advantage (indicative of right-hemisphere dominance) in the mental rotation task had lower testosterone levels. Overall these findings suggest that higher salivary testosterone levels may be associated with reduced right-hemisphere dominance for spatial tasks and reduced left-hemisphere dominance for verbal tasks, consistent with what would be expected from Geschwind and Galaburda's theory. However, it is noteworthy that a similar study conducted by Gadea, Gómez, González-Bono, Salvador and Espert (2003) found no significant relationships between testosterone levels, handedness, and cerebral lateralization assessed by dichotic listening. A cautionary note in the interpretation of these studies is that the association between fetal testosterone concentration and circulating levels of testosterone during adulthood has not been clearly established, and thus it is difficult to draw firm conclusions from these studies.

A number of studies in this area have obtained more direct measures of prenatal testosterone exposure, and investigated their relationship to indices of cerebral lateralisation obtained in childhood. Lust et al. (2010) measured testosterone levels in samples of amniotic fluid extracted between 16 and 18 weeks gestation for 54 children (25 girls, 29 boys). At six years of age, the children completed a dichotic listening task for number pairs. There was a positive relationship between amniotic-fluid testosterone concentration and the extent of the REA on the dichotic listening task. Grimshaw, Byrden and Finegan (1995) also correlated testosterone concentrations in amniotic fluid, taken between 14 and 20 weeks gestation, with dichotic listening performance and handedness measured at age 10 in 53 children (25 girls, 28 boys). Among females, a higher testosterone concentration was associated with stronger right handedness and a greater REA. Similar relationships were not found among the boys. Together, these findings suggest that higher concentrations of amniotic testosterone are associated with increased left-hemisphere dominance for language, consistent with the predictions of the callosal hypothesis.

Thus there appears to be some evidence that higher concentrations of testosterone are associated with more pronounced left hemisphere dominance for language, as predicted by Witelson and colleagues (Witelson 1991; Witelson & Nowakowski 1991). However, this pattern of findings contradicts the Geschwind and Galaburda (1987) hypothesis that higher fetal testosterone is associated with reduced or reversed cerebral lateralisation for language. Perhaps the existing evidence on the relationship between testosterone exposure and language lateralization is unreliable, given that few studies have used more direct measures for sampling the prenatal hormonal environment, such as the testosterone concentration in amniotic fluid or umbilical cord blood.

However, it is also important to explore the alternate possibility: that these findings are a true reflection of the underlying biology and that increased levels of fetal testosterone lead to more pronounced left-hemisphere lateralisation for language. Witelson and colleagues proposed that increased exposure to fetal testosterone increases typical lateralisation (i.e. more left-lateralised). However, the implications that increased left hemispheric lateralisation for language might have on language development is not clear. The callosal hypothesis was not developed to explain differences in language impairment and development. Studies examining neurological development *in utero* will clarify the effects of exposure to higher concentrations of fetal testosterone on neurological development. Future research in this area is likely to benefit from the use of more direct measures of both prenatal testosterone exposure (e.g. amniocentesis and umbilical cord blood) and cerebral lateralisation (e.g. neuroimaging).

Fetal testosterone exposure and autism spectrum disorders

The literature reviewed supports a relationship between atypical cerebral lateralisation and language impairment, and that this association holds for the autism population. While the evidence linking fetal testosterone exposure and atypical lateralisation are less consistent, there is some evidence for this proposal. The remainder of this chapter will examine hypotheses and empirical evidence linking fetal testosterone exposure and language impairment in autism.

One hypothesis gaining increasing attention in the scientific literature is the Extreme Male Brain (EMB) theory, proposed by Baron-Cohen (2002, 2003). According to the EMB theory, autism is an extreme form of the male cognitive profile, in which affected individuals show an enhanced ability to understand systems in terms of rules ('systemising') and a restricted ability to identify and understand another person's emotions and thoughts ('empathising'). The EMB theory was initially based on the observation of a gender difference in the prevalence of the condition; autism affects approximately four times as many males as females (Lord, Schopler, & Revicki 1982). Additional evidence for this position comes from findings that individuals with autism perform poorly on empathising tasks, such as understanding subtle emotional expressions, in which females typically show superior performance to males (Baron-Cohen, Wheelwright, Hill, Raste & Plumb 2001), but perform better on systemising tasks, such as the Embedded Figures Test, in which males typically outperform females (Jolliffe & Baron-Cohen 1997). With regard to biological mechanisms, Baron-Cohen proposed that prenatal testosterone exposure may be involved in the aetiology of the condition (Baron-Cohen 2002, 2003; Baron-Cohen, Knickmeyer & Belmonte 2005). Testosterone, the most biologically potent of all sex-steroids, is a small lipophilic molecule that is able to pass the blood-brain barrier and cell membranes, and bind with androgen receptors found in the cytoplasm of cells. Once androgen receptor and testosterone (or its metabolite dihydrotestosterone) molecules are bound, this structure is able to enter the nucleus, where it binds to DNA and affects transcription. Baron-Cohen (2002) proposed that the extreme form of the male brain – autism – may derive, at least in part, from elevated exposure to testosterone *in utero*; because males are exposed to greater levels of fetal testosterone, they are at greater risk for autism.

Accumulating empirical research using a variety of methodologies has sought to evaluate the ideas presented by Baron Cohen. Some of this research has utilized the second-to-fourth digit (2D:4D) ratio as an indicator of fetal testosterone concentrations. Exposure to higher levels of fetal testosterone prenatally is thought to promote the development of the fourth digit, while oestrogen promotes the growth of the second digit (Manning 2002). On average, males have a longer fourth digit relative to their second digit, while women have comparable second and fourth digit lengths (Manning, Stewart, Bundred & Trivers 2004). This sex difference has been observed as early as the first trimester (Galis, Ten Broek, Van Dongen & Wijnaendts 2010; Malas, Dogan, Hilal Evcil & Desdicioglu 2006). A lower 2D:4D ratio is associated with enhanced levels of a range of male-typical characteristics, such as aggression (Bailey & Hurd 2005; Coyne, Manning, Ringer & Bailey 2007; McIntyre et al. 2007), and spatial ability (Kempel et al. 2005; Manning & Taylor 2001; Peters, Manning & Reimers 2007; van Anders & Hampson 2005). A lower 2D:4D ratio has also been found among children with autism, and is also associated with greater levels of autistic-like traits in the general population (de Bruin, Verheij, Wiegman & Ferdinand 2006; Manning, Baron-Cohen, Wheelwright & Sanders 2001).

Other research relevant to the EMB theory has investigated children exposed to atypical testosterone environments *in utero*, such as those with CAH. Postnatal studies of girls with CAH have identified an increase in male-typical characteristics such as toy preference (e.g. cars and blocks; Berenbaum & Hines 1992; Hines 2004), aggression (Berenbaum & Resnick 1997), and enhanced spatial ability (Hampson, Rovet, & Altmann 1998; Resnick, Berenbaum, Gottesman, & Bouchard 1986). Furthermore, girls with CAH have also been found to exhibit increased autistic-like traits, measured by the Autism-spectrum Quotient (AQ), compared to matched controls (Knickmeyer, Baron-Cohen, et al. 2006). It is important to note that the increased scores on the AQ fell below the level that is associated with the possibility of a clinical diagnosis among the general population (Baron-Cohen, Wheelwright, Skinner, Martin, & Clubley 2001).

Ingudomnkul, Baron-Cohen, Wheelwright and Knickmeyer (2007) investigated the prevalence of disorders associated with elevated rates of testosterone among females with an autism spectrum disorder (ASD). Higher rates of a range of conditions were observed, including polycystic ovary syndrome, hirsutism, severe acne, and menstrual dysfunctions, such as irregular menstrual cycle and dysmenorrhoea. A further series of studies have found that girls with ASD (Knickmeyer, Wheelwright, Hoekstra & Baron-Cohen 2006) or high-levels of autistic-like traits (Whitehouse, Maybery, Hickey & Sloboda 2011) are more likely to experience delayed menarche, which is also thought to be associated with exposure to elevated levels of prenatal testosterone.

This brief summary of evidence from studies examining 2D:4D, CAH and other disorders associated with elevated testosterone, provides some support for a link between fetal testosterone exposure and higher levels of autistic-like behavioural characteristics. Language difficulties are a central feature of autism, and increasing research has investigated the association between fetal testosterone and language development.

Fetal testosterone and language development

Language development is known to vary between sexes, with males typically acquiring skills later and at a slower rate than females (Zubrick, Taylor, Rice & Slegers 2007). Experimental studies have found that, even within the first 12 months of life, males show less engagement in a range of communicative behaviours, such as joint attention (Olafsen et al. 2006) and dyadic interaction (Lutchmaya, Baron-Cohen & Raggatt 2001). Meta-analyses have also revealed that males are at increased risk for familial developmental language disorders (DLD; Whitehouse 2010). The presence of these sex differences has been attributed to intrinsic differences in capacity rather than differences in parenting (Huttenlocher, Haight, Bryk, Seltzer & Lyons 1991). For example, a recent epidemiological study found no significant influence of several maternal (education, employment) and family (structure, functioning) characteristics on language delay among 2-year-old children (Zubrick et al. 2007). Fetal testosterone may be one biological mechanism that underpins sex-differences in early language development.

A number of studies have investigated the language abilities of females with CAH. Resnick, Berenbaum, Gottesman, and Bouchard (1986) found that girls with CAH performed significantly worse than unaffected siblings on a range of expressive language tasks. Other studies have reported that females with CAH performed worse than age-matched control participants on synonym and verbal fluency tests (Helleday, Bartfai, Ritzén & Forsman 1994), and are at greater risk than the general population for learning and language disabilities (Plante, Boliek, Binkiewicz & Erly 1996). However, while these findings suggest that exposure to higher concentrations of fetal testosterone may affect postnatal behaviour, it is possible that cognitive differences in females with CAH may be associated with other causes of neurodevelopmental disruption in this population, such as 'salt-wasting'[3] (Kelso et al. 2000).

Other studies have investigated the association between 2D:4D ratio and language development ability. Luxen and Buunk (2005) found that a lower 2D:4D ratio (purportedly reflecting higher testosterone exposure) was significantly associated with lower verbal IQ for both sexes. Another study found no significant relationship between verbal ability and 2D:4D ratio in 39 adults (Kempel et al. 2005). Brosnan (2008) also reported no association between 2D:4D ratio and literacy in school children, when both sexes were analysed together. However, a significant association was found when females were investigated separately (but not males). While these findings appear to suggest an influence of fetal testosterone on language ability, the validity of the 2D:4D measure has been called into question. Hickey et al. (2010), for example, found no significant association between

3. Salt-wasting refers to the process of excretion of sodium-chloride in the urine. Individuals with CAH who suffer a salt-wasting crisis can suffer from episodes of hyponatremia or hypotension that permanently affect brain function (Kelso, Nicholls, Warne & Zacharin 2000; Nass & Baker 1991)

Table 1. Summary of the studies examining the relationship between fetal testosterone and language using direct measures

Study	Number of participants	Age of participants	Measures		Findings
			Testosterone	Language	
Finegan et al. (1992)	28 girls 30 boys	4 years	Amniotic Fluid	Language Comprehension	Significant inverse relationship
Lutchmaya, Baron-Cohen & Raggatt (2001)	40 girls 47 boys	2 years	Amniotic Fluid	Vocabulary	Significant inverse relationship
Knickmeyer, Baron-Cohen, Raggatt & Taylor (2005)	23 girls 35 boys	4 years	Amniotic Fluid	Speech Syntax Pragmatic Language	No sex differences
Auyeung et al. (2009)	31 girls 43 boys	Between 6 and 10 years	Amniotic Fluid	Verbal IQ	No significant relationship
Whitehouse et al. (2012)	395 girls 372 boys	1, 2 & 3 years	Umbilical cord serum	Language delay	Significant inverse relationship for males only

testosterone concentrations measured in either maternal blood during pregnancy or umbilical cord blood at birth, and the 2D:4D ratio in female offspring. It is therefore important to interpret findings in this area with caution.

Five studies examining three cohorts have used more direct measures to investigate the effects of fetal testosterone on language development (see Table 1). In four of these studies, fetal testosterone measures were obtained from amniotic fluid taken in the second trimester of pregnancy, with the fifth measuring testosterone levels in umbilical cord blood. Finegan et al. (1992) investigated the cognitive profile of typically developing children at age 4 years, and found a significant inverse association between amniotic testosterone concentrations and measures of language comprehension, classification, counting, and number facts in girls but not boys. However, fetal testosterone levels were not associated with expressive language skills in either sex.

The Cambridge Fetal Testosterone Project has examined the association between fetal testosterone levels (measured from amniotic fluid at 18 weeks pregnancy) and various aspects of childhood language development. When offspring of the pregnancies were 18 and 24 months of age, parents completed the Oxford Communication Development Inventory, in which they were asked to indicate which words their child could say. At both time-points, there was a significant inverse relationship between testosterone concentration and expressive vocabulary size when both sexes were analysed together (with sex controlled for). However, there were no significant relationships when males and females were investigated separately (Lutchmaya, Baron-Cohen & Raggatt 2001), which may reflect the poor statistical power when the already small sample (n = 87) was further divided by sex.

When offspring were 4 years of age, parents of 58 children (35 male, 23 female) completed the Children's Communication Checklist (CCC; Bishop 1998). At a behavioural level, males had significantly lower (worse) scores than females on the restricted interests and quality of relationships subscales. In addition, when sex was controlled for, higher testosterone levels were significantly associated with lower quality of social relationships and more restricted interests across both sexes (Knickmeyer, Baron-Cohen, Raggatt & Taylor 2005). However, no sex differences were observed for subscales assessing speech, syntax or pragmatic language subscales, and therefore the association between amniotic testosterone and language capability was not further investigated. Most recently, when children from the Cambridge cohort (n = 74: 43 male, 31 female) were between 6 and 10 years of age, verbal ability was measured using the Wechsler Abbreviated Scale of Intelligence (WASI). No sex differences were found on the Verbal IQ scores, and these scores did not correlate with testosterone concentrations when both sexes were analysed together (Auyeung et al. 2009). Again, it is possible that the lack of significant findings for language measures in these two studies reflects a lack of statistical power due to small samples sizes.

Finegan et al. (1992) and the Cambridge Fetal Testosterone Project utilized amniocentesis to estimate fetal testosterone concentrations. While amniotic fluid provides a more direct measure of fetal testosterone exposure than 2D:4D, this technique is not without limitations. Amniotic samples provide a proxy measure of blood hormone concentration in the fetus by gauging the level of testosterone that has entered the amniotic fluid via fetal urination or diffusion through the fetus's skin (Nagami, McDonough, Ellegood & Mahesh 1979). While the samples of amniotic fluid are thought to relate to the levels of testosterone in fetal blood, the exact relationship remains unclear. In addition, amniocentesis is performed only when there is a legitimate medical reason (e.g. advanced maternal age), and thus samples are unlikely to be representative of the broader population.

More recently, Whitehouse et al. (in press) utilized a different technique, examining the relation between testosterone concentrations measured from umbilical cord blood and language delay in early childhood. Seven hundred and sixty-seven (395 males; 372 females) children were assessed for language delay at one, two and three years of age. It was found that males exposed to high levels of prenatal testosterone were at an increased risk for clinically significant language delay in early childhood. Interestingly, increasing testosterone concentrations reduced the risk of language delay in females. These findings suggest that exposure to high levels of prenatal testosterone is a risk factor for language delay in males, but may be a protective factor for females. However, again, there are limitations of the methodological approach utilized in this study. Umbilical cord samples measure circulating testosterone concentrations late in gestation, which may not correlate highly with testosterone levels earlier in gestation, when important stages of neurodevelopment are known to occur (Collaer & Hines 1995).

In summary, research to date has provided some evidence of an association between fetal testosterone and language development (both structural and pragmatic), though the studies are not without limitations. Studies of CAH samples have generally provided evidence consistent with the claim that higher fetal testosterone is associated with reduced language and verbal ability. However, studies using the 2D:4D ratio as a proxy indicator of fetal testosterone exposure are less consistent in supporting this association. The studies that have used more direct measures of fetal testosterone have provided mixed results (see Table 1). In particular, the Cambridge Fetal Testosterone Project provided evidence of an initial relationship between amniotic testosterone and spoken vocabulary when the children were two; however at both follow-ups, no relationships between amniotic testosterone levels and language or communication measures were observed. This pattern of results may suggest that the relationship between fetal testosterone and language development may weaken as children get older, perhaps due to influences of the environment. However, this suggestion is not consistent with the findings of Finegan et al. (1992), who reported a significant relationship between testosterone levels and language measures when children were 4 years old. Taken together, the findings reviewed in this section suggest that a relationship between elevated fetal testosterone and restricted development of language and other communication skills may exist. Future research using alternative methodologies with different participant cohorts and larger sample sizes will provide valuable data in this area.

Limitations and conclusions

The purpose of this review was to examine the relationships between atypical cerebral lateralisation, language impairment and fetal testosterone exposure, with a focus on autism. While often limited by the use of indirect methods for determining cerebral lateralisation and for assessing the influence of fetal testosterone exposure, the available research provides evidence of associations between atypical cerebral lateralisation and language impairment, and between fetal testosterone and language development. However, the nature of any relation between fetal testosterone and cerebral lateralisation still remains unclear.

Since it is unethical to manipulate hormone levels for human fetuses, most researchers have relied on proxy measures and methodologies, such as the 2D:4D ratio, and clinical populations, such as CAH. However, both of these approaches have limitations; in particular, the 2D:4D ratio may not be an entirely accurate measure of the in utero hormone environment (Hickey et al. 2010) and people with CAH may be influenced by factors of the condition other than elevated fetal testosterone exposure. Even the more direct measures of fetal testosterone (e.g. measurements taken from amniocentesis and umbilical cord blood) have limitations. Furthermore, the commonly used measures of cerebral lateralisation – handedness and dichotic listening – are not consistently associated with more direct measures of language lateralisation derived from neuroimaging (Jäncke & Shah 2002; Whitehouse & Bishop 2008). In addition, the gold standard neuroimaging techniques (e.g. Wada and fMRI) can be invasive and costly to run, and so are often only viable when used with small samples.

Despite these limitations, there appears to be a degree of empirical evidence for relation between atypical cerebral lateralisation, language impairment, and fetal testosterone. There is some evidence for increased rates of atypical cerebral lateralisation for language in children and adults with autism. In particular, most of the studies investigating children with autism using neuroimaging techniques have reported that they exhibit less pronounced left-hemisphere lateralisation for language. Future research directly comparing individuals with autism to other developmental disorders characterised by language impairment (e.g. specific language impairment) will determine whether atypical patterns of lateralisation underlie all language impairment, not merely autism.

The research investigating the link between fetal testosterone and language development shows that higher fetal testosterone levels tend to be associated with reduced language skill. However, future research should investigate the validity of this relationship with more direct measures of fetal testosterone and with more representative samples from the general population. One alternative is to sample maternal blood at critical points during pregnancy, which has had promising results in other areas (e.g., gender typed behaviour; Hines et al. 2002; Udry 1994, 2000; Udry, Morris & Kovenock 1995), but has not yet been used to investigate language development.

Finally, the literature on the relationship between atypical cerebral lateralisation and fetal testosterone has reported varied results. There is little research supporting a link between higher concentrations of fetal testosterone and a particular pattern of atypical cerebral lateralisation. If higher fetal testosterone is associated with impaired language development, and language impairment in autism is associated with reduced left-hemisphere dominance for language, it follows that higher fetal testosterone should be related to reduced left-hemisphere dominance for language. However, only two studies have used more direct measures of fetal testosterone to date, and both of these utilised dichotic listening as the measure of cerebral lateralisation. No study has used both a more direct measure of fetal testosterone, such as sampling using amniocentesis or umbilical cord blood, and a neuroimaging technique to measure cerebral lateralisation.

To date, most research examining the EMB theory has focused on the behavioural symptoms of autism, such as enhanced systemising. However, if a relationship is found between fetal testosterone exposure and language development, perhaps through the mechanism of cerebral lateralisation, the EMB theory will be extended in its ability to explain the aetiology of autism. In addition, if this relationship is substantiated, it may have implications for links to other developmental disorders that involve language impairment and may facilitate early identification and intervention for several disorders, such as specific language impairment (Whitehouse & Bishop 2008) and cerebral palsy (Bishop, Brown & Robson 1990).

In conclusion, there is preliminary evidence for the relationship between language impairment in autism and atypical cerebral lateralisation, and for the effect of fetal testosterone exposure on language development. However, empirical data supporting the relationship between fetal testosterone and atypical cerebral lateralisation is tenuous, and this association requires more extensive research. If a clear relationship between fetal testosterone and atypical cerebral lateralisation could be established, it would have important implications for the aetiology of autism and other developmental disorders characterised by language impairment.

References

Arnold, A.P., & Gorski, R.A. (1984). Gonadal steroid induction of structural sex differences in the central nervous system. *Annual Review of Neuroscience, 7*(1), 413–442.

Auyeung, B., Baron-Cohen, S., Ashwin, E., Knickmeyer, R., Taylor, K., & Hackett, G. (2009). Fetal testosterone and autistic traits. *British Journal of Psychology, 100*, 1–22.

Bailey, A.A., & Hurd, P.L. (2005). Finger length ratio (2D:4D) correlates with physical aggression in men but not in women. *Biological Psychology, 68*(3), 215–222.

Baltaxe, C.A.M. (1977). Pragmatic deficits in the language of autistic adolescents. *Journal of Pediatric Psychology, 2*(4), 176–180.

Baron-Cohen, S. (2002). The extreme male brain theory of autism. *Trends in Cognitive Sciences, 6*(6), 248–254.

Baron-Cohen, S. (2003). *The Essential Difference: The Truth about the Male and Female Brain.* New York, NY: Basic Books.

Baron-Cohen, S., Knickmeyer, R.C., & Belmonte, M.K. (2005). Sex differences in the brain: Implications for explaining autism. *Science, 310*(5749), 819–823.

Baron-Cohen, S., Wheelwright, S., Hill, J., Raste, Y., & Plumb, I. (2001). The test revised version: A study with normal adults, and adults with Asperger syndrome or high-functioning autism. *The Journal of Child Psychology and Psychiatry and Allied Disciplines, 42*(2), 241–251.

Baron-Cohen, S., Wheelwright, S., Skinner, R., Martin, J., & Clubley, E. (2001). The autism-spectrum quotient (AQ): Evidence from Asperger syndrome/high-functioning autism, males and females, scientists and mathematicians. *Journal of Autism and Developmental Disorders, 31*(1), 5–17.

Barry, R.J., & James, A.L. (1978). Handedness in autistics, retardates, and normals of a wide age range. *Journal of Autism and Developmental Disorders, 8*(3), 315–323.

Berenbaum, S.A., & Hines, M. (1992). Early androgens are related to childhood sex-typed toy preferences. *Psychological Science, 3*(3), 203–206.

Berenbaum, S.A., & Resnick, S.M. (1997). Early androgen effects on aggression in children and adults with congenital adrenal hyperplasia. *Psychoneuroendocrinology, 22*(7), 505–515.

Bishop, D.V.M. (1998). Development of the children's communication checklist (CCC): A method for assessing qualitative aspects of communicative impairment in children. *Journal of Child Psychology and Psychiatry, 39*(6), 879–891.

Bishop, D.V.M., Brown, B.B., & Robson, J. (1990). The relationship between phoneme discrimination, speech production, and language comprehension in cerebral-palsied individuals. *Journal of Speech and Hearing Research, 33*(2), 210–219.

Blackstock, E.G. (1978). Cerebral asymmetry and the development of early infantile autism. *Journal of Autism and Developmental Disorders, 8*(3), 339–353.

Boddaert, N., Belin, P., Chabane, N., Poline, J.-B., Barthelemy, C., Mouren-Simeoni, M.-C., Brunelle, F., Samson, Y. & Zilbovicius, M. (2003). Perception of complex sounds: Abnormal pattern of cortical activation in autism. *American Journal of Psychiatry, 160*(11), 2057–2060.

Boddaert, N., Chabane, N., Belin, P., Bourgeois, M., Royer, V., Barthelemy, C., Mouren-Simeoni, M.-C., Philippe, A., Brunelle, F., Samson, Y., & Zilbovicius, M. (2004). Perception of complex sounds in autism: abnormal auditory cortical processing in children. *American Journal of Psychiatry, 161*(11), 2117–2120.

Brancucci, A., Babiloni, C., Babiloni, F., Galderisi, S., Mucci, A., Tecchio, F., Zappasodi, F., Pizella, V., Romani, G.L., & Rossini, P.M. (2004). Inhibition of auditory cortical responses to ipsilateral stimuli during dichotic listening: Evidence from magnetoencephalography. *European Journal of Neuroscience, 19*(8), 2329–2336.

Brancucci, A., Babiloni, C., Vecchio, F., Galderisi, S., Mucci, A., Tecchio, F., Romani, G.L. & Rossini, P.M. (2005). Decrease of functional coupling between left and right auditory cortices during dichotic listening: An electroencephalography study. *Neuroscience, 136*(1), 323–332.

Brosnan, M.J. (2008). Digit ratio as an indicator of numeracy relative to literacy in 7-year-old British schoolchildren. *British Journal of Psychology, 99*(1), 75–85.

Capps, L., Kehres, J., & Sigman, M. (1998). Conversational abilities among children with autism and children with developmental delays. *Autism, 2*(4), 325–344.

Clark, M.M., Tucker, L., & Galef, J.B.G. (1992). Stud males and dud males: intra-uterine position effects on the reproductive success of male gerbils. *Animal Behaviour, 43*(2), 215–221.

Clark, M.M., vom Saal, F.S., & Galef Jr, B.G. (1992). Intrauterine positions and testosterone levels of adult male gerbils are correlated. *Physiology & Behavior, 51*(5), 957–960.

Cohen-Bendahan, C.C.C., Buitelaar, J.K., van Goozen, S.H.M., & Cohen-Kettenis, P.T. (2004). Prenatal exposure to testosterone and functional cerebral lateralization: a study in same-sex and opposite-sex twin girls. *Psychoneuroendocrinology, 29*(7), 911–916.

Colby, K.M., & Parkison, C. (1977). Handedness in autistic children. *Journal of Autism and Developmental Disorders, 7*(1), 3–9.

Collaer, M.L., & Hines, M. (1995). Human behavioral sex differences: A role for gonadal hormones during early development? *Psychological Bulletin, 118*(1), 55–107.

Cornish, K., & McManus, I. (1996). Hand preference and hand skill in children with autism. *Journal of Autism and Developmental Disorders, 26*(6), 597–609.

Coyne, S.M., Manning, J.T., Ringer, L., & Bailey, L. (2007). Directional asymmetry (right-left differences) in digit ratio (2D:4D) predict indirect aggression in women. *Personality and Individual Differences, 43*(4), 865–872.

Dane, S., & Balci, N. (2007). Handedness, eyedness and nasal cycle in children with autism. *International Journal of Developmental Neuroscience, 25*(4), 223–226.

Dawson, G., Finley, C., Phillips, S., & Galpert, L. (1986). Hemispheric specialization and the language abilities of autistic children. *Child Development, 57*(6), 1440–1453.

Dawson, G., Warrenburg, S., & Fuller, P. (1982). Cerebral lateralization in individuals diagnosed as autistic in early childhood. *Brain and Language, 15*(2), 353–368.

de Bruin, E.I., Verheij, F., Wiegman, T., & Ferdinand, R.F. (2006). Differences in finger length ratio between males with autism, pervasive developmental disorder- not otherwise specified, ADHD, and anxiety disorders. *Developmental Medicine & Child Neurology, 48*(12), 962–965.

De Fossé, L., Hodge, S.M., Makris, N., Kennedy, D.N., Caviness, V.S., McGrath, L., Steele, S., Ziegler, D.A., Herbert, M.R., Frazier, J.A., Tager-Flusberg, H., & Harris, G.J. (2004). Language-association cortex asymmetry in autism and specific language impairment. *Annals of Neurology, 56*(6), 757–766.

Eales, M.J. (1993). Pragmatic impairments in adults with childhood diagnoses of autism or developmental receptive language disorder. *Journal of Autism and Developmental Disorders, 23*(4), 593–617.

Elkadi, S., R. Nicholls, M.E., & Clode, D. (1999). Handedness in opposite and same-sex dizygotic twins: testing the testosterone hypothesis. *NeuroReport, 10*(2), 333–336.

Escalante-Mead, P.R., Minshew, N.J., & Sweeney, J.A. (2003). Abnormal brain lateralization in high-functioning autism. *Journal of Autism and Developmental Disorders, 33*(5), 539–543.

Even, M.D., & Vom Saal, F.S. (1992). Seminal vesicle and preputial gland response to steroids in adult male mice is influenced by prior intrauterine position. *Physiology & Behavior, 51*(1), 11–16.

Finegan, J.-A. K., Niccols, G.A., & Sitarenios, G. (1992). Relations between prenatal testosterone levels and cognitive abilities at 4 years. *Developmental Psychology, 28*(6), 1075–1089.

Flagg, E.J., Cardy, J.E.O., Roberts, W., & Roberts, T.P.L. (2005). Language lateralization development in children with autism: Insights from the late field magnetoencephalogram. *Neuroscience Letters, 386*(2), 82–87.

Gadea, M., Gómez, C., González-Bono, E., Salvador, A., & Espert, R. (2003). Salivary testosterone is related to both handedness and degree of linguistic lateralization in normal women. *Psychoneuroendocrinology, 28*(3), 274–287.

Galis, F., Ten Broek, C., Van Dongen, S., & Wijnaendts, L. (2010). Sexual dimorphism in the prenatal digit ratio (2D:4D). *Archives of Sexual Behavior, 39*(1), 57–62.

Geschwind, N., & Galaburda, A.M. (1987). *Cerebral Lateralisation: Biological Mechamisms, Associations and Pathology.* Cambridge, MA: The MIT Press.

Grimshaw, G.M., Bryden, M.P., & Finegan, J.-A.K. (1995). Relations between prenatal testosterone and cerebral lateralization in children. *Neuropsychology, 9*(1), 68–79.

Hampson, E., Rovet, J.F., & Altmann, D. (1998). Spatial reasoning in children with congenital adrenal hyperplasia due to 21-hydroxylase deficiency. *Developmental Neuropsychology, 14*(2), 299 - 320.

Helleday, J., Bartfai, A., Ritzén, E.M., & Forsman, M. (1994). General intelligence and cognitive profile in women with congenital adrenal hyperplasia (CAH). *Psychoneuroendocrinology, 19*(4), 343–356.

Helleday, J., Siwers, B., Ritzén, E.M., & Hugdahl, K. (1994). Normal lateralization for handedness and ear advantage in a verbal dichotic listening task in women with congenital adrenal hyperplasia (CAH). *Neuropsychologia, 32*(7), 875–880.

Herbert, M.R., Harris, G.J., Adrien, K.T., Ziegler, D.A., Makris, N., Kennedy, D.N., Lange, N.T., Chabris, C.F., Bakardjiev, A., Hodgson, J., Takeoka, M., Tager-Flusberg, H. & Caviness Jr., V.S. (2002). Abnormal asymmetry in language association cortex in autism. *Annals of Neurology, 52*(5), 588–596.

Herbert, M.R., Ziegler, D.A., Deutsch, C.K., O'Brien, L.M., Kennedy, D.N., Filipek, P.A., Bakadjiev, A.I., Hodgson, J., Takeoka, M., Makris, N. & Caviness Jr., V.S. (2005). Brain asymmetries in autism and developmental language disorder: A nested whole-brain analysis. *Brain, 128*(1), 213–226.

Hickey, M., Doherty, D.A., Hart, R., Norman, R.J., Mattes, E., Atkinson, H.C., & Sloboda, D.M. (2010). Maternal and umbilical cord androgen concentrations do not predict digit ratio (2D:4D) in girls: A prospective cohort study. *Psychoneuroendocrinology, 35*(8), 1235–1244.

Hines, M. (2004). *Brain Gender*. Oxford: OUP.

Hines, M., Golombok, S., Rust, J., Johnston, K.J., & Golding, J., The Avon Longitudinal Study of Parents and Children Study Team. (2002). Testosterone during pregnancy and gender role behavior of preschool children: A longitudinal, population study. *Child Development, 73*(6), 1678–1687.

Hugdahl, K., Brønnick, K., Kyllingsbrk, S., Law, I., Gade, A., & Paulson, O.B. (1999). Brain activation during dichotic presentations of consonant-vowel and musical instrument stimuli: A ^{15}O-PET study. *Neuropsychologia, 37*(4), 431–440.

Hugdahl, K., Carlsson, G., Uvebrant, P., & Lundervold, A.J. (1997). Dichotic-listening performance and intracarotid injections of amobarbital in children and adolescents: Preoperative and postoperative comparisons. *Archives of Neurology, 54*(12), 1494–1500.

Huttenlocher, J., Haight, W., Bryk, A., Seltzer, M., & Lyons, T. (1991). Early vocabulary growth: Relation to language input and gender. *Developmental Psychology, 27*(2), 236–248.

Ingudomnukul, E., Baron-Cohen, S., Wheelwright, S., & Knickmeyer, R. (2007). Elevated rates of testosterone-related disorders in women with autism spectrum conditions. *Hormones and Behavior, 51*(5), 597–604.

Jäncke, L., & Shah, N.J. (2002). Does dichotic listening probe temporal lobe functions? *Neurology, 58*(5), 736–743.

Jolliffe, T., & Baron-Cohen, S. (1997). Are people with autism and Asperger syndrome faster than normal on the embedded figures test? *Journal of Child Psychology and Psychiatry, 38*(5), 527–534.

Jung, P., Baumgärtner, U., Bauermann, T., Magerl, W., Gawehn, J., Stoeter, P., & Treede, R.-D. (2003). Asymmetry in the human primary somatosensory cortex and handedness. *NeuroImage, 19*(3), 913–923.

Kelso, W.M., Nicholls, M.E.R., Warne, G.L., & Zacharin, M. (2000). Cerebral lateralization and cognitive functioning in patients with congenital adrenal hyperplasia. *Neuropsychology, 14*(3), 370–378.

Kempel, P., Gohlke, B., Klempau, J., Zinsberger, P., Reuter, M., & Hennig, J. (2005). Second-to-fourth digit length, testosterone and spatial ability. *Intelligence, 33*(3), 215–230.

Kimura, D. (1961). Cerebral-dominance and the perception of verbal stimuli. *Canadian Journal of Psychology, 15*(3), 166–171.

Kleinhans, N., Müller, R.-A., Cohen, D.N., & Courchesne, E. (2008). Atypical functional lateralization of language in autism spectrum disorders. *Brain Research, 1221*, 115–125.

Knaus, T.A., Silver, A.M., Kennedy, M., Lindgren, K.A., Dominick, K.C., Siegel, J., & Tager-Flusberg, H. (2010). Language laterality in autism spectrum disorder and typical controls: A functional, volumetric, and diffusion tensor MRI study. *Brain and Language, 112*(2), 113–120.

Knaus, T.A., Silver, A.M., Lindgren, K.A., Hadjikhani, N., & Tager-Flusberg, H. (2008). fMRI activation during a language task in adolescents with ASD. *Journal of the International Neuropsychological Society, 14*(06), 967–979.

Knickmeyer, R.C., Baron-Cohen, S., Fane, B.A., Wheelwright, S., Mathews, G.A., Conway, G.S., Brook, C., & Hines, M. (2006). Androgens and autistic traits: A study of individuals with congenital adrenal hyperplasia. *Hormones and Behavior, 50*(1), 148–153.

Knickmeyer, R.C., Baron-Cohen, S., Raggatt, P., & Taylor, K. (2005). Foetal testosterone, social relationships, and restricted interests in children. *Journal of Child Psychology and Psychiatry, 46*(2), 198–210.

Knickmeyer, R.C., Wheelwright, S., Hoekstra, R., & Baron-Cohen, S. (2006). Age of menarche in females with autism spectrum conditions. *Developmental Medicine & Child Neurology, 48*(12), 1007–1008.

Le Bihan, D., Mangin, J.-F., Poupon, C., Clark, C.A., Pappata, S., Molko, N., et al. (2001). Diffusion tensor imaging: Concepts and applications. *Journal of Magnetic Resonance Imaging, 13*(4), 534–546.

Lewin, J., Kohen, D., & Mathew, G. (1993). Handedness in mental handicap: investigation into populations of Down's syndrome, epilepsy and autism. *The British Journal of Psychiatry, 163*(5), 674–676.

Lohmann, H., Dräger, B., Müller-Ehrenberg, S., Deppe, M., & Knecht, S. (2005). Language lateralization in young children assessed by functional transcranial Doppler sonography. *NeuroImage, 24*(3), 780–790.

Lord, C., & Paul, R. (1997). Language and communication in autism. In D. J. Cohen & F. R. Volkmar (Eds.), *Handbook of Autism and Pervasive Development Disorders* (2nd ed.). New York NY: John Wiley & Sons.

Lord, C., Schopler, E., & Revicki, D. (1982). Sex differences in autism. *Journal of Autism and Developmental Disorders, 12*(4), 317–330.

Loveland, K.A., Landry, S.H., Hughes, S.O., Hall, S.K., & McEvoy, R.E. (1988). Speech acts and the pragmatic deficits of autism. *Journal of Speech and Hearing Research, 31*(4), 593–604.

Loveland, K.A., & Tunali, B. (1993). Narrative langauge in autism and the theory of mind hypothesis: A wider perspective. In S. Baron-Cohen, H. Tager-Flusberg, & D.J. Cohen (Eds.), *Understanding Other Minds: Perspectives from Autism.* Oxford: OUP.

Lust, J.M., Geuze, R.H., Van de Beek, C., Cohen-Kettenis, P.T., Groothuis, A.G.G., & Bouma, A. (2010). Sex specific effect of prenatal testosterone on language lateralization in children. *Neuropsychologia, 48*(2), 536–540.

Lutchmaya, S., Baron-Cohen, S., & Raggatt, P. (2001). Foetal testosterone and vocabulary size in 18- and 24-month-old infants. *Infant Behavior and Development, 24*(4), 418–424.

Luxen, M.F., & Buunk, B.P. (2005). Second-to-fourth digit ratio related to Verbal and Numerical Intelligence and the Big Five. *Personality and Individual Differences, 39*(5), 959–966.

Malas, M.A., Dogan, S., Hilal Evcil, E., & Desdicioglu, K. (2006). Fetal development of the hand, digits and digit ratio (2D:4D). *Early Human Development, 82*(7), 469–475.

Markoulakis, R., Scharoun, S.M., Bryden, P.J., & Fletcher, P.C. (2012). An examination of handedness and footedness in children with high functioning autism and Asperger syndrome. *Journal of Autism and Developmental Disorders, 42*(10), 2192–2201.

Manning, J.T. (2002). *Digit Ratio: A Pointer to Fertility, Behavior, and Health.* New Brunswick, NJ: Rutgers University Press.

Manning, J.T., Baron-Cohen, S., Wheelwright, S., & Sanders, G. (2001). The 2nd to 4th digit ratio and autism. *Developmental Medicine & Child Neurology, 43*(3), 160–164.

Manning, J.T., Stewart, A., Bundred, P.E., & Trivers, R.L. (2004). Sex and ethnic differences in 2nd to 4th digit ratio of children. *Early Human Development, 80*(2), 161–168.

Manning, J.T., & Taylor, R.P. (2001). Second to fourth digit ratio and male ability in sport: implications for sexual selection in humans. *Evolution and Human Behavior, 22*(1), 61–69.

Mathews, G.A., Fane, B.A., Pasterski, V.L., Conway, G.S., Brook, C., & Hines, M. (2004). Androgenic influences on neural asymmetry: Handedness and language lateralization in individuals with congenital adrenal hyperplasia. *Psychoneuroendocrinology, 29*(6), 810–822.

McIntyre, M.H., Barrett, E.S., McDermott, R., Johnson, D.D.P., Cowden, J., & Rosen, S.P. (2007). Finger length ratio (2D:4D) and sex differences in aggression during a simulated war game. *Personality and Individual Differences, 42*(4), 755–764.
Medland, S.E., Duffy, D.L., Wright, M.J., Geffen, G.M., Hay, D.A., Levy, F.,Van-Beijsterveldt, C.E.M., Willemsen, G., Townsend, G.C, White, V., Hewitt, A.W., Mackey, D.A., Bailey, J.M., Slutsky, W.S. Nyholt, D.R., Treloar, S.A., Martin, N.G. & Boomsma, D.I. (2009). Genetic influences on handedness: Data from 25,732 Australian and Dutch twin families. *Neuropsychologia, 47*(2), 330–337.
Medland, S.E., Loehlin, J.C., & Martin, N.G. (2008). No effects of prenatal hormone transfer on digit ratio in a large sample of same- and opposite-sex dizygotic twins. *Personality and Individual Differences, 44*(5), 1225–1234.
Merke, D.P., & Bornstein, S.R. (2005). Congenital adrenal hyperplasia. *The Lancet, 365*(9477), 2125–2136.
Moffat, S.D., & Hampson, E. (2000). Salivary testosterone concentrations in left-handers: An association with cerebral language lateralization? *Neuropsychology, 14*(1), 71–81.
Mueller, S.C., Temple, V., Oh, E., VanRyzin, C., Williams, A., Cornwell, B., Grillon, C., Pine, D.S., Ernst, M., & Merke, D.P. (2008). Early androgen exposure modulates spatial cognition in congenital adrenal hyperplasia (CAH). *Psychoneuroendocrinology, 33*(7), 973–980.
Müller, R.A., Behen, M.E., Rothermel, R.D., Chugani, D.C., Muzik, O., Mangner, T.J., & Chugani, H.T. (1999). Brain mapping of language and auditory perception in high-functioning autistic adults: A PET study. *Journal of Autism and Developmental Disorders, 29*(1), 19–31.
Müller, R.A., Chugani, D.C., Behen, M.E., Rothermel, R.D., Muzik, O., Chakraborty, P.K., & Chugani, H.T. (1998). Impairment of dentato-thalamo-cortical pathway in autistic men: language activation data from positron emission tomography. *Neuroscience Letters, 245*(1), 1–4.
Nagami, M., McDonough, P., Ellegood, J., & Mahesh, V. (1979). Maternal and amniotic fluid steroids throughout human pregnancy. *American Journal of Obstetrics and Gynecology, 134*, 674–680.
Nass, R., & Baker, S. (1991). Androgen effects on cognition: Congenital adrenal hyperplasia. *Psychoneuroendocrinology, 16*(1–3), 189–201.
Nass, R., Baker, S., Speiser, P., Virdis, R., Balsamo, A., Cacciari, E., Loche, A., Dumic, D., & New, M. (1987). Hormones and handedness. *Neurology, 37*(4), 711.
Natsopoulos, D., Koutselini, M., Kiosseoglou, G., & Koundouris, F. (2002). Differences in language performance in variations of lateralization. *Brain and Language, 82*(2), 223–240.
Olafsen, K.S., Rønning, J.A., Kaaresen, P.I., Ulvund, S.E., Handegård, B.H., & Dahl, L.B. (2006). Joint attention in term and preterm infants at 12 months corrected age: The significance of gender and intervention based on a randomized controlled trial. *Infant Behavior and Development, 29*(4), 554–563.
Orton, S. (1929). A physiological theory of reading disability and stuttering in children. *New England Journal of Medicine, 199*(21), 1046–1052.
Peters, M., Manning, J., & Reimers, S. (2007). The effects of sex, sexual orientation, and digit ratio (2d:4d) on mental rotation performance. *Archives of Sexual Behavior, 36*(2), 251–260.
Plante, E., Boliek, C., Binkiewicz, A., & Erly, W.K. (1996). Elevated androgen, brain development and language/learning disabilities in children with congenital adrenal hyperplasia. *Developmental Medicine & Child Neurology, 38*(5), 423–437.

Prior, M.R., & Bradshaw, J.L. (1979). Hemisphere functioning in autistic children. *Cortex, 15*(1), 73–81.

Pujol, J., Deus, J., Losilla, J.M., & Capdevila, A. (1999). Cerebral lateralization of language in normal left-handed people studied by functional MRI. *Neurology, 52*(5), 1038.

Redcay, E., & Courchesne, E. (2008). Deviant functional magnetic resonance imaging patterns of brain activity to speech in 2-3-year-old children with autism spectrum disorder. *Biological Psychiatry, 64*(7), 589–598.

Resnick, S.M., Berenbaum, S.A., Gottesman, I.I., & Bouchard, J.T.J. (1986). Early hormonal influences on cognitive functioning in congenital adrenal hyperplasia. *Developmental Psychology, 22*(2), 191–198.

Rosenzweig, M.R. (1951). Representations of the two ears at the auditory cortex. *American Journal of Physiology – Legacy Content, 167*(1), 147–158.

Ryan, B.C., & Vandenbergh, J.G. (2002). Intrauterine position effects. *Neuroscience & Biobehavioral Reviews, 26*(6), 665–678.

Soper, H.V., Satz, P., Orsini, D.L., Henry, R.R., Zvi, J.C., & Schulman, M. (1986). Handedness patterns in autism suggest subtypes. *Journal of Autism and Developmental Disorders, 16*(2), 155–167.

Surian, L. (1996). Are children with autism deaf to gricean maxims? *Cognitive Neuropsychiatry, 1*(1), 55–72.

Tager-Flusberg, H. (1981). On the nature of linguistic functioning in early infantile autism. *Journal of Autism and Developmental Disorders, 11*(1), 45–56.

Tager-Flusberg, H., & Sullivan, K. (1995). Attributing mental states to story characters: A comparison of narratives produced by autistic and mentally retarded individuals. *Applied Psycholinguistics, 16*(3), 241–256.

Takeuchi, M., Harada, M., Matsuzaki, K., Nishitani, H., & Mori, K. (2004). Difference of signal change by a language task on autistic patients using functional MRI. *The Journal of Medical Investigation: JMI, 51*(1–2), 59–62.

Tapp, A.L., Maybery, M.T., & Whitehouse, A.J.O. (2011). Evaluating the twin testosterone transfer hypothesis: A review of the empirical evidence. *Hormones and Behavior, 60*(5), 713–722.

Tunturi, A.R. (1946). A study on the pathway from the medical geniculate body to the acoustic cortex in the dog. *American Journal of Physiology – Legacy Content, 147*(2), 311–319.

Udry, J.R. (1994). The nature of gender. *Demography, 31*(4), 561–573.

Udry, J.R. (2000). Biological limits of gender construction. *American Sociological Review, 65*(3), 443–457.

Udry, J.R., Morris, N.M., & Kovenock, J. (1995). Androgen effects on women's gendered behaviour. *Journal of Biosocial Science, 27*, 359–368.

van Anders, S.M., & Hampson, E. (2005). Testing the prenatal androgen hypothesis: measuring digit ratios, sexual orientation, and spatial abilities in adults. *Hormones and Behavior, 47*(1), 92–98.

van den Noort, M., Specht, K., Rimol, L.M., Ersland, L., & Hugdahl, K. (2008). A new verbal reports fMRI dichotic listening paradigm for studies of hemispheric asymmetry. *NeuroImage, 40*(2), 902–911.

Verhoeven, J.S., Rommel, N., Prodi, E., Leemans, A., Zink, I., Vandewalle, E., Noens, I., Wagemans, J., Steyaert, J., Boets, B., Van de Winckel, A., De Cock, P., Lagae, L., & Sunaert, S. (2011). Is there a common neuroanatomical substrate of language deficit between autism spectrum disorder and specific language impairment? *Cerebral Cortex*. DOI: 10.1093/cercor/bhr292.

Wetherby, A.M. (1986). Ontogeny of communicative functions in autism. *Journal of Autism and Developmental Disorders, 16*(3), 295–316.
Whitehouse, A.J.O. (2010). Is there a sex ratio difference in the familial aggregation of specific language impairment? A meta-analysis. *Journal of Speech, Language and Hearing Research, 53*(4), 1015–1025.
Whitehouse, A.J.O., & Bishop, D.V.M. (2008). Cerebral dominance for language function in adults with specific language impairment or autism. *Brain, 131*(12), 3193–3200.
Whitehouse, A.J.O., & Bishop, D.V.M. (2009). Hemispheric division of function is the result of independent probabilistic biases. *Neuropsychologia, 47*(8–9), 1938–1943.
Whitehouse, A.J.O., Mattes, E., Maybery, M.T., Sawyer, M.G., Jacoby, P., Keelan, J.A., & Hickey, M. (2012). Sex-specific associations between umbilical cord blood testosterone levels and language delay in early childhood. *Journal of Child Psychology and Psychiatry.*
Whitehouse, A.J.O., Mattes, E., Maybery, M.T., Sawyer, M.G., Jacoby, P., Keelan, J.A., & Hickey, M. (in press). Umbilical cord blood testosterone levels predict early langauge delay in males.
Whitehouse, A.J.O., Maybery, M., Hickey, M., & Sloboda, D. (2011). Brief report: Autistic-like traits in childhood predict later age at menarche in girls. *Journal of Autism and Developmental Disorders, 41*(8), 1125–1130.
Williams, D., Botting, N., & Boucher, J. (2008). Language in autism and specific language impairment: Where are the links? *Psychological Bulletin, 134*(6), 944–963.
Witelson, S.F. (1985). The brain connection: the corpus callosum is larger in left-handers. *Science, 229*(4714), 665–668.
Witelson, S.F. (1989). Hand and sex differences in the isthmus and genu of the human corpus callosum. *Brain, 112*(3), 799–835.
Witelson, S.F. (1991). Neural sexual mosaicism: Sexual differentiation of the human temporo-parietal region for functional asymmetry. *Psychoneuroendocrinology, 16*(1–3), 131–153.
Witelson, S.F., & Nowakowski, R.S. (1991). Left out axoms make men right: A hypothesis for the origin of handedness and functional asymmetry. *Neuropsychologia, 29*(4), 327–333.
Zubrick, S.R., Taylor, C.L., Rice, M.L., & Slegers, D.W. (2007). Late language emergence at 24 months: An epidemiological study of prevalence, predictors, and covariates. *Journal of Speech, Language and Hearing Research, 50*(6), 1562–1592.

Index